Technology Leadership in Teacher Education:
Integrated Solutions and Experiences

Junko Yamamoto
Slippery Rock University of Pennsylvania, USA

Chris Penny
West Chester University of Pennsylvania, USA

Joanne Leight
Slippery Rock University of Pennsylvania, USA

Sally Winterton
West Chester University of Pennsylvania, USA

Information Science REFERENCE

INFORMATION SCIENCE REFERENCE

Hershey · New York

Director of Editorial Content:	Kristin Klinger
Director of Book Publications:	Julia Mosemann
Acquisitions Editor:	Lindsay Johnston
Development Editor:	Dave DeRicco
Publishing Assistant:	Myla Harty
Typesetter:	Brittany Metzel
Production Editor:	Jamie Snavely
Cover Design:	Lisa Tosheff
Printed at:	Yurchak Printing Inc.

Published in the United States of America by
Information Science Reference (an imprint of IGI Global)
701 E. Chocolate Avenue
Hershey PA 17033
Tel: 717-533-8845
Fax: 717-533-8661
E-mail: cust@igi-global.com
Web site: http://www.igi-global.com/reference

Library of Congress Cataloging-in-Publication Data

Technology leadership in teacher education : integrated solutions and experiences / Christian Penny, Joanne Leight, and Sally Winterton, editors.

p. cm.

Includes bibliographical references and index.

Summary: "This book presents international authors, who are teacher educators, and their best practices in their environments, discussing topics such as the online learning environment, multimedia learning tools, inter-institutional collaboration, assessment and accreditation, and the effective use of Web 2.0 in classrooms"--Provided by publisher. ISBN 978-1-61520-899-9 (hardcover) -- ISBN 978-1-61520-900-2 (ebook) 1. Teachers--Training of. 2. Educational technology--Study and teaching. I. Penny, Christian, 1973- II. Leight, Joanne, 1965- III. Winterton, Sally.

LB1707.T448 2010

370.71'1--dc22

2009040562

British Cataloguing in Publication Data

A Cataloguing in Publication record for this book is available from the British Library.

List of Reviewers

Chris Penny, *West Chester University of Pennsylvania, USA*
Joanne Leight, *Slippery Rock University of Pennsylvania, USA*
Sally Winterton, *West Chester University of Pennsylvania, USA*
Mary C. Dalmau, *Victoria University, Australia*
Chinwe Ikpeze, *St. John Fisher College, USA*
Stella C. S. Porto, *University of Maryland University College, USA*
Lisa Marie Blaschke, *University of Maryland University College, USA*
Richard Altenbaugh, *Slippery Rock University of Pennsylvania, USA*
Padma Anand, *Slippery Rock University of Pennsylvania, USA*
Marty J. Park, *Office of Education Technology, Kentucky Department of Education, USA*

Table of Contents

Detailed Table of Contents

instruction. The types of assignments and the importance of effective instructor feedback and instructor visibility are examined in relation to course construction. Effective assessment techniques for online courses are also examined in the context of the knowledge and skills participants in such courses should display. The major thrust of the presented materials is the understanding that as presentation techniques change assessment techniques need change to be effective.

To positively foster teacher knowledge, skills and beliefs regarding technology integration, a teacher preparation program at a university in New Jersey, USA carried out the process of revising a face-to-face technology skill based course into a fully online one in which the focus changed to "teaching with technology." This chapter provides a detailed account of how the course was revised, and describes the challenges the authors faced. The solutions that came to the fore during this process are also provided. The chapter concludes with recommendations for other teacher educators who might be offering online educational technology courses to candidates of a similar population.

Research has shown that gender disparities exist in online communication. Understanding the factors that enable students to effectively communicate online and ultimately manage their own discussions has important learning and pedagogical implications. This study examined the communication and interactional processes of peer-directed online discussions. Gender disparities were found in communication styles and in the use of socioemotional content. Men were expository whereas messages posted by women were of an epistolary nature. Women used socioemotional content more than men. However, interactions, such as the extent to which men and women persisted in message threads as well as responded to one another, were comparable overall. Although not significant, women posted more messages of longer length but men received more replies to their messages. The findings have important pedagogical implications for educators who wish to engage students in peer-directed text-based asynchronous discussions.

Foreword

Stepping out of one's comfort zone and adapting to the trends that assist preservice teachers in providing quality instruction in this rapidly changing world of technology can challenge even the most dedicated teacher educator. As Jill Ashbaugh Earman suggests in this book, students who are entering schools at present have moved from a position of "digital immigrants" to "digital natives." Students are now entering school possessing technology skill sets that have altered the manner in which information is absorbed, processed, retained, and /or dismissed. Providing teacher educators with the tools necessary to equip preservice teachers with the skills needed to accommodate these "digital natives" requires an effort to remain current on new advances in technology that affect these methods.

The information provided in this book offers the practical application of technology in the learning environment, which can be modified to optimize the success of preservice teachers in the field. The chapters offer tried and tested implementations of technology by teacher educators, which will assist in providing preservice teachers with life-long skills that are adaptable to the advances in technology in the future. My position as an educator and "digital immigrant" in this world of changing technology provides a unique opportunity to witness the adaptability of the educational system's transition toward meeting the needs of their cliental in this new age.

This collection of experienced-based examples of teacher educator leadership in the field is a compilation of the processes used regarding what teacher educators think and do when adapting new technology. Developing online environments that assist students and professionals in distance learning opportunities offer many challenges to educators who recognize this growing trend in education. You will discover an ample amount of practical examples that will assist in the development of your own online program to meet your needs and the needs of your students.

Accountability in technology education is an important component to successfully document all aspects of instruction. Portfolios and accreditation standards are vital to maintain a successful program. These issues are addressed in a manner that is relevant to the expectations of all stakeholders and will assist in providing you with information adaptable to fit your needs.

Preparing preservice teachers to meet the needs of their students in the field through the use of technology is in growing demand. Modeling these practices in a manner that produces the transfer of knowledge and skill in these areas is the call to order for teacher educators if success in this area is to be realized. Whether a "digital immigrant" or "digital native," you will find this new journey informative.

Kioh Kim, Ph.D.
Northwestern State University
Natchitoches, Louisiana

Kioh Kim *is an Assistant Professor of Educational Technology at Northwestern State University (NSU) of Louisiana. His teaching and research interests include examining and developing potential applications of emerging technologies in the classroom, improving training which results in teachers' increased use of computer-based technology in their classroom, and developing effective online learning environments. Dr. Kim uses a variety of forms of subtle and obvious positive feedback in hopes that students not only learn better, but adopt similar modeling techniques in their own classrooms. Dr. Kim has considerable teaching experience with technology in South Korea and the United States. Dr Kim's teaching experiences include teaching English at the middle and high school levels, teaching at a college in South Korea, and teaching undergraduate and graduate educational technology courses at the University of Wyoming and NSU. Dr. Kim has written extensively including a book titled Appreciating Computer-Based Technology Use in Teacher Education Programs: A Case-Study Monograph (Chicago, IL: Discovery Association Publishing House). He enjoys living in Northwest Louisiana with his wife and two children.*

Preface

HOW THIS BOOK CAME ABOUT

Technology Leadership in Teacher Education, along with *Technology Implementation and Teacher Education*, was born from professional dialogue of scholars from around the world. I love going to international conferences and listening to ideas of experts from different areas. Ideas grow with interaction: sometimes I have coffee or lunch with scholars that I just met at a conference so I can learn more about their practices teaching philosophies, and important issues in their environments. Such conversation causes me to ponder this question: how can I successfully apply practices used in Austria, Netherlands, Japan, or Great Britain, to the context of the United States, the country in which I am teaching? This book aims to mimic the structure of such a process: international authors, who are teacher educators, present their best practices in their environments. They also imply how their cases can be generalized so that audience can think about how to adapt and implement what worked in the authors' environment into those of the readers.

Technology changes rapidly. Since the time span from a book proposal to the publication is about two years, books that focus on pedagogical issues rather than technological how-to tend to attract teacher educators. Also, an editor of an instructional technology book needs to have a keen sense of current and emerging trends. To grasp the trends, I skimmed through over 500 journal articles and conference proceedings covering the most recent three years. I composed the draft for the book proposal after identifying critical issues and trends. Then a group of teacher educators exchanged ideas about the draft and finalized our book proposal. While doing so, we decided to publish books for two different strands. One was for leadership in teacher education and the other was for teacher educators as reflective practitioners.

During fall 2008, I sent out emails to scholars who already published in relevant topics. The response was very encouraging. I especially enjoyed the process of reading their ideas via email or listening to them over the telephone. Authors asking for my feedback often motivated me to look for recent publications of their topics. Hence, there was a constant active exchange between authors and myself. Furthermore, reviewers and authors had very productive interaction during formative evaluation process: first during the chapter proposal stage, then during the chapter drafting stage. The process was double-blind reviewed, so I often acted as a mediator to pass on the comments and questions between the reviewers and the authors. Authors displayed a high degree of professionalism as they used formative feedback to make their chapters stronger. This is another example of professional dialogues refining ideas.

ORGANIZATION OF THIS BOOK

The first section of this book is structured around the topic of online learning environment. Jill Ashbaugh Earman compares digital immigrants and digital natives and their preferences for online activities, and offers suggestions for effective online course design for both. Ron Lombard addresses issues that online instructors need to know including retaining visibility, evidencing compassion to students, building communities, and knowing participants. Heejung An and Hilary Wilder share their journey to structure their online class according to the Technological Pedagogical Content Knowledge (TPACK) framework. William Gibbs and Ronan Bernas analyze the different online behavior according to gender.

The second section centers on multimedia learning tools. Prudence Cuper and Yi Gong discuss the use of video analysis for preservice teacher education. Jacqueline McLaughlin showcases the success story of connecting inservice and preservice teachers with inquiry-based science education.

The third section addresses inter-institutional collaboration. Shari Stockero discusses how a university can support inservice teachers' professional development through a blended course. Jacqueline Mumford and Elizabeth Juelich-Velotta share their implementation of service learning. Gloria Latham and Julie Faulkner reflect upon their challenges and successes for creating and running a virtual school.

The fourth section focuses on assessment and accreditation. Natalie Johnson-Leslie talks about creating an electronic evidence room using College LiveText. Lesia Lennex, Brianna Swetnam, and Heather Flynn also share their experience about creating an electronic evidence room, but through surveys from stakeholders. Jeremy Dickerson, Howard Coleman, and Dennis Kubasko talk about their five-year process of institutionalizing electronic portfolio.

The fifth section covers Web 2.0. Ron Lombard and Stella Porto point to the effective use of Web 2.0 in classrooms. Terry Herman mentions strategies and concerns for data Web mashups. The final section addresses trends in technology education. Robert N. Ronau, Christopher R. Rakes, Margaret Niess, Lauren Wagener, David Pugalee, Christine Browning, Shannon O. Driskell, and Susann Mathews provide broad view of emerging research frameworks of instructional technology. Kevin Biesinger and Kent Crippen summarize practical recommendations for technology educations for teachers.

Acknowledgment

I would first like to thank my co-editors for their enthusiasm, professionalism, and support.

Technology Leadership in Teacher Education: Integrated Solutions and Experiences
Chris Penny, *West Chester University of Pennsylvania, USA*
Joanne Leight, *Slippery Rock University of Pennsylvania, USA*
Sally Winterton, *West Chester University of Pennsylvania, USA*

Technology Implementation and Teacher Education: Reflective Models
Ronald Lombard, *Chatham University, USA*
Joseph Kush, *Duquesne University, USA*
Jay Hertzog, *Slippery Rock University of Pennsylvania, USA (retired)*

They worked well as a team to co-develop the two books, and then to review and to fine-tune the respective books.

This book could not have been made possible without a group of dedicated reviewers. Their expertise and dedication ensured the quality and the integrity of the double-blind review process.

Mary C. Dalmau, *Victoria University, Australia*
Chinwe Ikpeze, *St. John Fisher College, USA*
Stella C. S. Porto, *University of Maryland University College, USA*
Lisa Marie Blaschke, *University of Maryland University College, USA*
Richard Altenbaugh, *Slippery Rock University of Pennsylvania, USA*
Padma Anand, *Slippery Rock University of Pennsylvania, USA*
Marty J. Park, *Office of Education Technology, Kentucky Department of Education, USA*
Lawrence Tomei, *Robert Morris University, USA*

I would also like to thank Dr. Richard Altenbaugh of Slippery Rock University of Pennsylvania. This book and Technology Implementation and Teacher Education: Reflective Models, were the first books that I edited. I depended on his experience as a journal editor when I wrote rejection messages that encouraged authors to keep up with their scholarship even though their chapters did not appear in the books. Finally, I would like to thank Mr. Tyler Heath and Ms. Julia Mosemann of IGI-Global for the tireless support they have provided.

Junko Yamamoto, Editor
August 2009, Slippery Rock, Pennsylvania

Section 1
Online Environment

Chapter 1
Online Learning Engages Students of the Digital Age

Jill A. Ashbaugh Earman
Duquesne University, USA

ABSTRACT

Technology capabilities are rapidly growing in the world of education. As distance education applications are being designed to be more user-friendly, online learning opportunities are becoming more of a reality in secondary schools and institutions of higher education, with students enrolling in online and blended courses. Many of the early and current distance learners are "digital immigrants," that is, they are not well-versed in technology systems and need to adjust to a whole new way of learning to succeed in the online environment. However, future students enrolling in online courses will be "digital natives," students who have grown up surrounded by the ever-evolving technology of the digital age. Digital natives acquire and process information in ways that are far different than previous generations, requiring educators to re-think the design and delivery of relevant curriculum. This chapter will discuss the phenomenon of digital natives and immigrants, current practices and perceptions, and a successful model of online learning in an upper elementary school classroom.

INTRODUCTION

Technology capabilities are rapidly growing in the world of education. As online course management software applications are being designed to be more user-friendly, online learning opportunities are becoming more of a reality in secondary schools and institutions of higher education. In the fall 2005 term, almost 3.2 million students were enrolled in at least one online course at the post-secondary level, representing an increase of 35 percent over the previous year (Allen & Seaman, 2006). By the fall of 2007, that number had increased to almost four million students (Allen & Seaman, 2008). During the 2005-2006 school year, 63.1 percent of school districts in the United States had students enrolled in online or blended courses (Picciano &

DOI: 10.4018/978-1-61520-899-9.ch001

Seaman, 2007). Only two years later, that number had increased to 75% (Picciano & Seaman, 2009).

A variety of training opportunities have been employed to prepare instructors to meet the unique demands of the online learning environment, however a new phenomenon has emerged that requires further inquiry. Many of the early and current distance learners are "digital immigrants," that is, they are not well-versed in technology systems and need to adjust to a whole new way of learning to succeed in the online environment. According to Cross (2006):

In 2006, virtually everyone in the U.S. over the age of 30 or so has become an immigrant in their own country – digital immigrants. In this definition, being an immigrant means being new to the digital culture, not knowing of or understanding the nuances on which a culture is built. In essence, a large group of Americans is bicultural... Speaking the same technological language exists within the larger digital culture much like speaking a language is part of any other culture. To function fully in any culture, one must speak the language. (p. 52)

The dilemma in designing online learning opportunities is that a large portion of current and future students enrolling in online courses will be "digital natives," students who have "spent their entire lives surrounded by and using computers, videogames, digital music players, video cams, cell phones, and all the other toys and tools of the digital age" (Prensky, 2001, p. 1). Prensky posits that as a result of growing up immersed in a technology environment, digital natives acquire and process information in ways that are far different than previous generations. Being digital natives means that the nuances of the culture are accessible and make sense to them. As Oblinger (2004) points out:

There is a growing body of evidence that students have developed a different set of attitudes and aptitudes as a result of growing up in an IT and media-rich environment. While this may provide great advantages in areas such as their ability to use information technology and to work collaboratively, it may create a disconnect between their expectations and the learning environments they find in colleges and universities. (p. 15)

The relationships between technology and pedagogy must be scrutinized in order to improve the curriculum for the digital age (Giroux, 1994). It is imperative that online programs are designed to meet the needs of the learners. In order to further explore the idea of developing appropriate online learning environments, this chapter will discuss current practices and perceptions of online learning within the context of the phenomenon of digital natives and immigrants. A case study describing a successful model of online learning in an upper elementary school classroom will demonstrate that a rigorous and relevant curriculum can be provided that meets the learning preferences of digital natives.

BACKGROUND

Digital immigrants typically choose online learning environments due to the flexibility, convenience, and accessibility of the courses. Adults appreciate being able to do their coursework from their homes or offices. Asynchronous learning environments allow them access to their learning at any time, from anywhere there is Internet access. Even when course participants meet in a synchronous environment, such as a chat room, they still have the convenience of not having to travel to a college campus to attend class. These digital immigrants generally value online courses that mirror the content and delivery of face-to-face courses (Greenberg, Vojir, & Whitney, 2000). They are not interested in the graphics, video, 3-D immersive simulations and other technology innovations that can be provided by the high-tech world. Traditionally, online courses are not designed for digital natives. They are geared to the needs of focused, self-disciplined, and motivated adult learners (Guernsey, 1998).

According to O'Lawrence (2006), adult learners possess certain characteristics that influence their participation in online learning opportunities:

- They possess a variety of prior learning and work experiences.
- They can integrate new concepts with their prior knowledge while picking up new ideas from their colleagues with similar work experiences.
- They enjoy and desire practical applications, because the co-hoc nature of most of these programs draws prospective students from the same way of life and work-related similarities.
- They learn best by having control over their learning environment and have the opportunity to showcase their talents in group and special projects.
- They enjoy the ability to participate voluntarily in the learning experience. (p. 48)

When an online course can meet these needs, adult learners are more inclined to enroll in and complete the course. Adults readily recognize whether or not their learning needs are being considered and met. If a course does not support one or more of these needs, the adult learner is more likely to be disengaged and eventually drop out of the course (Chyung, 2001).

Digital natives want to be engaged by the technology in ways that are unavailable or not possible in conventional settings (Clarke, 2005). They enjoy the interactivity of 3-D immersive environments, which allows for a variety of experiences that cannot be duplicated in a traditional classroom. They like the rich media tools that allow them to create their own learning and manipulate the online environment. Currently, very little of what children do in school actually takes into account their technological capabilities. According to Prensky (2005/2006):

Our young people generally have a much better idea of what the future is bringing than we do. They're already busy adopting new systems for communicating (instant messaging), sharing (blogs), buying and selling (eBay), exchanging (peer-to-peer technology), creating (Flash), meeting (3D worlds), collecting (downloads), coordinating (wikis), evaluating (reputation systems), searching (Google), analyzing (SETI), reporting (camera phones), programming (modding), socializing (chat rooms), and even learning (Web surfing). (p. 10)

Obviously, there exists a disconnect between how digital natives are learning, taught largely by digital immigrant instructors, and how they are living their lives.

In order to better address the constructivist approach to learning for digital natives, research suggests that pedagogy must shift from teacher-centered instruction to experiential learning. Carstens and Beck (2005) describe how the digital natives who are entering the workforce now, or who will be soon, are much different than their predecessors, because of the time they have spent playing video games. These people learn and behave differently, and business and industry will need to redefine their training models to meet the needs of their new generation of workers.

Educational games are slowly being introduced as serious tools for learning. Because they can easily be incorporated into an online learning environment, games are a practical and relevant way to reach digital natives in a format that holds their attention. According to Carstens and Beck (2005), "Games reinforce certain beliefs about the self, how the world should work, how people relate to one another and finally, about the goals of life in general. Games create a self-centered universe where the player is running the show, and can manipulate other people and objects to his or her will" (p. 23). Eighty percent of managers under the age of 34 say that they have significant experience with video games.

There are several parallels between gaming environments and how young people learn:

- **Activates prior learning:** Games require facts. Players must use previously learned information and learn new facts to move on to higher levels of gameplay.
- **Context:** Context is important in games. Knowing what information or techniques to apply in which situation enables greater success.
- **Feedback and assessment:** Games provide ample feedback on the player's progress. Online help can provide just-in-time remediation, as well.
- **Transfer:** Games require transfer of learning from other venues – life, school, and other games. Being able to see the connection and transfer existing learning to a unique situation is part of gameplay.
- **Experiential:** Games are inherently experiential. Those who play games engage multiple senses. For each action, there is a reaction. Feedback is swift. Learning is often by trial and error: hypotheses are tested and users learn from the results.
- **Social:** Games are often social environments, sometimes involving large distributed communities. (Oblinger, 2004, p. 8)

Games help children to develop the mindset that there are many pathways to solve a problem or approach a task, and any can be tried with a low risk of failure. Competition is engrained in digital natives. In general, they are quick decision makers and prefer to complete a project alone as opposed to depending on others. These qualities make them better prepared to deal with the changing paradigm of the global workforce, therefore educational programs should reflect their unique qualities. For example, the skills being taught should have value to the learner and should be immediately applicable. Risk in a safe environment should be encouraged. Learning should not feel like formal education, should be interactive, and should be more peer-focused than teacher-centered.

In summary, the literature suggests that to be successful in an online learning environment, students must be responsible, self-disciplined, and motivated to do well (Perez Cereijo, 2006). However, certain characteristics about how digital natives and digital immigrants learn best will require educators to determine how to design online learning environments that best suit the needs of both groups. While adult learners still think of learning in terms of the traditional classroom setting, and want their online experience to imitate it, the digital natives are wired to learn in the world or high-tech, and their needs must be considered for the future of online education.

Current Online Program Design Elements and Pedagogical Practice

Online instruction is rapidly gaining ground in the world of distance education. Web-Based Tools, such as BlackBoard, WebCT, and Moodle, offer students several modes of interaction with a course. Through the use of these tools, students can learn content, engage in synchronous and asynchronous peer and instructor communication, and participate in classes taught online in real-time. Discussion boards offer students the ability to share and discuss ideas, building on one another's thoughts. Wikis provide a place to build communities of knowledge on any given topic, and participants can use this type of space for the planning and preparation of entire projects. Virtual classrooms allow for synchronous learning to take place, as in a traditional classroom, but without the need to attend class on a campus. In a virtual classroom, students and instructors can speak to one another, communicate through text, write and draw on a virtual whiteboard, and provide visual aides such as PowerPoint presentations, concept webs, and video. Complete courses can now be offered using web-based tools. Courses designed for delivery through the Internet are growing in prevalence each year, especially for adult education and corporate training (Hall, Watkins, & Ercal, 2000).

Advocates of online learning have stated that it is an efficient means of instruction with the ability to individualize for unique needs. In addition, emphasis is placed on individual responsibility and determination of learning goals and outcomes. (Navarro & Shoemaker, 2000). Virtual learning environments provide the means to incorporate constructivist learning, as students are encouraged to create meaning by building ideas and concepts together. This has been shown to be an important component of pedagogy for digital natives. Ewing, Dowling, and Courts (1998) identified six constructivist premises as important to the online learning environment:

- Learning is contextual.
- Learning demands active engagement.
- Learning is collaborative.
- Learning incorporates autonomy and control.
- Learning includes personally preferred modes of learning.
- Learning results in individually meaningful constructions. (p. 4)

A sense of community in online courses is an essential element of the design. Students who feel connected to the learning environment and their peers tend to be more satisfied and do not drop out of online courses. This is one reason why some degree-granting programs utilize the cohort method and encourage bonding between the students (Ouzts, 2006). Mimirinis and Bhattacharya (2007) found that collaboration and communication within a virtual learning environment are critical for deep learning to occur. Networks of learners should be an essential part of online courses. Better learning outcomes are realized when groups of learners work together toward a common goal and focused discussion groups are part of the course design.

Communication is another important factor that must be considered when designing online environments. Both digital natives and digital immigrants need various kinds of communication throughout an online course. In fact, communication was the number one factor identified by Ortiz-Rodriquez, Teig, Irani, Roberts, and Rhoades (2005) as contributing to the quality of online instruction. They demonstrated that many types of communication are essential to students' success. Students experience the most success in a class where there is positive communication with the instructor and with the other students. This communication can take on many forms, including synchronous discussion of concepts and ideas, asynchronous discussion boards, constructive feedback, and even availability of help from technical staff. Of all of these, students cited feedback as the most important form of communication in an online course.

The use of video should be considered when designing an online course. Video choice is an element that is difficult to mimic in a classroom setting, but can be applied to an online course with ease. Some learning styles are positively correlated with certain types of videos used for instruction (Yoder, 1994). Students who prefer practical application of ideas, concrete experiences, and active participation favor interactive video as part of the course delivery. Interactive video gives them opportunities to apply the information that they learn in authentic tasks. Reflective learners who prefer more abstract conceptualization favor linear video in their coursework. These students do not feel the need to immediately use what they learn, but rather need time to reflect upon and internalize the new concepts. It is vital that the instructor considers the types of learners in the course when utilizing video components.

The instructor should consider the type of learner enrolled in the course when choosing the activities. Digital natives want to be immersed in stimulating activities that make use of digital content and need to have choices of the available tools to complete the learning tasks. However, digital immigrants like their online environment to mirror the bricks-and-mortar classroom that they remember. Arbaugh and Benbunan-Fich (2006) explored the relationship between teaching methods in online learning environments and student learning and satisfaction in an MBA program. The students enrolled in this program would be considered digital immigrants. This study looked at objectivist and constructivist epistemology and individual and group activities. Findings indicated that the andragogy and activity-type most preferred by this group was the objectivist approach with group activities. Students rated the objectivist methods and collaboration significantly higher in their perceived learning and satisfaction than any of the other combinations of approaches. This study supports the idea that digital immigrants want their online learning to simulate the traditional classroom. In a study of graduate nursing students, DeBourgh (2003) found that student satisfaction overall was highest when pedagogical strategies that promote transformational learning were used. For these students, it was not enough to learn new material; they expected to have a meaningful change in their lives as a result of the newly acquired skills and knowledge.

Simulations are gaining ground as important components in the online environment. Laff (2007) discussed the serious use of games for training purposes for military, medical, and emergency personnel. The goal of simulations is to learn and practice in computer-generated real-life situations. For example, a military simulation may guide its participants through the process of negotiating in a hostile environment, planning and implementing strategies, and navigating in unfamiliar terrain. A medical student, using a simulation, could practice surgical skills over and over, until they become perfected. Emergency personnel could participate in maneuvers such as hostage situations, safe implosion of buildings, and search and rescue. In a school setting, students may become avatars in a virtual world, solving myriad social, economic, health, safety, and environmental problems through collaboration with other students' avatars. Games can be totally immersive, and trainees and students alike can learn through trial and error in a safe environment before applying their skills in the real world.

The current pedagogy and design elements in online learning environments are as varied as the learners they attract. It is imperative that instructors discover by which means their particular audiences will learn best. While digital immigrants desire online environments that mimic a traditional classroom setting, digital natives want to be fully immersed in the virtual world of learning.

Students' and Instructors' Perceptions and Preferences

Students' overall perceptions of distance learning are that it is convenient and collaborative. Students are able to complete their coursework from their home or office, and they can work with other students from all over the world (Svetcov, 2000). Students report that the benefits of online learning are that there is no commute, the location is flexible, they have easy access to a university, there is individualized attention from the instructor, and they have more time to consider their answers before responding to questions. For some students in remote locations, the lack of a commute to participate in online learning contributes greatly to their success. Even for people kept busy by family and work commitments, the ability to plan their coursework around their lives, without having to drive to class, is important. For business people who are often out-of-town and for military personnel stationed in isolated locations, the flexible location allows for participation that would be impossible in a traditional setting. A study by Sankaran and Bui (2001) concluded that students who work full-time and who live the furthest from the university had a higher preference for taking courses in an online environment than any other group. Distance education allows students who are busy with work and life commitments, and who live some distance from a university, the chance to pursue courses and a college degree. In addition, when working asynchronously, students have time to reflect and formulate in-depth answers and analysis that is simply not possible in a face-to-face environment (Matthews, 1999).

Students have noticed that in virtual learning environments, they often receive individualized attention and feedback from their instructors. This has been noted as one of the most important motivating factors for online learners. Graduate students, presumably digital immigrants, who are new to online learning, have better success in online courses that are led by an instructor, as opposed to those that incorporate independent learning only. This supports the premise that they want their online environments to mirror the traditional classroom. Timely feedback is essential to their success and motivation as well. Especially when doing independent work, students must experience frequent feedback on their progress in order to feel a connection to the class. The same study also found that in the early stages of a student's online work, problem-based courses with intensive student-instructor interaction were preferred by students. This type of learning environment helped students to become familiar with the tools of the online environment with ongoing and frequent support. With growing self-assurance, they became prepared for more independent work. As students progressed through the online program, web-based modules supported by less instructor interaction were just as effective as the earlier courses, since students had gained confidence in their abilities and independence in the online environment (Jiang, Parent, & Eastman, 2006).

The match or mismatch between the design of the online learning environment and a student's learning style and maturity level, as well as his self-efficacy for working in the online course, are strong determinants of his perceptions of his online courses. The relationship of learning styles to graduate students' perceptions of asynchronous online coursework was reported by Fearing and Riley (2005). Visual, auditory, and kinesthetic learning styles of the digital immigrants, along with their perceptions of online courses, were assessed. In general, students expressed positive opinions about taking online coursework in an asynchronous format, even though the majority of participants had a kinesthetic learning style. The authors concluded that mature students who pursue advanced degrees will take courses by convenient methods, such as online, even though the work is not in their favored learning style. They surmised that the students experienced success because they developed and used good computer skills. This supports the Jiang, Parent, and Eastman (2006) study in which students became more inclined to do well with independent work, after they developed a belief in their abilities to work in the online environment. In another study, students' perceptions of the quality of a course, access to the instructor, reliability of the technology, and their own self-efficacy with the course material were strong factors in influencing a choice to enroll in an online course (Tabatabaei, Schrottner, & Reichgelt, 2006). This study also found that there were no significant differences between the perceptions of part-time and full-time students on these factors.

An online instructor must be committed to interacting with the students in several ways. Wong's (2005) study of the perceptions of students regarding interaction with instructors in an online environment yielded some recommendations to help establish and maintain the human connection. Students suggested holding virtual office hours in a chat room. As shown in other studies as well, students require feedback and communication with their instructors. Gaining support on campus from an instructor may be as difficult as going to class on campus for some students, so dedicated hours reserved for interaction in a chat room can alleviate this concern. Students also suggested conducting scheduled chat sessions with anyone in the class who wished to participate, in order to discuss questions, problems, and projects. The synchronicity of the chat sessions helps students to collaborate in real-time and to feel a sense of connectedness with their classmates. Also addressing the need for a connection with the others in their class, students suggested including student and instructor photographs and biographies on the class website. This is especially important when there is no face-to-face contact among the class members. Some environments make use of real-time video through web cameras, but most synchronous classrooms rely exclusively on audio and text communication. Further demonstrating the need to be connected with their classmates, online learners wanted to use all kinds of communication, such as the telephone, chat rooms, discussion boards, and email, and some would consider holding a few face-to-face meetings during the course term.

Being digital immigrants, many instructors have voiced concerns about the quality of educational experiences that can be delivered through online courses. There is a concern about the ability of the university to provide adequate technical support at a distance. There is also a belief that adult learners are less able to use technology than digital natives, and instructors will struggle to teach in the online world (Lefor, Benke, & Ting, 2003). While these concerns may show some validity through the early years in the development of online environments, through training and support educators will continue to enhance their skills at offering appropriating online activities, and students will continue to adapt to the virtual environment. Furthermore, as more and more digital natives reach the age of university enrollment, the belief that students are not able to use technology well enough to succeed in online courses will diminish.

Another concern often posed by instructors is that distance learning cannot measure up to traditional classroom learning. Addressing that notion, O'Lawrence (2006), citing Diaz, stated:

> *...this type of question is premised on the implicit, yet rarely mentioned assumption, that traditional education is the ideal mode of educational delivery and thus can serve as the gold standard against which all other forms of alternative education should be measured. Diaz refers to the assumption as untenable, simply because it is impossible to determine whether one class method is better than another without first agreeing on the criteria for such a determination. (p.48)*

In other words, it has not been shown that traditional classroom instruction has any advantage over online education in terms of student achievement. There is a growing body of evidence to show that there are no significant differences in the quality of learning between traditional and online courses. In a 2005 study, Lao and Gonzales found differing points of view among the professors they interviewed. While some agreed that online education was inferior to traditional instruction, others felt that both served students equally well. All agreed that timely feedback was important. Half of the professors felt that preparing for online courses took too much time, and that they were not adequately trained in the technology to provide online education. This study concluded that online environments can be just as conducive to learning as a face-to-face classroom, and that instructors must consider their approach to teaching and utilize all of the available technology tools to enhance the learning process.

In general, student perceptions of online learning are positive. Presently, most students engaging in online learning are digital immigrants, who appreciate the convenience and flexibility of the online format. Distance learning allows them to fit their learning into their work and family lives without the same amount of disruption that a traditional campus program entails. Since instructors in online environments are also digital immigrants, it is no surprise that online instruction tends to mimic the traditional classroom. This is the preferred online environment for adult learners.

Online learning is still getting mixed reviews from instructors. Some view it as the hallmark of the future, and are working diligently to incorporate pedagogy and design to address the needs of their students. Others are not convinced of the importance of online learning and view the preparation as too time-consuming. Ongoing training and support of these digital immigrant instructors will be paramount to their success as online course facilitators.

For the digital natives who are now getting their first experiences with online learning, they appreciate being able to use the ubiquitous technologies with which they have lived their whole lives. Stepping through the doorway to school should not mean taking a step back in time, but rather a leap into the digital age. More and more, educators are realizing that their students are different from students of the past, and need a whole new, engaging way of learning.

A Moodle Model for Online Learning

Experienced educators understand that as students change, teaching methods must change as well. It is not unusual for students to enter classrooms with more technology experience than their teachers. This is what led 29-year veteran teacher Mr. J. Kevin Freeberg to begin to explore ways of reaching youngsters on their own turf. In 2007, the Indiana Area School District, in which Freeberg teaches sixth grade, offered to the faculty a workshop on using Moodle, a free online course management system. Freeberg joined the workshop and never looked back. Struck by the ease in which online components could be developed and implemented, Freeberg parlayed the one-day workshop and several follow-up work sessions into a wealth of knowledge about Moodle that he willingly shares with his colleagues, but admits, "There is always something left to learn (J. K. Freeberg, personal communication, March 31, 2009). "

Freeberg recommends his successful training and implementation model to others. Training consists of the teacher and students learning how to use Moodle, but implementation, actually using Moodle to learn, is the goal. To begin, he advises learning as much as possible from an experienced Moodle user. By attending an introductory workshop, Freeberg not only learned specific elements of Moodle that he could begin using immediately with his class, but by viewing samples of others' work was also able to envision the big picture of how Moodle could be used to restructure his lessons to engage students.

"Piece by piece, try something with kids," advises Freeberg. Although Moodle is intended to be used for distance learning, he suggests trying out new components with the students and teacher present in the same room. That way, the teacher can guide the students and see what they are doing, and the students can see what the teacher's computer screen looks like as well. "We talk a lot about Internet safety. They know I can see a log of everything they do." Following a successful classroom trial, Freeberg has the students attempt the same type of assignment from their home computer. For those who lack computer resources in their homes, the school, local library, and university labs can be accessed.

After introducing individual components to students, such as retrieving documents, linking to websites and videos, taking quizzes, participating in forums and chats, and constructing an interactive glossary, units of study can be created in which all of the students' work is completed using Moodle. Freeberg constructed a unit on the Roaring Twenties that the students completed this year. The Moodle site contained text that students could read; a forum in which to take notes, post links, and respond to others; quizzes and tests; a wiki to create group projects; links to external websites containing pictures, videos, simulations, and primary documents; and a student-created glossary, which highlights the defined terms throughout every other document on the Moodle site, providing a link to the glossary for students needing clarification of terms.

Using the Moodle site, Freeberg is able to differentiate instruction to meet the diverse needs of the students in his classroom. By using a pre-test, Freeberg determines where a student should enter the online unit: at the beginning for all of the background knowledge, somewhere in the middle to fill in gaps, or jumping immediately to enrichment activities. Although every student must meet the objective of the unit, their paths through the material can be markedly different. Where one student may like to read text and examine primary documents, another may prefer to watch video and participate in lively discussion boards. Some students enjoy expressing their ideas through factual essays or creative writing, while others make use of the wide variety of digital tools Freeberg provides, like concept webs, slide shows, movies, and podcasts. Having students engage in the digital content means that Freeberg serves as a facilitator of learning, rather than a bell-to-bell lecturer. This lesson design allows him the freedom to devote more time to a few students who struggle, providing them with the one-on-one attention they need.

With over 47,000 hits to his Moodle site this year, Freeberg and his students are experiencing the success of learning Moodle and of learning *with* Moodle. He explains the advantages of using the online course management software. Most important, the students find the Moodle units engaging. Students who were reluctant to participate in class readily contribute to online forums and the community of knowledge that is built by the students. This, in turn, provides them with the confidence that comes from success, and they begin to contribute more during face-to-face learning. Further, Moodle allows entire units to be completed without paper and pencil, empowers students to work at their own pace to explore in depth the topics that are of most interest to them, and permits the teacher to provide more content than is ever possible in a classroom lesson. Simply stated by Freeberg, "It hooks them. It has rejuvenated my teaching."

FUTURE RESEARCH DIRECTIONS

Technology is rapidly changing, and as it does, it holds the potential to change the form and function of education. It is this author's hope that educators can begin to become proactive in their use of current and emerging technologies, to help their students be on the cutting edge of appropriate tools to stimulate their creative thinking and problem solving abilities. Future research is needed in the area of developing online learning environments for digital natives, specifically to suggest the best ways to use current and emerging technologies to increase student achievement and teach the skills that will be necessary for students to have a successful and productive future. Further, research needs to be conducted to develop appropriate training models for teachers, so that they may provide the education that digital natives require.

CONCLUSION

Clearly, there are similarities and differences in the pedagogical practices that will best suit the needs of digital natives and digital immigrants in the online learning environment. Virtual learning environments are easily adaptable to all kinds of learning needs, and it is imperative that educators discover which methods work best with their differing audiences. Current programs are varied in their approaches to instruction, ranging from completely independent courses to completely synchronous delivery.

As shown in the review of the literature, success in an online course depends foremost on the responsibility, self-discipline, and motivation of the student. Beyond that, there are practices that instructors may employ to address the unique learning needs of their particular students. Digital immigrants are more likely to do well in courses that address their need for an environment that mirrors a conventional classroom setting, with direct instruction, timely feedback, direct application of their learning, and traditional assessments. Digital natives, on the other hand, require a more constructivist approach to learning. They need to feel that they are a part of a larger community of learners working together to solve problems and build knowledge. They require active engagement, collaboration, and control over their learning. They are motivated by the rich and varied multimedia tools, 3-D graphics, and immersive simulations that are only available to them in a virtual environment.

Great strides are already being made in some online environments, as instructors prepare to address the changing and varied needs of their students. It will be a challenge to provide an optimal learning environment, as students enrolling in online courses will continue to be a mix of digital immigrants and digital natives, with more and more natives enrolling in the years to come. Support and training for the instructors will be a benefit to everyone involved, and careful ongoing scrutiny of pedagogy and design will be paramount to students' success in future online learning environments. As demonstrated by Freeberg, when an instructor is willing to learn how to take advantage of the technology tools that are available, ultimately the students are the beneficiaries.

REFERENCES

Allen, I. E., & Seaman, J. (2006). *Making the grade: Online education in the United States, 2006.* Retrieved April 2, 2009, from http://www.sloan-c.org/publications/survey/pdf/making_the_grade.pdf

Allen, I. E., & Seaman, J. (2008). *Staying the course: Online education in the United States, 2008.* Retrieved April 2, 2009, from http://www.sloan-c.org/publications/survey/pdf/staying_the_course.pdf

Arbaugh, J. B., & Benbunan-Fich, R. (2006). An investigation of epistemological and social dimensions of teaching in online learning environments. *Academy of Management Learning & Education, 5*, 435–447.

Carstens, A., & Beck, J. (2005). Get ready for the gamer generation. *TechTrends, 49*, 22–25. doi:10.1007/BF02763643

Chyung, S. Y. (2001). Systematic and systemic approaches to reducing attrition rates in online higher education. *American Journal of Distance Education, 15*(3), 36–50. doi:10.1080/08923640109527092

Clarke, O. (2005). Engaging the digital natives in learning. *Primary & Middle Years Educator, 3*(3), 20–25.

Cross, T. L. (2006). Digital immigrants, natives, and "tweeners": A glimpse into the future for our students with gifts and talents. *Gifted Child Today, 29*(3), 52–53.

DeBourgh, G. (2003). Predictors of student satisfaction in distance delivered graduate nursing courses: What matters most. *Journal of Professional Nursing, 19*, 149–163. doi:10.1016/S8755-7223(03)00072-3

Ewing, J. M., Dowling, J. D., & Courts, N. (1998). Learning using the World Wide Web: A collaborative learning event. *Journal of Educational Multimedia and Hypermedia, 8*, 3–22.

Giroux, H. (1994). *Disturbing pleasures: Learning popular culture.* New York: Routledge.

Greenberg, E., Vojir, C., & Whitney, F. (2000). *Listening to MAPP online voices: Learning and teaching over the Internet*. Aurora, CO: University of Colorado Health Sciences Center.

Guernsey, L. (1998). Distance education for the notso-distant. *The Chronicle of Higher Education, 44*, A29–A30.

Hall, R. H., Watkins, S. E., & Ercal, F. (2000, April). *The horse and the cart in web-based instruction: Prevalence and efficacy*. Paper presented at the Annual Meeting of the American Educational Research Association, New Orleans, LA.

Jiang, M., Parent, S., & Eastman, D. (2006). Effectiveness of web-based learning opportunities in a competency-based program. *International Journal on E-Learning, 5*, 353–360.

Laff, M. (2007). Serious Gaming: The trainer's new best friend. *T + D, 61*, 52-57.

Lao, T., & Gonzales, C. (2005). Understanding online learning through a qualitative description of professors and students' experiences. *Journal of Technology and Teacher Education, 13*, 459–474.

Lefor, P. J., Benke, M., & Ting, E. (2003). Information technology and adult learners at Empire State College. *New Directions for Student Services, 102*, 35–42. doi:10.1002/ss.87

Matthews, D. (1999). The origins of distance education and its use in the United States. *T.H.E. Journal, 27*(2), 54–67.

Mimirinis, M., & Bhattacharya, M. (2007). Design of virtual learning environments for deep learning. *Journal of Interactive Learning Research, 18*, 55–64.

Navarro, P., & Shoemaker, J. (2000). Performance and perceptions of distance learners in cyberspace. *American Journal of Distance Education, 14*(2), 15–35. doi:10.1080/08923640009527052

O'Lawrence, H. (2006). The influence of distance learning on adult learners. *Techniques, 81*(5), 47–49.

Oblinger, D. G. (2004). The next generation of educational engagement. *Journal of Interactive Media in Education, 8*, 1–18.

Ortiz-Rodriguez, M., Teig, R. W., Irani, T., Roberts, T. G., & Rhoades, E. (2005). College students' perceptions of quality in distance education: The importance of communication. *Quarterly Review of Distance Education, 6*, 97–184.

Ouzts, K. (2006). Sense of community in online courses. *The Quarterly Review of Distance Education, 7*, 285–296.

Perez Cereijo, M. V. (2006). Attitude as predictor of success in online training. *International Journal on E-Learning, 5*, 623–639.

Picciano, A. G., & Seaman, J. (2007). *K-12 online learning: A survey of U.S. school district administrators.* Retrieved April 2, 2009, from http://www.sloan-c.org/publications/survey/pdf/K-12_Online_Learning.pdf

Picciano, A. G., & Seaman, J. (2009). *K-12 online learning: A 2008 follow-up survey of U.S. school district administrators.* Retrieved April 2, 2009, from http://www.sloan-c.org/publications/survey/pdf/k-12_online_learning_2008.pdf

Prensky, M. (2001). Digital natives, digital immigrants. *Horizon, 9*(5), 1–2. doi:10.1108/10748120110424816

Prensky, M. (2005/2006). Listen to the natives. *Educational Leadership, 63*(4), 8–13.

Sankaran, S. R., & Bui, T. (2001). Impact of learning strategies and motivation on performance: A study in web-based instruction. *Journal of Instructional Psychology, 28*, 191–199.

Svetcov, D. (2000). The virtual classroom vs. the real one. *Forbes, 166*(7), 50–52.

Tabatabaei, M., Schrottner, B., & Reichgelt, H. (2006). Target populations for online education. *International Journal on E-Learning, 5*, 401–414.

Wong, P. (2005). Online and face-to-face students' perceptions of teacher-learner interactions: A preliminary examination. *Distance Leanring, 2*(5), 1–7.

Yoder, M. (1994). Preferred learning style and educational technology: Linear vs. interactive video. *Nursing & Health Care, 15*(3), 128–132.

Chapter 2
The Nuts and Bolts of Online Course Planning

Ron Lombard
Chatham University, USA

ABSTRACT

Materials presented deal with major aspects of planning an effective online course that can create an environment which will serve as a learning community. A review of misassumptions often made about online courses provides an introduction to the steps required make online courses effective. Issues covered include the knowledge and skills required from the instructor and participants for success in learning and instruction. The types of assignments and the importance of effective instructor feedback and instructor visibility are examined in relation to course construction. Effective assessment techniques for online courses are also examined in the context of the knowledge and skills participants in such courses should display. The major thrust of the presented materials is the understanding that as presentation techniques change assessment techniques need change to be effective.

INTRODUCTION

During the 2005-2006 school year over 500,000 K-12 students participated in an online course and more than one-third of public school districts offered virtual learning opportunities (Powell & Patrick, 2006). With this continued and increasing growth in virtual learning comes a need for qualified teachers who are effective in a virtual environment (Kyong & Bonk).Institutions of higher education have increasingly embraced online education, and the number of students enrolled in distance programs is rapidly rising in colleges and universities throughout the United States. In response to these changes in enrollment demands, many states, institutions, and organizations have been working on strategic plans to implement online education. At the same time, misconceptions and myths related to the difficulty of teaching and learning online, technologies available to support online instruction, the support and compensation needed for high-quality instructors, and the needs of online students create challenges

DOI: 10.4018/978-1-61520-899-9.ch002

for the creators of vision statements and planning documents.

In 2004 a research firm (Edu-ventures) released a report that put the number of students enrolled in online courses at close to one million, doubling the number from just two years earlier. The report predicts another 500,000 or more students will enroll in online courses over the next two years. The company estimates that by the end of 2008, students enrolled in courses entirely online will constitute more than 15 percent of the total number of students enrolled at degree-granting institutions in the United States (Carnevale, 2005). Sloan consortium reported in 2006 that 53.6% of surveyed colleges and universities see online courses as major part of plan for future. That future is now. The need for the development of online courses and the need for educators to employ skills in applying technology and producing effective online courses must be reviewed (Oblinger & Hawkins, 2005).

It is based on this level of growth and the need for creating effective online course that this chapter presents a basic guide to aid instructors of online courses to deal with issues and problems that arise. Having created and taught online courses for the past seven years the writer offers knowledge learned from mistakes made and insights of lessons learned. This chapter presents insights and suggestions dealing with aspects of the formation, administration, assessment and suggestions for online courses. The goal is the creation of a guide for online courses that function as real communities of learning in which both the students and instructor are highly engaged in the learning process. Emphasis is placed on the nuts and bolts of course planning and activities with suggestions that will aid instructors in setting up their own online courses.

Background

The organization of this chapter will explore misassumptions about online courses, what the instructor needs to know, and what skills and knowledge students need to have for success in such a learning environment. In the context of course administration the materials will review traditional tools for effective course presentation and new tools that will enhance all aspects of the course. There are a number of misassumptions about online courses that provide a guide to viewing what makes courses effective and presents materials in an organized manner that need to be reviewed. The role of the instructor in course construction and presentation in the context of visibility, understanding of and dealing effectively with student problems, both leading to the creation of a positive community of learning needs to be examined. Likewise, the skills, knowledge, attitudes, and technological abilities of class participants must be reviewed to create a framework for a course compatible to participants' individual needs and learning styles. The issue of effective assessment modalities is also reviewed in the context of online courses. These are the areas that serve as the nuts and bolts in the creation and holding together of online courses. Each factor must be considered so the correct nuts and bolts are selected for the creation and maintaining of an effective online course.

Misassumptions about Online Courses

There are a number of major misassumptions about online courses to review prior to considering methods to enhance courses, since these misassumptions impact on the major views of the value of online courses. One misassumption is that online courses are easier and require less time and effort than traditional courses. Research related to online courses suggest that nothing could be further from the truth. In many cases it requires more time to complete aspects of online courses and students on the average should be willing and able to commit to four to fifteen hours per week per course. Potential online students and instructors need to view online courses as a more convenient way to take course and not an easier way. The misassumption related to the issue of the depth of online courses is related to the first misassumption and allows critics of online courses to use this misassumption as an expression of weakness in courses. Another misassumption is that online courses only provide cursory or surface examinations of the subject matter and require the same level of skills from participants. To deal with this concern the instructors must plan courses that evoke higher levels skills of critical thinking and decision making. Projects and other major assessment tools in such courses must require that students apply newly learned knowledge and skills demonstrating the ability to make connections between reflective decisions and problem solving. The writing aspect of online courses also should place emphasis on the ability of learners to share ideas and insights over time and space, as in real life. Effective communication is a major skill needed in any area and since online courses call for a high level of written communication, students must demonstrate this skill at a high level of competency (Littlefield, 2007).

Another misassumption arises in the context the lack of face to face contact between faculty and students. Defenders of the online approach are quick to point out the use of discussion forums can create an environment that forces students to be more participatory in the class. Hiltz & Wu (2003) have carried out research demonstrating that the instructor plays an important role to motivate effective online discussions; more online guidance, more structured discussion topics and considerable time devotion are required for instructors.

It is important to point that this defense is based on an assumption that the instructor creates well planned discussion inquires and makes a sustained effort to reply to student responses. These replies are made in a manner that stimulates further discussions of responses, a skill the instructor needs to develop for courses to be really successful. Online forums and discussions support the major belief that before most individuals will commit thoughts to writing a great deal of reflection takes place when those thoughts are shared with others in the class. This belief, that reflections are enhanced by having students write responses, is a key factor that supports the online process. Markel (2001) Points out that the resulting kinds of learning from these processes are not a regurgitation of a lecture or reading. It is a negotiated interpretation of knowledge with student ownership. The learning is deeper and students refine their thinking and their voice through a reflective process.

A final misassumption is that online courses are not accepted by other institutions and are regarded as sub-standard in comparison to traditional courses. On the contrary, online courses are gaining acceptance and in some cases where the outcome of the course centers on a demonstration of working with others over distance it is preferable. Finally, completion of an online course demonstrates a student's abilities in relation to self-motivation and use of flexibility in the context of time (Littlefield, 2007).

What Online Instructors Need To Know

If one of the goals of an online course is to create a community of learning that calls for active participation and collaboration, there are specific suggestions for instructors to enhance their "visibility online". One of the ways this can be accomplished is to make instructor presence personal. The instructor achieves familiarity by releasing some personal information in terms of interests creating an environment that is open yet structured. The inclusion of photos allows students to place a name with a face and this works both ways with both students and instructors posting images. Introductions from course participants provide an environment in which the instructor and participants exchange some personal information creating an open environment allowing for expression of ideas. Introductions allow students an opportunity to find common interests among class members. Instructors need to be aware that their expectations for the course and for student performance form a model for student participation and attention to deadlines. Instructors provide a positive model by providing responses and feedback in a timely and insightful manner. Instructors must inform students that they have reviewed students' assignments and must keep in touch with students by posting personalized messages. Instructors can also take quotes from student comments and discussion forums when posting discussions. Announcements must be updated and those that are no longer relevant need to be deleted since clutter can cause confusion, Instructors can also post announcements and then send each student an email about the announcement to insure that each student receives personal notification of important topics (Baker, 2001; Woods & Ebersole, 2003).

At the beginning of the online course students must be informed of the instructor's expectations. One approach the instructor can implement is the posting of timelines or calendars online with specific dates and times for completing assignments for the course. This posting guides the students and they plan for effective use of time. This information can be posted in the course syllabus and also as a calendar. By presenting due dates in a different colored font, instructors insure that vital information is readily available for students. If the instructor conducts a podcast at the beginning of the course, students receive an introduction to the course and also make a personal connection with the instructor. The podcast also serves as a way for the instructor to provide specific instructions for the students (Savery, 2005).

The instructors need to make themselves available for dealing with issues for individual students. By setting office hours and utilizing chatting, the instructor gives the participants a set time by which they can communicate to deal with specific problems or questions related to the course. It is a good idea to post the times for such chat sessions at the start of the course allowing participants to plan for individual exchanges Personal contact could be required at the start of the course to make sure all participants and the instructor are on the same page. Later the communication can be made optional for participant. It is also a good idea for the instructor to log exchanges to refer to at a later time if a question or problem arises related to exchanges or instructions. Keeping a record of exchanges between the instructor and students is a wise move in terms of demonstrating a sincere effort to work with students having difficulties. Making an effort to remove bandwidth limitations to allow for the use of short video clips to serve as introductions to the course will go a long way in enhancing visibility and creating a feeling of real social presence for all participants. If such capability is available for the instructor, employing the process will help to meet the needs of students who learn best by visual stimulus.

The instructor can follow specific suggestions to insure that students are able to recognize expectations for the course. These suggestions enhance the level of instructor visibility and provide students with opportunities to ask questions related to the expectations for an online course. The posting of a "frequently asked questions" (FAQ) area, shared by all participants provides a commons area for determining the level at which participants demonstrate understanding of course expectations. The instructor can review postings and provide responses while becoming aware of concerns and problems as they arise. It is important for the instructor to display visibility here. Allowing participants to both post questions and offer comments also provides opportunities for participants to share insights and assume some ownership for the course. Participants can also provide suggestions to each other and to the instructor in some cases offering suggestions that improve aspects of the course. This can be a real aid to the instructor when issues related to technology of differing platforms comes up and participants with similar platforms can offer insights and suggestions that might not be immediately apparent to the instructor. Another helpful suggestion involves the creation of a commons area for participants to participate in exchanges not directly related to course assignments. The creation of a participant lounge where classmates can network provides an area where discussions can take place and not clutter up assignment discussion forums with non-course related information. The instructor should limit visibility in this area as it should be a place that participants can view as their own (Rourke, Anderson, Garrison, & Archer, 1999).

Administration of the online course requires that the instructor keeps the course organized and moving forward toward specific goals. Most important, the course must have a very high level of specificity. In this context the instructor needs to prepare the syllabus carefully and thoroughly and post it on the Learning Management System (LMS) so it is easily accessible by students. A well-conceived syllabus answers learner questions before they are asked. The syllabus must be proactive in terms of course assignments and expectations. The instructor needs to prepare a document that explains the "Do's and Don'ts" of the online class. This includes rules for netiquette, for comments in the discussion forums, and for communicating concerns to the instructor. Some instructors have students send an email message acknowledging that they have read the Class Rules and agree to abide by them. The instructor should use different formats for online resources and label each clearly (pdf, htm, doc, and ppt). Participants then select which format is most useful to them. The instructor provides information and links to specific applications such as Adobe Reader for pdf files.

The instructor can employ the capabilities of the LMS to control access to course materials. A selective release function manages files so that new instructional material is made available to the student only when mastery of previous material has been demonstrated. Depending on the sophistication of the LMS this may or may not be feasible. The purpose of this function is to allow the student to progress at an individual pace while ensuring that the instructional objectives have been achieved.

Displaying Compassion and Understanding For Student Problems

Instructors must display compassion and understanding of problems that confronts students in an online course. Some of the problems in the online course that evoke understanding and compassion by the instructor involve the computer and network technologies and the level of skills and knowledge of technology students bring to the course. Students can over estimate personal skills in utilizing technology or the ability of their equipment to meet the technical requirements of the course. The reaction of the instructor to these issues must demonstrate levels of both understanding and compassion in the context of participants' problems with equipment or skills with technology.

The instructor must take action to deal with these issues before their weight impacts on the course in a negative manner. Introductory requirements and assignments provide insight of individual levels of technical competence and identify students who may require additional supports. Individual students can contact the instructor in private personal way to share a lack of technical knowledge. This will provide the student will guidance without alerting other students to the problem and embarrassing the student. Problems similar to those that arise in the face to face classroom like family emergencies will arise and guidelines for dealing with these need to be addressed in the beginning of the course. The syllabus should provide some freedom for the instructor to meet these issues. The ability to deal with issues in private manner is important and gives the instructor the ability to make decisions that may have been unforeseen at the start of the course. Demonstrating understanding and compassion of student problems of a personal nature must be apparent throughout the course even though the instructor never meets face to face with students. The online environment should not lessen the interaction levels between all course participants or effect the decisions of the instructor. Displaying levels of understanding and compassion for individuals' concerns and problems of a personal nature are actions that must be exercised throughout the online course to allow development of an effective community of learning (Swan, 2004).

Creating an Effective Online Learning Community – Building Blocks For a Successful Course

The instructor provides an adequate amount of time between assignments to allow for the assessment of participants' levels of understanding before progressing on to deeper levels of cognitive materials. The strategy of providing smaller and more frequent assessments and spreading of assessment activities across the course will provide participants with a feeling of comfort in terms of course development. This will also provide participants with additional opportunities to process course concepts and content. The timeframes of the course need to allow for this ability to grasp the courses major concepts and skills. Trying to cover too much too fast with little time for reflection can be a totally ineffective approach. Individual student interactions include recognition of work that reflects a real understanding of materials. This is particularly true in the format of chat or forum discussions. In these formats instructors carry out questioning of student responses and assignments to bring about reflection in the context of applying theory to application and creation of products. With these goals in mind, it very effective to utilize a culminating activity that calls for application of individual skills and knowledge. Lapointe & Reisetter (2008) propose that clearly that online learning can support autonomy, through the creation of products. This is possible because the nature of this medium allows a number of choices about when and how to learn content. Likewise, a student's need for competence is supported by numerous opportunities to digest content and meet course goals. This type of activity allows participants to demonstrate levels of understanding and allows participants an opportunity to recognize their own growth in the context of the course.

Effective online learning is not passive. A collaborative approach allows for high levels of interactivity and is often employed to enhance the constructivist approach. Participants collaborating in common time can be facilitated if they are working on a common project or are participating in a common thread in a discussion or conversation about a topic. Researchers of aspects of motivation emphasize a student's need to belong to a learning community in order to achieve optimal learning (Baumeister & Leary, 1995; Osterman, 2000; Ryan & Deci, 2000). The projects, assignments, and discussions allow participants to assume the major role in the learning process with the instructor assuming a facilitative approach by providing resources and guidance for effective student centered learning (Northedge, 2002).

A suggested approach to organizing the online application is a sequence of units of study, which can be presented online as a learning sequence comprised of self-contained modules. The selection of a specific organizational approach depends on length and complexity of content being covered. A module can function at the level of a unit or a chapter. In any case, text headings serve as conceptual organizers for topics and subtopics within a module. This provides a structure that participants are familiar with and aids in exchanges between the participants and the instructor in terms of specific area for a course. The format helps in keeping all participants in the course on the same page. The more self-contained modules are, the easier they can be moved in the sequence of instruction or chosen for other customizations with content from other sources. These serve as self-contained lessons such as definitions or examples. Discrete learning objects and modules permit maximum flexibility in constructing courses, but it critical to functionally connect information as well. This interrelation of information creates a structure much like a text that utilizes advanced organizers like learning objectives, module openers and closers, discussion questions or critical thinking questions, overviews, summaries or reviews, and glosses for technical terms. All modules must have learning objectives, making clear what students should know or be able to do after interacting with the unit. These learning objectives and advanced organizers should be linked with various documents and other resources that will aid the participants in working through the lessons and meeting the requirements of the objectives (Wijekumar, 2005).

By laying out the modules and objectives in the context of a connective tissue, a well organized course can be formulated. The length of modules will be dependent on the depth of in which the material is to be presented and level of technicality. Since most online courses are presented in the time frame of a semester, modules are usually presented over the period of a week. The modules will be much like chapters in a text, except that the technology that can be employed in an online course should allow for the inclusion of interactions and use of media for presentation of materials. The media selected for inclusion must be chosen with the thought toward the pedagogy approach that best fits the needs of the objectives. The content of the module includes resources that will provide the background for students to gain an understanding of the objectives of the module. Keeping the resources centered on the objectives of the module is the key to providing participants with a sense of direction in the context of course development. It is essential to provide an organizational framework for the modules and the course so that clarity of purpose for assignments and materials displays the connection to objectives. Web-based instruction suggests an increasing communication among learners, including reconceptualizing learning from a one-time fixed term to an on-going event that is intermingled with the actual work processes. As part of the process of mastering content, significant learning often occurs as the result of learner-to-learner communication. Logically, meaningful learning is more likely to occur when learners have access to a supportive community that encourages knowledge building and social reinforcement (Moller, Wellesley, Huett, 2008).

Skills and Knowledge of Online Participants

The basic skills required for online participants includes telecommunication skills, use of emails, uploading and downloading attachments and hyperlinks, use of zip-files, and uploading procedures for specific Learning Management Systems (LMS). Knowledge of an individual's computer operating system, recognition that there will be difference between Apple and PC platforms and, most importantly an understanding of the speed of one's Internet setup is aspects of technical knowledge that play a major role in the course. If any plug-in is required the participants will need knowledge in these areas as well. It would save a lot of problems if instructions for and a guide is made available to students who may have concerns or problems with technical aspects of the course. Another suggestion is to provide a non-threatening assignment at the start of the course that requires the application of these skills to allow both the student and the instructor an opportunity to assess and discuss any concerns or problems. Once the problems of technology are dealt with, then the instructor can address the really important demands of the course, in terms of the participants' ability to collaborate and communicate in an effective manner.

A multi-year study reviewed the major skills, needs and expectations of both instructors and participants providing insights into areas of course construction. Identified are the following conclusions: the availability of multiple tools added flexibility to the learning environment. The selected technology tools must appeal to multiple participant learning styles. Both collaboration and reflection elements are needed to play a major role in the course. A course can be constructed in which a learning community is created with all the required elements in place to ensure a level of success (Menchaca & Bekele, 2008).

The emphasis placed on effective communication of ideas within limited presentation modalities is heightened in the online format. A solution to this is to take into account differing participants' styles of communication and provide a number of presentation opportunities allowing options for presentation formats. Rather than rely only on narrative feedback from participants such response opportunities could include power point presentations, participant created podcasts, and discussion forum responses that display both presentation skills to summarize materials and abilities to display listening skills in the context of other participants' responses. In any discussions or responses it is also important for participants to be aware of the importance of netiquette to enhance communications. The basic rules to remember include;

- Adhere to the same standards of behavior that you would in face to face conversations
- Make sure to take into account other participants' time and bandwidth capabilities
- Respect the privacy of others
- Be willing to take into account other participants have the right to express differing opinions
- Mistakes will be made since we are dealing with humans
- Do not express anything that totally disregards the feeling of others
- Recognize the fact that not everyone has the same bandwidth to deal with normal attachments and graphics
- Remember anything put online can be public, at the very least by course participants, and some information participants may not wish to share.

Keeping in mind that the whole point of discussion forums is for participants to express individual views makes it important to accept the fact that participants will express points of views or insights that may not be totally acceptable to all participants. This must be viewed as an opportunity to listen to what others have to say and add to the learning experience of the online process. If a point of view does appear to be questionable, a discussion is more beneficial than an attack on the participant's position and can lead to insights by other participants. If positions still seem questionable, the beauty of the forum is the ability to provide attachments to support the one's point of view. This sharing of additional sources opens a whole new perspective in some cases and students centered learning can take place. Participants, being human, also will make mistakes in posting and presenting materials. Participants need to be tolerant of mistakes and request a clarification rather than posting negative statements about responses. In the context of bandwidth, the factor of time plays a major role in an effective flow in the course. It is always best to make statements and responses brief and to the point and to decide if the time required for down loading is worth the interruption of course flow. Being brief takes into account that all participants wish to feel they have an adequate opportunity to express views and no one participants needs to feel the need to be the center of the entire conversation (Shea, 2004).

The personal characteristics of online participants play a major role in the level of success in an online course. These characteristics are internal attributes of participants and need examination in the context of retention of a participant in online courses. Terrell (2008) suggests the most outstanding of the attributes for online classes include:

- Self-motivation either intrinsic or extrinsic
- Independence
- Task oriented
- Good time management capabilities
- High level of reading comprehension skills in particular in following instructions
- Above average communication and writing skills

The importance of the characteristic of self-motivation is supported by the understanding that most online participants have had little past experience in a learning environment that does not provide face to face interaction with an instructor to check on progress. The motivation that participants need to stay actively engaged in the course is dependent on how much feedback participants require. If participants are deeply interested in understanding the material being presented, intrinsic motivation is an effective driving force. If, however, participants are motivated primarily by grades, external motivation is the driving force and the instructor needs to provide feedback as often as possible to supply the motivation required to maintain a level of engagement. The importance of being task oriented and having good time management capabilities is of major importance since the typical online course is not self-paced. In most cases there are deadline for assignments even though the class does not meet at a constant established time. This requires the establishment of a personal schedule to cover materials and complete assignments and a level of self-discipline and independence that is above that of most traditional courses environments. Following instructions is connected to effective time management since getting things correct the first time will save a great deal of time throughout the entire course. Following directions is also connected to effective reading skills since the ability to comprehend instructions and understand written assignments is a skill required for success in online courses.

A number research projects have been conducted to examine the relationship between online participants' attributes and success in online courses. The studies were conducted in response to the trend of many students to drop out of online courses and to identify personal attributes of these students. The strongest connections between dropping an online course and personal attributes were found in the areas of past academic success, patterns of dropping out at the beginning of a course, offering of orientation prior to entering an online course, higher reading scores on standardized tests, and the level of experience with technology. It is only common sense that students who have developed problems with academic success would also display the same lack of success in an online course. Likewise, why would an online course be different, if a pattern has been established in dropping out of courses? The orientation factor, however, illustrates the importance of motivation of the student since in most cases the orientation was an optional experience. Participants in online courses who took advantage of the orientation were more successful in the courses. Students made individual decisions to either take part or not take part in the orientation demonstrating the importance of task orientation and self-motivation. The higher level of experience participants had with technology in the context of prior online courses also has a positive impact on future online success. The standout ability and attribute for success in online courses is related to reading comprehension levels. This is an important factor to be aware of in that it suggests the point that the basic skill of reading must be established for success in online courses. This drives home the point that the skills that have been basic in our educational system for years will continue to impact student success even in the context of increasing use of technology for the teaching and learning processes. Without basic skills, technology will make little difference as a teaching or learning tool. This finding is the most valuable lesson to be learned from the research related to success in online courses (Wojciechowski & Palmer, 2005).

Online course require that participants adjust to at least two overlying concepts that might not be as prevalent in traditional course. These two areas deal with participants being active defenders of their ideas and values combined with an open-mindedness allowing for viewing materials from various perspectives and becoming comfortable with a student –centered approach that calls for collaborative problem solving. Reviewing elements of the first aspect, the participants will be placed in position in which calls for a defense of their positions in a written format demonstrating a real understanding and organization of thoughts about their individual values. And since this is an expectation for all participants the exchange of perspectives should allow for the possibility of participants to widen their views about various elements covered in the course. Since communication is the means by which individuals will be required to demonstrate effective skills, it is vital that participants can communicate effectively in writing and organize presentations in a clear and concise manner. The second area, acceptance of a student-centered approach and collaboration, forces participants to accept new learning approaches. Students assume responsibility for the major aspects of both the teaching and learning processes. This will require students to employ aspects of problem solving approaches. The problem-solving aspect is linked to real-world situations and calls for collaboration over time and distance which for many participants is a new concept. Adjusting to this new type of learning environment composed of so many different approaches and expectations can be difficult for newcomers to online courses and these adjustments need to be taken into account when observing participant work throughout the course.

APPROACHES TO EFFECTIVE ONLINE ASSESSMENT

Any course, either face to face or online, requires tools for accountability in relation to mastery of materials and observable levels of understanding. To provide accountability, testing and assessments are utilized to serve as tools to measure the levels of participants' ability to demonstrate mastery of knowledge and to provide evidence of participants' ability to apply content knowledge to solving problems in the context of that knowledge. Testing measures the knowledge level mastered by participants. While the assessment process focuses on measuring the abilities in terms of application of that knowledge, online courses place a great deal of emphasis on collaboration and communication. The assessment process needs to be viewed not as an end but as a means to complete the learning process (Volderwell, et. al. 2007).

The major problems with assessments and testing in online course center on the lack of ability to monitor course participants in a traditional sense. Academic honesty becomes an issue since the instructor cannot be positive the work received is being submitted by a specific course participant. Likewise, the issue of time differs from face to face and online courses. Traditional courses in general have set time limits of testing durations and the settings in which testing takes place. Traditional testing also does not allow for the use of extensive resources to be utilized while the examination takes place. But when assessment takes place online, the instructor would have no idea what types of resources the participant may be utilizing while taking part in the assessment. Instructors who place no credence on results from open-book assessments will find this as an unacceptable weakness in online assessment. These issues all give rise to a fear that the expected levels of accountability in the context of assessment security cannot be maintained in an online setting. If this assumption is accepted many of the assessment proof used to support participant accountability in the context of the course could be viewed as weak at best (Khare & Lam, 2008). To deal with these issues it is apparent that the use of and types of assessments must be reviewed and examined for online courses. This review of assessment modality in an online environment must take place since any major changes in the way materials are presented is counter-balanced by the need to change the way we assess materials in this environment.

Online courses create an environment in which both constructivist and situated learning are excellent teaching and learning techniques. The constructivist approach focuses on the aspects of inquiry and analysis as learning avenues for knowledge mastery. This approach also places great emphasis on the participant's desire to learn not to receive a positive grade but because of a desire to extend a level of knowledge (Wolsey, 2008). The constructivist approach is paired with the situated learning approach calling for the use of knowledge to be applied to real life situations in most online courses. This is an approach different from many traditional courses because it requires higher level application skills and higher level thinking skills on the part of course participants. The instructor must offer an extension of time for assessments if they are to be completed in a comprehensive, reflective fashion. The online environment is excellent for this approach since it allows for participant differences in the context of need for time to complete assignments in a location that provides a level of comfort acclimated for the individual (Khare & Lam, 2008). The time required to truly reflect on content and to respond the questioning in the context of course content does require participant responses that display a level of understanding and reflection. This means that expectations for discussion responses and completed assignments are higher in many cases than in traditional courses. This changes the assessment modality, in that the questions asked and the prompts for the discussion forums must call for a demonstration of a deeper understanding and the ability to apply content and knowledge to real life situations. The assessments become protracted in nature since the expectations become higher (Wolsey, 2008).

To deal with the problems discussed at the start of this section, the following insights are offered to deal with each of the problems related to assessment. In the context of academic honesty, the suggestion is made that instructors take time to become familiar with the writing style of course participants. Through close observation of threaded discussion responses the instructor would be able to recognize any major changes in responses presented by individual participants. This should deal with the issue of knowing who is really doing the work in the online course. It must be understood, however, that student writing skills will become enhanced throughout the course and the instructor must remain aware of participants work throughout the course. The issue of time can be dealt with through most learning management systems by controlling the amount of time the testing aspect of the course will be left open to responses. This can even be controlled in such a manner for online courses that takes into account different time zones of participants. The important aspect in relation to time for assessments must be linked to goals of the course. If the test is only looking for a demonstration of context knowledge such adaptations will meet the needs of the course. But, if the goal of the assessment is to assess deeper levels of understandings of course materials a protracted assessment approach allowing adequate time for reflection and review of content is prove to be more effective. This belief of need time for reflection holds true with both written assignments and with discussion forum materials. The availability of resources to be utilized during the assessment process concern needs to be reviewed in the context of situated learning. In the context of real life authentic assessment is the format that could provide a judgment as to the level of a participant's ability to organize and apply content knowledge to deal with content related issues. If we want to assess in this type of environment, we need to take into account that in real life situations individuals do refer to resources and cannot be expected to retain every separate piece of content. The fact that online participants know what types of resources would serve best and where to find specific information demonstrates that they would be able to do the same in an authentic situation if it arose (Gaytan, 2005).

A review of the literature about online courses and the specific goals and objectives for participants aside from the basic mastery of content information displays similarities in the context of preparing participants for applying knowledge and skills. The common application skills for online courses appear to match with more open-ended types of assessments. The skills being assessed are

- Development of strategic / critical thinking
- Analysis and interpretation of information / data
- Decision making skills based on a cycle of analysis – reflection - solution – implementation of action plan
- Integration of knowledge and learning to deal with course objectives (Kahre & Lam, 2008).

These skills match with the suggested pattern of assessment for formative data leading to a comprehensive examination to serve as a summative evaluation for measuring student mastery of content and skills in the course (Vonderwell, Liang, Alderman, 2007). Many of the devises used for assessment in online courses are geared toward the formative aspect of assessment to determine if participants are really meeting the level of understanding required for success in the course. Instructor analysis on postings and responses on course discussion forums is an excellent example of this approach. The forum needs to be directed by content application questions and participants must receive specific feedback to serve as a guide in terms of formative assessment. The forum with participant response, questions, and collaboration provide an excellent window in which to view participant application of content knowledge and reflections connected to the major course objectives (Wolsey, 2008).

Gaytan (2005) presents the view that these types of assessments appear to offer the best means of assessment in an online course fall in to the categories of:

- **Authentic Assessment:** based on real world performance of participants to demonstrate application of content knowledge
- **Performance Assessments:** that reflects skills of participants in action in the context of the learning process and where emphasis is placed on long term vs. short term memory
- **Portfolio Assessment:** where all final products of the course can be collected for review in the context of growth and development displayed by participants as they progress through the course

The specific articles to be assessed by these types of assessment are generally fall into four areas:

- **Asynchronous Discussions:** This area of assessment calls for structure to be effective by the use of assigned roles for some participants in such discussions and posting protocols which make clear the expectations for discussion forums. Content understanding, collaboration, and participation are the specific areas to be measured in these forums (Vonderwell, et al., 2007).
- **Case Studies:** The use of case studies as a background for assessment of both skills and knowledge is an excellent means by which to examine participants' abilities to deal with analytical aspects of content from the course. The case study approach for assessment allows observation of the

participant passing through the processes of evaluating a specific situation, interpreting data, applying and integrating what has been learned through the course, and the creation of logical positions based on supporting content choices and recommendations (Khare & Lam, 2008).

- **Project Completion:** The use of project-based assessments to evaluate participants work offers a great deal of potential since it is closely related to the case study approach but allows more flexibility in terms of choosing project that are connected to the major content topic of the course.

All of these assessment items reviewed above require structure for results to have any validity. The major suggested structure for such assessment is the utilization of specific rubrics that measures participants' work in the context of all the expectations for the course. Feedback from the rubric needs to review all criteria and keep participants informed as to what particular strengths and weakness are observed. The rubric will be a key measuring tool for all the above mentioned assessment modalities. The feedback provided through these rubrics is of major importance and instructors need to put major thought into its creation (Wolsey, 2008).

- **Traditional Testing:** This form of assessment still has its place in the assessment process and it can be controlled and monitored at least to some degree. To check on participants' knowledge of content this approach is still effective and quick. But if the goals are for review of real levels of understanding this approach will fall short.

SUGGESTIONS FOR FUTURE RESEARCH

There is still a need to research the strategies that will be implemented for an effective online course and most important a review of how prepared instructors and participants are to enter the environment of online courses. Research centering on the so-called "born digital" generation in terms of success in online courses also needs to be carried out in the future. Assessment modalities for online courses needs a great deal more research with emphasis on the use the use of rubrics for effective assessment.

CONCLUSION

While the implementation of online courses has grown, more training is required by both instructors and participants to increase the level of success and retention in the online environment. The role of the instructor changes to become a coach and facilitator and the skills of the participants grow in the context of application of knowledge. One problem that needs to be addressed when planning for an effective online environment is the creation of a balance between the structure of such a course and the autonomy for participants to view assignments and content from differing perspectives. The structure of the course clarifies expectations for participants, while the autonomy allows participants to go beyond a simple review of course content. It is also very surprising that so little research has been carried out in relation to effective assessment techniques for online courses. The research on online courses must continue as the capabilities of the technology increases and more participants come into online courses with a deeper background in effective use of technology.

REFERENCES

Baker, J. D. (2001). The effects of instructor immediacy and student cohesiveness on affective and cognitive learning in the online classroom. (Doctoral dissertation, Regent University, 2001). *Dissertation Abstracts International, 62*, 06. 2081 UMI No. 3018333.

Baumeister, R. F., & Leary, M. R. (1995). The need to belong: Desire for interpersonal attachments as a fundamental human motivation. *Psychological Bulletin, 117*(3), 497–529. doi:10.1037/0033-2909.117.3.497

Carneval, D. (2005, June 28). Online Courses Continue to Grow Dramatically. *Chronicle of Higher Education*, 14-26. Retrieved September 2, 2008 from http://chronicle.com/prm/daily/2005/06/2005062802t.htm

Gaytan, J. (2005). Effective Assessment Techniques for Online Instruction. *Information Technology. Learning and Performance Journal, 23*(1), 25–36.

Hiltz, R., & Wu, D. (2003). *Online Discussions and Perceived Learning*. Retrieved May 2009, from http://www.alnresearch.org/Data_Files/articles/full_text/wu_Hiltz(2003).pdf

Khare, A., & Lam, H. (2008). Assessing Student Achievement and Progress with Online Examinations: Some Pedagogical and Technical Issues. *International Journal on E-Learning, 7*(3), 383–403.

Kyong, J. K., & Bonk, C. J. (2006). The Future of Online Teaching and Learning in Higher Education. *EduCause Quarterly, 29*(4). Retrieved October 23, 2008 from http://net.eduause.edu/ir/library/pdf/eqm0644.pdf

LaPointe, L., & Reisetter, M. (2008). Belonging Online: Students' Perceptions of the Value and Efficacy of an Online Learning Community. *International Journal on E-Learning, 7*(4), 641–666.

Littlefield, J. (2008). Top 5 Distance Learning Myths. *About.com*. Retrieved October 30, 2008, from http://distancelearn.about.com/od/distancelearning101/a/5Myths.htm

Markel, S. (2001). Technology and Education Online Discussion Forums: It's in the Response. *Online Journal of Distance Learning Administration, 4*(2), 63–74.

Menchaca, M., & Bekele, T. A. (2008). Learner and instructor identified success factors in distance education. *Distance Education, 29*(3), 231–253. doi:10.1080/01587910802395771

Moller, L., Foshay, W. R., & Huett, J. (2008). The Evolution of Distance Education: Implications for Instructional Design on the Potential of the Web. *TechTrends, 52*(3), 70-76. Retrieved April 2009, from http://ncolr.org/jiol/issues/viewarticle.cfm?volID=4&IssueID=15&ArticleID=73

Northedge, A. (2002). Teaching by Distance Learning. In McKeachie, W. J. (Ed.), *Teaching Tips* (11th ed., pp. 258–267). Boston, MA: Houghton-Mifflin.

Oblinger, D., & Hawkins, B. (2008). We don't Need to Worry about E-Learning Anymore. *EduCause Review, 40*(4), 14-15. Retrieved September 30, 2008 from http://connect.educause.edu/Library/EDCAUSE+REVIEW/The Mythab outELearning/40560?time=1237616004

Osterman, K. F. (2000). Students' need for belonging in the school community. *Review of Educational Research, 70*(3), 323–367.

Rourke, L., Anderson, T., Garrison, D., & Archer, W. (1999). Assessing social presence in asynchronous text-based computer conferencing. *Journal of Distance Education, 14*(2), 14-28. Retrieved November 1, 2008, from http://cade.athabascau.ca/vol14.2/rourke_et_al.html

Ryan, R. M., & Deci, E. L. (2000). Intrinsic and extrinsic motivations: Classic definitions and new directions. *Contemporary Educational Psychology*, *25*(1), 54–67. doi:10.1006/ceps.1999.1020

Savery, J. R. (2008). BE VOCAL: Characteristics of Successful Online Instructors. [from http://www.ncolr.org/jiol]. *Journal of Interactive Online Learning*, *4*(2), 141–159. Retrieved October 15, 2008.

Shea, V. (2004). Netiquette. *Albion Books*. Retrieved November 15, 2008 from http://www.albion.com/catNetiquette.html

Swan, K. (2004). Relationships between Interactions and Learning in Online Environments. *Sloan-C Effective Practices Site*. Retrieved October 4, 2008, from http://www.aln.org/effective/index.asp

Terrell, S. (2008). Consider Learner Characteristics, Learning Conditions in Course Design. *Magna Resources for Higher Education September*. Retrieved November 30, 2008, from http://www.magnapubs.com/issues/magnapubs_ff/5_22/news/601829-1.html

Vonderwell, S., Liang, X., & Alderman, K. (2007). Asynchronous Discussions and Assessment in Online Learning. *Journal of Research on Technology in Education*, *39*(3), 309–329.

Wijekumar, K. (2005). Creating Effective Web-Based learning Environments: Relevant Research and Practice. *Innovate, 1*(5). Retrieved, December 29, 2008, from http://www.innovateonline.info/index.php?view=article&id=26

Wojciechowski, A., & Palmer, L. B. (2005). Individual Student Characteristics: Can Any Be Predictors Of Success In Online Classes? *Online Journal of Distance Learning Administration, 8*(2). Retrieved December 20, 2008, from http://www.westga.edu/~distance/ojdla/summer82/wojciechowski82.htm

Wolsey, T. (2008). Efficacy of Instructor Feedback on Written Work in an Online Program. *International Journal on E-Learning*, *7*(2), 311–330.

ADDITIONAL READING

Abbott, L. (2005). The Nature of Authentic Professional Development during Curriculum-Based Telecomputing. *Journal of Research on Technology in Education*, *37*(4), 379–398.

Allen, E., & Seaman, J. (2008). *Staying the course: Online education in the United States. (Technical Report)*. Needham, MA: Sloan Consortium.

Carr-Chellman, A. A. (2006). Desperate technologists: Critical issues in e-learning and implications for higher education. *Journal of Thought*, *41*(1), 95–119.

Charlene, A Dykman, Charles K Davis. (2008). Online Education Forum - Part Three A Quality Online Educational Experience. *Journal of Information Systems Education*, *19*(3), 281–290.

Dawson, S. (2006). A study of the relationship between student communication interaction and sense of community. *The Internet and Higher Education*, *9*, 153–162. doi:10.1016/j.iheduc.2006.06.007

Dick, W., Carey, L., & Carey, J. O. (2005). The Systematic Design of Instruction (6,h ed.). Boston, MA: Allyn and Bacon.

Doyle, William, R. (2009). Online Education: The Revolution That Wasn't. *Change*, *41*(3), 56–59. doi:10.3200/CHNG.41.3.56-58

Greco, Gina. (2009). Teaching Online: 2 Perspectives--A Reaffirmation of Why I Became an Educator. *The Chronicle of Higher Education.* 55, (38), p. A.33.

Hirschheim, R. (2005). The Internet-Based Education Bandwagon: Look Before You Leap. *Communications of the ACM, 48*(7), 97–101. doi:10.1145/1070838.1070844

Lewis, C. C., & Abdul-Hamid, H. (2006). Implementing effective online teaching practices: Voices of exemplary faculty. *7wiovafive. Higher Education, 57*(2), 83–98.

Mitchem, K., Fitzgerald, G., Hollingsead, C., & Koury, K. (2008). Enhancing Case-Based Learning in Teacher Education Through Online Discussions: Structure and Facilitation. *Journal of Interactive Learning Research, 19*(2), 331–350.

Natarajan, M. (2006). Use of Online Technology for Multimedia Education. *Information Services & Use, 26*(3), 249–256.

Roblyer, M. D. (2006). *Integrating Educational Technology into Teaching* (4th ed.). Upper Saddle River, NJ: Pearson Education, Inc.

Singh, P., & Pan, W. (2004). Online education: Lessons for administrators and instructors. *College Student Journal, 38*, 302–308.

Snyder, M. (2009). Instructional-Design Theory to Guide the Creation of Online Learning Communities for Adults. *TechTrends, 53*(1), 48–57.

Spellings, M. (2006). *A Test of Leadership: Charting the Future of U.S. Higher Education. Jessup.* MD: U.S. Dept. of Education - Education Publications Center.

Stagg, S. P., & Slotta, J. (2009). Saying Yes to Online Learning: A First-Time Experience Teaching an Online Graduate Course in Literacy Education. *Literacy Research and Instruction, 48*(2), 120–137. doi:10.1080/19388070802226303

Swan, K. (2001). Virtual interaction: Design factors affecting student satisfaction and perceived learning in asynchronous online courses. *Distance Education, 22*, 306–331. doi:10.1080/0158791010220208

Tallent-Runnels, M. K., Thomas, J. A., Lan, W. Y., Cooper, S., Ahern, T. C., & Shaw, S. M. (2006). Teaching courses online: A review of the research. *Review of Educational Research, 76*(1), 93–115. doi:10.3102/00346543076001093

Vonderwell, S., & Zachariah, S. (2005). Factors that influence participation in online learning. *Journal of Research on Technology in Education, 38*(2), 213–230.

Waltonen-Moore, S., Stuart, D., Newton, E., Oswald, R., & Varonis, E. (2006). From Virtual Strangers to a Cohesive Online Learning Community: The Evolution of Online Group Development in a Professional Development Course. *Journal of Technology and Teacher Education, 14*(2), 287–312.

Wong, A. F., Choon-Lang, Q., Divaharan, S., Woon-Chia, L., Peer, J., & Williams, M. D. (2006). Students' and Teachers' Perceptions of Computer-Supported Project Work Classroom Learning Environments. *Journal of Research on Technology in Education, 38*(4), 449–479.

Wuensch, Karl L, Wuensch, Shahnaz Aziz, Ozan, Erol, & Kishore, Masao, M H N Tabrizi. (2008). Pedagogical Characteristics of Online and Face-to-Face Classes. *International Journal on E-Learning, 7*(3), 523–533.

Zhao, Y. (2007). Social studies teachers' perspective of technology integration. *Journal of Technology and Teacher Education, 15*(3), 311–333.

Zhao, Y., Pugh, K., Sheldon, S., & Byers, J. (2002). Conditions for classroom technology innovations. *Teachers College Record, 104*(3), 482–515. doi:10.1111/1467-9620.00170

Chapter 3
Implementing an Online Educational Technology Course in a Teacher Preparation Program:
Challenges and Solutions

Heejung An
William Paterson University, USA

Hilary Wilder
William Paterson University, USA

ABSTRACT

To positively foster teacher knowledge, skills and beliefs regarding technology integration, a teacher preparation program at a university in New Jersey, USA carried out the process of revising a face-to-face technology skill based course into a fully online one in which the focus changed to "teaching with technology." This chapter provides a detailed account of how the course was revised, and describes the challenges the authors faced. The solutions that came to the fore during this process are also provided. The chapter concludes with recommendations for other teacher educators who might be offering online educational technology courses to candidates of a similar population.

INTRODUCTION

In order to support teacher candidates in becoming practitioners capable of understanding and applying technology integration in their future classrooms, research suggests that pre-service teachers should be prepared to teach *with* technology, rather than just learning *about* technology (Glazewski & et. al., 2001; Doolittle & Hicks, 2003; Mason et al., 2000; Mishra & Koelher, 2008; Wenglinsky, 2005). To address this pedagogical issue, the teacher preparation program at William Paterson University, New Jersey, USA, revised its technology course requirement, moving it from one focusing on only the acquisition of technology skills to one in which elementary school teacher candidates were encouraged to use a range of Information and Communication Technologies (ICT) to teach various types of subject matter

DOI: 10.4018/978-1-61520-899-9.ch003

content, while also promoting student-centered technology integration to ensure their future K-12 students meet state and/or federal mandates for technological literacy. This is clearly important in the U.S. since the National Educational Technology Standards for Teachers (ISTE, 2008) exemplify uses of technology to maximize teaching effectiveness as well as to advance students' technological literacy. It is also important to note that teachers need to know how to use assistive technologies to maximize the effectiveness of the instructional experiences for all students.

The objectives of this chapter are three-fold. The first is to describe the rationale and theoretical underpinnings for developing an online educational technology course that addressed these aims, along with the collaborative strategies employed to successfully implement the online educational technology course. In describing this, we address the challenges encountered and how we attempted to solve them in order to bring the plan to fruition. The second objective is to report our findings, in order to show the effectiveness of this endeavor. Lastly, we will provide some lessons learned that might be applicable to other teacher preparation programs with similar student populations.

THEORETICAL BACKGROUND

Teaching about Technology and with Technology

In the United States, there has been a strong push to integrate technology into teacher preparation programs. Yet, even though the student to computer ratio has been raised up to 3.8:1, numerous research studies have indicated that technology is not being integrated into school curricula successfully (Wells & Lewis, 2006). For instance, Brown and Warschauer (2006) have reported that "... even with the latest emphasis on technology, many public school districts are faced with an unwelcome surprise. After spending millions of dollars to connect their schools and their students to the Internet, their newly installed computers often sit unused" (p. 600). Furthermore, even when technology is incorporated into the curriculum, it is often used for efficiency oriented tasks, such as word processing, rather than more educative purposes (Cuban, 2001).

This problem is partly due to the way in which educational technology courses are taught in teacher education programs. Research has shown that many programs tend to offer a single educational technology course focusing only on basic technology skills training (Kay, 2006), rather than technology across the curriculum to promote higher-order thinking and problem-solving skills. As a result, many students feel unprepared to enter classrooms ready to use technology in meaningful ways (Brown & Warschauer, 2006). That being said, there has been little clarity regarding what knowledge teachers need to know to effectively integrate technology into their teaching practice. To address this concern about how to best focus on technology integration in teacher preparation programs as a way of thinking about the knowledge teachers should obtain in order to integrate technology into their teaching effectively, Mishra and Koelher (2006) introduced the Technological Pedagogical Content Knowledge (TPACK) framework. This conception is not entirely new, rather it has been extended from Shulman's (1986) work describing pedagogical content knowledge, emphasizing the importance of "the central role of content and pedagogy in uses of educational technology" (Bull et al., 2007). In this conception, Mishra and Koelher (2008) stressed that an analysis of teaching and learning with technology requires an understanding of the complex set of interrelationships among pedagogy, content, and technical knowledge. Thus, instead of seeing these as three distinct knowledge bases, - Technological Knowledge (TK), Pedagogical Knowledge (PK), and Technology (TK) - they emphasized the interactions between and among these three forms of knowledge. That is, there are interactions between PK and CK which bring about Pedagogical Content Knowledge (PCK); TK and CK taken together bring about Technological Content Knowledge (TCK); the intersections of Technology and Pedagogy bring about Technological Pedagogical Knowledge (TPK); the interactions of all three bodies among knowledge Technology, Pedagogy, and Content, bring about Technological Pedagogical Content Knowledge (TPACK). Technological Knowledge (TK): Knowledge of the skills required to utilize a technology effectively. More detailed information about TPACK can be found at http://www.tpck.org. The definitions of each of the aforementioned forms of knowledge are as follows (Mishra, & Koehler, 2008).

- **Technology Knowledge (TK):** Knowledge about technologies (e.g., Blackboard, Internet, digital video).
- **Content Knowledge (CK):** Knowledge about the actual subject matter that is to be learned/taught.
- **Pedagogical Knowledge (PK):** Knowledge of the processes and practice or methods of teaching and learning and how it encompasses overall educational purposes, values and aims.
- **Pedagogical Content Knowledge (PCK):** Knowledge of pedagogy that is applicable to the teaching of specific content.
- **Technological Content Knowledge (TCK):** Knowledge that involves understanding of the manner in which technology and content are reciprocally related to each other.
- **Technological Pedagogical Knowledge (TPK):** Knowledge that emphasizes the existence, components and capabilities of various technologies as they are used in teaching and learning settings.
- **Technological Pedagogical Content Knowledge (TPACK):** Knowledge that emphasizes the dynamic, transactional relationship between these three knowledge components.

However, it is important to note that at the same time, it is often emphasized that even though technologies should not be positioned or taught as stand-alone tools, research indicates that one of the primary frustrations teachers experience during technology integration efforts is their own lack of computer knowledge and experience (Hanks, 2002; Mehlinger & Powers, 2002).

Digital Divide

Since 2001, the No Child Left Behind Act (USDOE, 2001) has required that students achieve technological literacy by Grade 8. However, efforts to assess this and hold districts accountable for meeting this mandate have only recently been put in place (eSchool News, 2008). In the meantime, across the U.S. (DeBell & Chapman, 2003) and around the world (Trucano, 2005) the digital divide still exists in the use and access to information and communication technologies in education. Students' exposure to technological literacy, even in highly developed U.S. states like New Jersey, has been uneven, with affluent districts providing rich technology-integrated instruction (as well as students having access to technology in their homes) and less affluent district making it a lower priority. As such, in order to ensure students' technological literacy (especially if they do not have the technology available outside of school (Fox & Livingston, 2007)), teachers and administration must be fully behind these efforts and prepared to implement them, in addition to having the actual technology and infrastructure available. Unfortunately, from our own experience, many of the students who enter our program come from neighboring urban districts which do not have these fully-supported programs in place, thus creating a chicken-and-egg problem.

Usage of Online Courses in Teacher Preparation Programs

In recent years, online courses and programs have gained a great deal of popularity in teacher preparation programs, primarily because students find this instructional modality to be very convenient. For example, Hudson (2006) examined preservice teachers' perceptions of online science instruction and found that most students perceived that the primary perceived advantage was flexibility in learning. In their study, this flexibility included: maintaining lifestyle and working arrangements, catering to individual learning modes, accessing web-based resources and assessment examples at any time, and more open communication with faculty and peers. Perceived disadvantages included the issue of self-discipline for completing the course requirements, the uncertainty of ICT skills needed for completing assessment tasks and the variability of support during lectures. Although there has been concern over the quality and effectiveness of alternate route programs in general, and online programs specifically (Baines, 2006), it is clear that the use of online technologies will continue to grow in professional development programs and provide lifelong learning opportunities for teachers.

AN ONLINE EDUCATIONAL TECHNOLOGY COURSE FOCUSING ON TEACHING WITH TECHNOLOGY

Background and Challenges

Although we have long required an educational technology course as part of the K-8 initial certification program at William Paterson University, in the past this course was viewed as an add-on, designed to be taken during the student teaching semester and predominantly taught by adjuncts. Since there was no pre-requisite for this course, many students had only minimal technology experience. The bulk of the class was therefore spent teaching basic technology skills (which tended to be developed only as standalone TK) for students who were often exhausted and overwhelmed with student teaching. It was obvious to most (including the students) that this was a case of "too little, too late," recognizing that: a) the technology skills and techniques they were finally learning would have been useful to them throughout their college experience; and b) they were not getting much in the way of TPK, TCK, or TPACK.

In 2005, as part of a state-mandated overhaul of our teacher preparation programs, the course was revised to be taken when students first entered the program and subsequently delivered online via the Blackboard Course Management System. An underlying goal was to move the focus away from acquiring a prescribed set of technology skills toward teaching with technology to develop TPACK (Mishra & Koelher, 2006), so that teacher candidates could begin developing knowledge and the capability to integrate technology in meaningful ways into their content and pedagogy, especially as a means to promote future student-centered activities that would facilitate higher-order thinking and collaboration (Doolittle & Hicks, 2003; Mason et al., 2000; Wenglinsky, 2005). Besides this focus shift regarding the course content, there were other goals that we hoped to accomplish through this online course: a) help the teacher candidates become aware of how learning can occur with/through technology; and b) help these future teachers become comfortable and experienced in using online distance-learning technologies for their own professional development and lifelong learning. That is, students were expected to consider themselves as self-regulated learners who would thrive with this form of instruction.

However, as the course was revised, we also faced new challenges. First, there was a realization that while the technological literacy of incoming students had steadily improved, due to the introduction of recent state K-12 technology standards, many (particularly from financially disadvantaged districts) still arrived unprepared. Switching to an online format, focusing on teaching with technology (with no hands-on lab) made us very aware of the digital divide occurring in K-12 school settings in the US that many of our students came out of. This lack of previous exposure to basic and contemporary digital tools made it much harder for us to provide meaningful educational technology courses which looked at ways in which the tools could be used for pedagogical purposes (Ferris, Roberts, & Skolnikoff, 1997; Gomm, 2003; Ross & Banister, 2004). As such, many students entering our programs did not have the computer skills needed to focus on teaching/learning with technology, rather than teaching/learning about technology.

Second, we wanted a course which would clearly model the objectives articulated in TPACK. In this regard, we sought to design and develop a course which fully integrated technology in helping students understand pedagogy and content knowledge. In other words, we wanted the course to include assignments and exercises that required purposeful and relevant technology usage for problem solving, creativity, collaboration/communication, and analysis, as well as assessment and professional development.

Third, there was a challenge in persuading all of the adjuncts to embrace the online modality. After all, before the revisions, this course was originally taught in a face-to-face environment by many adjuncts (at least four sections per semester, with many being off-site). We thus needed to enable all of the instructors to find a good balance between consistency and flexibility when teaching online, in terms of using the materials, as well as how to teach online.

Fourth, it was a challenge providing technical support, since the course ran completely online, and the instructors faced new limitations in helping their students with technical problems and questions that arose. (e.g., Blackboard content management system problems, and using various types of software for their assignments).

Solutions and Recommendations

In order to solve the aforementioned first challenge, a two–staged curriculum was designed. That is, before the teacher candidates took the educational technology course (CIEE213: Teaching in a Global Technological World) in the first semester of the program offered by the Teacher Education program, at the College of Education, we set up a prerequisite. In executing this, we collaborated with the Computer Science department to provide an introductory technology skills course (CS-215: Computer and Information Technology for Educators) along with the ability to test out of it by passing a challenge exam. This was intended to ensure that students in our online educational technology course were able to focus on technology integration and pedagogy, while also being ready to complete all of the assignments that were expected of them. CS-215 was offered in a hands-on computer lab and was designed around the entry-level criteria recommended in the original National Educational Technology Standards for Teachers (ISTE, 2000). By requiring CS-215 (or alternatively, passage on a test-out proficiency exam), the educational technology course could then be designed to focus exclusively on students' skills and knowledge to use technology in their K-12 teaching and to create technology-learning experiences for their K-12 students. Once students fulfilled this entry requirement (either by taking the basic technology course, or testing out of it) and were accepted into the program, they were expected to take the online CIEE-213 course along with the introduction to education course, CIEE213.

To meet the 2nd challenge mentioned above, this online educational technology course focused on teaching *with* technology and on the concepts of technology integration to foster K-12 students' technological literacy; rather than focusing on specific technology training as in the previous version of this course (which was based on hands-on computer lab sessions). This online course was also developed in collaboration with a faculty member from the Special Education department who had expertise in assistive technology. In this way, the course was able to incorporate TPK to meet the varied needs of our diverse learners. By sequencing the course early in the education program, students were further able to use basic TPCK in the content-based "methods" courses they were to take later in the program. In addition to helping students gain the knowledge, skills and dispositions for using technology to supplement and/or increase the effectiveness of their instruction, a major goal of the course was to get the students to understand their role in helping their learners become technologically literate. Additionally, in order to achieve the goals in helping teacher candidates become aware of how learning can occur with/though technology and become self-regulated learners, the instructors modeled effective use of technology to design and deliver instruction. In this course, for example, comprehensive course materials and assignments were designed and developed ahead of time and presented as part of a very structured syllabus in the Blackboard Learning Management System – not a haphazard process.

Figures 1 and 2 outline the detailed course modules in sequence as well as the assignments, with detailed descriptions. Out of 15 weeks during the semester, most modules were designed to be taught during one week, except module 5 which was for 2 weeks. As shown in Figure 1, none of the course modules focused on technology, itself, as a distinct area of subject matter. Rather, they focused on how teachers could incorporate technology into their classrooms. Furthermore, all of the assignments were designed to provide students with the opportunity to use technology for collaboration/communication, problem solving, creativity analysis, and assessment, as listed in Figure 2. Each module was also designed to build up to the major assignments. Throughout the course, there were major assignments along with 9 discussions. All of the discussion questions were designed and posted by the authors, except the group discussion for which students addressed the discussion questions for the assigned topic. There were certain weeks out of the 15 in which no particular discussion questions were required, so that students could focus on the major assignments, but an ongoing discussion schedule was used to ensure that students were keeping up with

Figure 1. The module sequence of the online educational technology course

Module	Topics
1	What is educational technology - enhancing teaching with technology
2	Assistive Technology (AT): - Assistive tech overview - Low tech and high tech for special needs learners - Individualized education plan (IEP) classifications
3	Universal Design for Learning (UDL): - Universal Design for Learning overview - Principles of UDL
4	Evaluating educational technology
5	Social, Ethical, Legal and Human issues
6	Technological literacy: what do students need to know about technology?
7	Integrating technology literacy into Language Arts & Social Studies instruction
8	Integrating technology literacy into Math & Science instruction
9	Technology-integrated unit plan
10	WebQuest
11	Assessing and evaluating learning with technology
12	Electronic portfolios
13	Using technology for professional development
14	Reflections

Figure 2. Online educational technology course assignments

Assignments	Descriptions	Technologies used	Instructional goals
Discussions	Nine discussion sessions. These focused on technology media as a way to enhance teaching, assistive technology to enhance learning, technology literacy standards as part of what 21st century students need to know, and technology integration into core content areas. The detailed discussion questions are attached in Appendix A)	Blackboard forums	Using Technology for collaboration communication
Educational Technology Evaluation	Evaluate and describe an educational software program, including the type of program, the ways you might use it and the underlying learning theory. An educational software program can be anything that was designed to teach k-12 students (it can be a CD-ROM, video, or web- based program, etc.) This would include programs like KidPix or MathBlasters, but not application programs like Word or PowerPoint (although the latter are now used in schools, they were designed for personal business productivity purposes, and as such, have no inherent underlying pedagogical focus). Evaluation should include criteria for developmental and instructional appropriateness for all (regular, special needs, and limited English language) learners. At a minimum, the evaluation should cover the items listed on Blackboard	Word processing program such as Microsoft Word	Technology evaluations based on the appropriateness to specific instructional needs TK, TPK, TCK
Technology Grant Proposal	Use PowerPoint or a similar program to create a simple grant proposal presentation which shows how you would spend $5,000 on technology for any one of the following scenario classes of regular and inclusion students: • 1st grade class- 20 students: 2 ELL, 3 ADHD, 4 with below average fine motor skills. There are 2 iMacs and 1 printer in this classroom, which are both 2 years old and connected to the internet • 3rd grade class- 23 students: 3 ELL, 5 ADHD, 2 with minor visual challenges. There is 1 pc and 1 printer in this classroom, both are 6 years old. There are Ethernet connections in the classroom for connection to the Internet • 5th grade class- 25 students: 6 ELL, 2 ADHD, 1 with minor auditory challenges. There is 1 pc and 1 printer in this classroom, both are 3 years old. The building has a wireless network to connect to the internet In addition to saying how money will be sent, the proposal should also include a rationale (why money is being spent the way you are proposing). Minimum slides required: 1. a title slide with your name 2. a slide with a few bullets explaining why you need the purchase 3. a slide for each proposed equipment/software to be purchased including: o reason for purchasing this item (what specific academic standards/goals will it help your students achieve) o price o manufacturer o a picture of the equipment (with citation to where the picture came from) 4. a final budget total slide: add up everything - it should come to under $5,000.00 (and no, you don't get to keep the extra money 5. a wrap-up slide with a few bullets for anticipated results from this purchase (how this will solve the problems shown on the 2nd slide) See attached sample presentations and over the next few sessions, start researching possible technologies and collecting information. Be creative and have fun 'spending' 5 grand.	Multimedia presentation program such as Microsoft PowerPoint Internet search for items to be purchased	Using technology for problem solving TK, TPK
Cross-curricular unit plan integrating technologies	The activities in the unit plan should address the New Jersey Core Curriculum Content Standard (NJCCCS) 8.1 and NETS-S standards. The objectives of the unit plan should address two or more of the core content areas (math, science, social studies, language arts). This should include two or more activities in which students also meet standards for basic computer skills and tools and application of productivity tools as defined by 8.1 and the NETS-S performance indicators. You may pick whatever grade and main core content area you want, but should also include ways to adapt the unit plan for diverse learners	Word processing program such as Microsoft Word	Using technology for creativity TK, TPK, TCK, TPCK
Grading Spreadsheet for unit plan	Work on the grading part of your unit plan and use it to create a "grading spreadsheet" application based on your rubric. Make up names and scores for at least 3 students and record grades for all of the activities you have included in your unit plan for them. The spreadsheet should automatically calculate a total score for each student and an average class score for each activity (Use appropriate functions). Graph the scores in a bar graph and think about how you could use this to modify your unit plan if these were real scores	Spreadsheet program such as Microsoft Excel	Using technology for analysis TK, TPK
Electronic Portfolio	Using the Blackboard Content E-Portfolio function to start your e-portfolio. This e-portfolio should at least include your 1) technology evaluation, 2) grant proposal, 3) unit plan and 4) grading spreadsheet, to be used as artifacts which demonstrate your ability to meet NJ teaching standards. Each or the four artifacts should have an annotation explaining why it shows evidence of the standard(s) you have selected it for. You are not expected to have your e-portfolio completed - just started, but feel free to add other assignments from other classes, and make a homepage that reflects your personality	Electronic portfolio tool embedded in the Blackboard Content Management System	Using technology for assessment and professional development TK

the class. With the exception of the discussions, all of the course modules and assignments were posted prior to the beginning of the course, so that students could read ahead and plan for time to work on assignments. In addition, students could start on and post drafts of major assignments on the Blackboard forum before the due dates for feedback from the professor and classmates. Students were also encouraged to share ideas, technologies they found, and tips in an effort to foster engagement and satisfaction in the *process* of carrying out the assignments as well as in the finished product. In short, we sought to ensure that we afforded continued engagement and attention in this online environment, so that they stay on track and maintain commitment.

To address the third aforementioned challenge, in the course design phase, the lead professor made a Blackboard master course shell that was accessible by all of the other instructors (who were usually adjuncts) and requested their input and feedback, and also requested that all of the adjuncts use the same materials as well as contribute to them as part of a collaborative effort. Since the lead professor's Blackboard master course shell was available to all of the other instructors, they were able to see how the lessons were carried out (e.g., providing constructive and prompt feedback, sending out weekly reminders and announcements with the Blackboard announcement functionality as well as additional ways to contact students via email). Furthermore, the lead professor observed the adjuncts' courses once a year (virtually, and/or by phone or person).

For the aforementioned fourth challenge, in order to teach more effectively in an online environment, we also collaborated with our university's Instruction and Research Technology (IRT) office to: a) provide in-person technology help for various projects that students had to complete during the CIEE213 online course; and b) offer in-person workshops for e-portfolio assignments, required in the CIEE213 course. Even though students took CS-215 or took the challenge exams, we thought they might still need technology help. Also, there was a new assignment included which was more geared toward educational applications (e.g., developing a developmental portfolio), which we found that students needed to know.

PROGRAM EVALUATION

To examine the impact of the online educational technology course, we conducted a study which looked at students' competency with technology, TPACK thinking, and technology integration understanding. In general, we found that the course was effective at providing students with an understanding of how technology, pedagogy, and content should be combined in their teaching as well as furthering students' technology competence and self-efficacy (Author 1 & Author 2, in submission, see the article for detailed results of the study). In addition, we looked at how students perceive themselves as online learners and whether this class modeled effective teaching with technology strategies. As presented in Figure 3, qualitative evaluations of the postings regarding the online educational technology course in the reflection forum suggested that the most perceived advantage of the online course was: a) flexibility; b) helping them to gain time management skills; and c) giving them experience using the computer.

However, it is important to note that these benefits would have been mentioned only if the instructor's facilitation strategy was effective. For example, student comments on the instructor were as follows:

I have taken two or three online classes in the past and no other teacher was as helpful as you. My other classes just expected you to know everything about taking an online class and did not offer to assist me in anyway. I really had to just figure out everything on my own back then. For this online class, you reached out to us a number of times. You were happy to help and did not even mind

Figure 3. Perceived advantage of the online course format

Theme	Example
Flexibility	"I honestly love online classes because it works around my work schedule. I find it easier for me to take online classes because of my busy schedule." "I really enjoyed being an online distance learner because I am very disciplined and organized and so it was nice to not have to be committed to going to a class at a certain time each week, but still be able to keep up with the workload and thoroughly learn the material."
Gaining time management skills	"...One plus of this class was that I really learned how good my time management skills were because it was up to me to fit this class into my schedule and get all of my work done." "I do know from previous online classes that they are more difficult than face-to-face classes, but I feel it forces you to use your time wisely."
Gaining experience using computers	"Taking online course gave me great experience using the computer and Internet; which is especially important nowadays."

meeting on campus to assist us in person. You were extremely helpful and very precise with your instructions for things which was a great help! You were always available for questions and to meet with students, and even though I live too far away to actually meet with you in person I felt more comfortable knowing that I could if I desperately needed to.

Professor's weekly reminders were very helpful.

As someone else mentioned I thought the way that you (professor) explained each and every assignment and gave examples was so very helpful because for me it helped give me an exact understanding of how the assignments needed to be completed. I also thought that you gave us plenty of time to complete assignment and never once did I feel rush to accomplish one.

I believe it all turned out great and there was a lot of communication between the professor and students and even student to student.

Even though the majority of students provided positive reflections about their online course experience, some students also indicated that there were disadvantages, due to the lack of face-to-face communication. For example, on student wrote,

Now that it is the end of the semester, I have to say that it wasn't that bad, but I think I prefer the interaction of an actual class. I missed having discussions with people right away and I felt like some of the energy might have been lost waiting for others to post responses.

Another student wrote,

Although I'd rather learn in a classroom environment, my experience as an online distance learner has been fine for the most part. I like to physically be in the classroom, and be able to participate and ask questions to the professor as it comes to my mind. Technology plays an important role in society today, but I don't think it should be incorporated as a class. .....Although I'm sure students do a lot of work online, I don't believe it is equal to a regular in-class college education.

Furthermore, since this online course was the first one offered in this teacher preparation program, it played a role in enabling other faculty to embrace the online format, by using Blackboard in their courses. For instance, after other senior faculty observed this course, they then started to consider using Blackboard, themselves (e.g., some faculty started using Blackboard to turn their face-to-face courses into blended ones; some faculty converted their existing courses into online ones; and some faculty started to develop entirely new online courses). In short, this online course provided a framework that other faculty members could consider in developing and teaching their own online courses.

FUTURE DEVELOPMENT AND RESEARCH DIRECTIONS

Research evidence suggests that student teachers' who learn to teach with technology should be contextually and socially situated in the school-based learning environment, rather than taught in isolation of it (Bullock, 2004; Dexter & Riedel, 2003). Stuhlmann (1998) suggested that the reinforcement and practice of using technology over time has an enormous impact on the teacher candidates' ability to transfer skills to other educational situations. Thus, changes in TPACK and beliefs may be impacted not only by taking educational technology courses, but by also developing the pedagogical skills needed to utilize technology effectively in real classroom settings. Therefore, we would like to conduct more research, to follow the teacher candidates through their practicum, their student teaching and their first-year teaching experiences, after competing CIEE213. Findings from this longitudinal research will provide valuable and detailed insights about these teacher candidates' competencies and beliefs on using educational technology, and how the teacher education program at William Paterson University's College of Education has shaped these pre-service teachers' views toward educational technology. In particular, this could also provide us with data on how experience and familiarity with an online course may facilitate future online professional development opportunities, which are especially important for lifelong learning.

Another area of future work is the continued incorporation of new and emerging Web 2.0 technologies (e.g. blogs, wikis, social networking applications) into the course. It is important to stress however, that any technology, new or old, should only be included if it is appropriate to what is being taught; we do not want to include the technology 'du jour' for technology's sake, but rather because it will give our students a deeper understanding of how technology can be used to promote learning.

CONCLUSION

In this chapter, the challenges we faced and the solutions we implemented have been described. The result of this effort was the transition of a face-to-face technology skills course into an online educational technology one focusing on teaching *with* technology. We believe that moving to an online format that emphasized the more integrative approach was extremely beneficial to our students and has thus enabled us to meet our goals. We also recommend that more teacher candidates in other programs be given an opportunity to learn via an online web instruction, since this instructional modality undoubtedly serve well as they become professional teachers.

In closing, when designing a teacher education program to prepare candidates to use and integrate technology, there are a number of decisions to be considered. Having this experience in our institution, we would like to offer to the readers who have similar students populations like our institutions, the following important considerations:

- Does the program expect that all candidates have a basic level of technological literacy? (either as an entry-requirement or as a pre-requisite to an educational technology course). This is especially important if the course is to be offered online, with no face-to-face hands-on component.
- Does the program have a stand alone educational technology component or should these higher-order TPK and TPCK skills be

integrated into the other education courses? The latter choice assumes that both students and the teacher education faculty members are proficient in lower-order, basic technology skills and that faculty members are prepared to revise their other education courses to incorporate educational technology into them. One alternative may be to offer a technology component for all of the education courses that would be delivered online, creating a hybrid course that combined in-class and online collaboration/communication, problem solving and analysis assignments in each of the core content and pedagogy courses.

- Does the institution have a center that could offer online students constant technical support? Even though students are usually considered to have basic technology skills, they often still need technology help and support. Make an agreement between the instructor/department and the department of computing services before implementing an online program.
- Who is going to teach the online courses? Even though the course is well-designed, the way in which the instructor actually facilitates the online course is of key importance. Since the instructor cannot see or hear the physical cues that are par for the course in face-to-face settings (verbal complaints, facial expressions, etc.) the pedagogical aims might be very different.

REFERENCES

An, H., & Wilder, H. (2010, April). Preparing elementary preservice teachers from a non-traditional student population to teach with technology. In submission Paper session presented at The *Annual Meeting of the American Educational Research Association*, Denver, Colorado.

Baines, L. (2006). Deconstructing Teacher Certification. *Phi Delta Kappan, 88*(4), 326–329.

Brown, D., & Warschauer, M. (2006). From the university to the elementary classroom: Students' experiences in learning to integrate technology in instruction. *Journal of Technology and Teacher Education, 14*(3), 599–62.

Bull, G., Park, J., Searson, M., Thompson, A., Mishra, P., Koehler, M. J., & Knezek, G. (2007). Editorial: Developing technology policies for effective classroom practice. *Contemporary Issues in Technology & Teacher Education, 7*(3). Retrieved from http://www.citejournal.org/vol7/iss3/editorial/article1.cfm.

Bullock, D. (2004). Moving from theory to practice: An examination of the factors that preservice teachers encounter as the attempt to gain experience teaching with technology during field placement experiences. *Journal of Technology and Teacher Education, 12*(2), 211–237.

Cuban, L. (2001). *Oversold and Underused, Computers in the Classroom.* Boston, MA: Harvard University Press.

DeBell, M., & Chapman, C. (2006). *Computer and Internet Use by Students in 2003 (NCES 2006–065).* U.S. Department of Education. Washington, DC: National Center for Education Statistics. Retrieved from http://nces.ed.gov/pubsearch/pubsinfo.asp?pubid=2006065

Dexter, S., & Riedel, E. (2003). Why improving preservice teacher educational technology preparation must go beyond the college's walls. *Journal of Teacher Education, 54*(4), 334–346. doi:10.1177/0022487103255319

Doolittle, P., & Hicks, D. (2003). Constructivism as a theoretical foundation for the use of technology in Social Studies. *Theory and Research in Social Education, 31*(1), 72–104.

eSchool News. (2008). *On the way: Nation's first tech-literacy exam*. Retrieved March 8, 2009, from http://www.eschoolnews.com/news/top-news/?i=55483

Ferris, A., Roberts, N., & Skolnikoff, W. (1997). Technology and preservice education: Models that work, models that don't. *Educational Technology Review*, *7*, 13–19.

Fox, S., & Livingston, G. (2007). Hispanics with lower levels of education and English proficiency remain largely disconnected from the internet. *Pew Internet & American Life Project: Latinos Online*. Retrieved March 8, 2009, from http://www.pewinternet.org/PPF/r/204/report_display.asp

Gomm, S. (2003). Computer Literacy Defined and Implemented as University Graduation Requirement. In C. Crawford et al. (Eds.), *Proceedings of Society for Information Technology and Teacher Education International Conference 2003* (pp. 941-944). Chesapeake, VA: AACE.

Hanks, R. F. (2002). Environmental and personal factors effecting K-12 teacher utilization of technology. Paper presented at the *National Educational Computing Conference*, San Antonio, Texas (ERIC Reproduction Service No. ED475934). Retrieved April 3, 2009, from http://www.eric.ed.gov

Hudson, P. (2006). Examining Preservice Teachers' Involvement in Online Science Education. *Journal of Interactive Learning Research*, *17*(4), 367–385.

International Society for Technology in Education. (2000). *NETS for teachers 2000 profiles*. Retrieved March 21, 2009, from http://www.iste.org/Content/NavigationMenu/NETS/ForTeachers/2000Standards/Profiles/NETS_for_Teachers_2000_Profiles.htm

International Society for Technology in Education. (2008). *NETS for teachers 2008*. Retrieved March 13, 2009, from http://www.iste.org/Content/NavigationMenu/NETS/ForTeachers/2008Standards/NETS_for_Teachers_2008.htm

Kay, R. (2006). Evaluating strategies used to incorporate technology into preservice education: A review of the literature. *Journal of Research on Technology in Education*, *38*(4), 383–408.

Mason, C., Berson, M., Diem, R., Hicks, D., Lee, J., & Dralle, T. (2000). Guidelines for using technology to prepare social studies teachers. *Contemporary Issues in Technology & Teacher Education*, *1*(1). Retrieved from http://www.citejournal.org/vol1/iss1/currentissues/socialstudies/article1.htm.

Mehlinger, H. D., & Powers, S. M. (2002). *Technology and teacher education: A guide for educators and policymakers*. Boston: Houghton Mifflin.

Mishra, P., & Koehler, M. J. (2006). Technological Pedagogical Content Knowledge: A new framework for teacher knowledge. *Teachers College Record*, *108*(6), 1017–1054. doi:10.1111/j.1467-9620.2006.00684.x

Mishra, P., & Koehler, M. J. (2008, March). *Introducing Technological Pedagogical Content Knowledge*. Paper presented at the Annual Meeting of the American Educational Research Association, New York City, NY.

Ross, C., & Banister, S. (2004). From high school to college: How prepared are teacher education candidates for technology integration? In C. Crawford et al. (Eds.), *Proceedings of Society for Information Technology and Teacher Education International Conference 2004* (pp. 228).

Stuhlmann, J. M. (1998). A model for infusing technology into teacher training programs. *Journal of Technology and Teacher Education*, *6*(2-3), 125–139.

Trucano, M. (2005). *Knowledge Maps: ICTs in Education*. Washington, DC: infoDev / World Bank. Retrieved from http://www.infodev.org/en/Publication.8.html

U. S. Congress. (1995). *Teachers and technology: Making the connections (GPO #052-003-0149-2). Office of Technology Assessment*. Washington, DC: U.S. Government Printing Office.

U.S. Department of Education. (2001). *Enhancing Education Through Technology Act of 2001*. Retrieved March 8, 2009, from http://www.ed.gov/policy/elsec/leg/esea02/pg34.html

Wells, J., & Lewis, L. (2006). *Internet access in U.S. public schools and classrooms: 1994-2005 (NCES 2007020)*. U.S. Department of Education. Washington, DC: National Center for Education Statistics. Retrieved November 1, 2007, from http://jtc.colstate.edu/vol2_2/pelling.htmhttp://nces.ed.gov/pubsearch/pubsinfo.asp?pubid=2007020.

Wenglinsky, H. (2005). *Using technology wisely: The keys to success in schools*. New York: Teachers College Press.

APPENDIX A

Nine Discussion Questions

1. ***Session 1:*** Choose an educational theorist (Piaget, Gardner, Dewey, Vygotsky, Noddings, Bruner, Freire, Montessori, Bloom, or any other theorist you can think of) and write about how you think their philosophy affected the way they might have used (or not used) technology/media to teach. Your response should be at least about 2 or 3 paragraphs long.

2. ***Session 2:*** Look through this week's readings and then write at least a one paragraph response regarding the following:

- What is assistive technology? - Please define it in your own words. Why is it necessary? Then, give an example of an assistive technology found in a school you are familiar with (for eg, as a student, teaching assistant, etc) and reflect on how you think this assistive technology might have been helpful for students with special needs. (e.g.: This is an example of an assistive technology http://www.brailler.com/ra.htm for a braille printer)

3. ***Session 3:*** How does a public learning space such as the Valley Road building at William Paterson University or a public school or library lend itself (or not lend itself) to the Universal Design for Learning principles (refer to the Principles at http://www.design.ncsu.edu/cud/about_ud/udprinciples.htm)? (Please give the name and address of the building you are evaluating). Give suggestions for improvements.

4. ***Sessions 5-6:*** You will be assigned to a group. Within your group, you will be assigned one of the following topics:

- Digital divide
- Copyright and cyber-ethics
- Privacy, security and cyber-safety
- Environmental impact of technology

You will be responsible for researching and summarizing that topic in your group discussion board and posing a question about it for group-mates to answer. Your question does not have to have a right or wrong answer but should get your group-mates thinking about the implications of this topic for education.

5. ***Session 7:*** What do you think about the NJ and NETS-S technology standards? Is there anything else that you feel needs to be modified or added? What are some barriers that might prevent your students from meeting these standards?

6. ***Session 8:*** Visit the Language Arts, Social Studies and AT resource web sites listed for this session. Then, pick a NJCCCS reading or writing performance indicator (ex NJCCCS 3.2.A.5 for Kindergarten) and social studies performance indicator (ex. NJCCCS 6.1.A.5 for grade k-2) and briefly describe a cross-curricular activity you might do to meet that standard which also meets the NJCCCS tech literacy and NETS-S standards (i.e. students learn to use a technology while they are learning about reading or writing). This does not need to be a complete lesson plan - look at the attached examples and be sure to include: 1) Language Arts and Social Studies Standard addressed2) Activity list3) Technology Literacy Standards (NJCCCS 8.1 and NETS-S) 4) Special Needs Adaptations

7. ***Session 9:*** Visit the math, science and AT resource web sites listed for this session. Pick a NJCCCS math performance indicator (ex. NJCCCS 4.4.A.2 for grade 3) and performance indicator (ex. NJCCCS 5.5.A.1 for grade 4) and briefly describe a cross-curricular activity you might do to meet that standard which also meets the NJCCCS tech literacy and NETS-S standards (i.e. students learn to use a technology while they are learning about math). This does not need to be a complete lesson plan -look at attached examples and be sure to include:

1. Math & Science Standards addressed
2. Activity list
3. Technology Literacy Standards (NJCCCS 8.1 and NETS-S)
4. Special Needs Adaptations

8. ***Session 11:*** Review a WebQuest on the Web. Share the WebQuest you have found. What did you like and/or dislike about it? If you were a designer of this WebQuest, what would you have added/modified in order to improve it? Why would it be worthwhile for other learners to visit the site you chose?

9. ***Session 14:*** Find a teacher resources web site and evaluate its helpfulness. Make sure you post the URL along with your comments, so that it can be shared with your classmates.

Chapter 4
Gender Differences in Online Communication of Teacher Preparation Students

William J. Gibbs
Duquesne University, USA

Ronan S. Bernas
Eastern Illinois University, USA

ABSTRACT

Research has shown that gender disparities exist in online communication. Understanding the factors that enable students to effectively communicate online and ultimately manage their own discussions has important learning and pedagogical implications. This study examined the communication and interactional processes of peer-directed online discussions. Gender disparities were found in communication styles and in the use of socio-emotional content. Men were expository whereas messages posted by women were of an epistolary nature. Women used socio-emotional content more than men. However, interactions, such as the extent to which men and women persisted in message threads as well as responded to one another, were comparable overall. Although not significant, women posted more messages of longer length but men received more replies to their messages. The findings have important pedagogical implications for educators who wish to engage students in peer-directed text-based asynchronous discussions.

INTRODUCTION

The use of text-based asynchronous computer mediated communication (CMC) in educational courses presents a number of advantages while, at the same time, it poses challenges for educators. Educational online discussions, for example, enable students to contribute at times convenient to them and to reflect on responses before submitting them. However, effectively implementing and managing discussions can be demanding. Instructors who attempt to read and respond to messages during an active conference may become inundated unless they use methods to manage dialogue and/or pedagogical techniques to accomplish the learning objectives. How to successfully manage discussions is a topic of interest to educators. Increasingly, they are capitalizing on the uniqueness of text-based CMC to provide students with opportunities to manage their own online communities of learning, where learners engage in

DOI: 10.4018/978-1-61520-899-9.ch004

dialogue with minimal instructor intervention. Not only are peer-directed activities potentially more manageable for instructors, they are advantageous from a learning perspective. The CMC environment engenders constructivist approaches such as collaborative learning and peer-directed activities that may promote learner-centeredness and self-direction (Murphy, Harvell, Sanders, & Lu Epps, 1999). For instance, students may be charged with initiating and sustaining discussion. Such responsibility will likely offer them insights into group interaction, information management, and peer-conflict; domains typically dealt with by instructors. These novel situations can stimulate discourse beneficial to learning (Fahy, 2003; Juler, 1990), expose students to diverse perspectives, and embolden their self-sufficiency.

Providing students increased autonomy to manage their own online discussions raises key questions such as (a) will rude or asocial behavior become more prevalent because discussions are not actively monitored by an instructor; (b) will individuals dominate and/or censor others or inhibit participation; and (c) will gender disparities be more pronounced. Research indicates that there are marked differences in male and female communication styles and the disparities generally do a disservice to women. Herring (2000) reports that compared to men, women post fewer messages, receive fewer replies, and, at times, are discouraged from participating. The extent to which such disparities affect communication in peer-directed discussions has important learning and pedagogical implications. The present study investigated the communications of men and women in peer-directed online discussions to more fully understand the role gender plays in activities that are managed primarily by students.

THEORETICAL FRAMEWORK

The researchers' rationale for analyzing male-female communication was predicated on two assumptions: (a) in CMC environments educators employ learner-centered approaches that afford students increased control over learning activities and ultimately their own learning. Students are often given responsibility for creating and sustaining online peer-directed discussions; (b) gender differences have been shown to exist in male-female online communication and interaction, which may profoundly affect communication. The dynamics of or interactional exchanges occurring within peer-directed discussions may exacerbate gender disparities.

THE ONLINE ENVIRONMENT AND GENDER

Mann and Stewart (2000) citing Lee (1996) state that because visual or non-verbal cues, so distinctive of face-to-face communication, are absent in CMC, biases that disenfranchise lower-status groups would be eliminated. Since gender is not revealed through visual channels some predicted that gender inequalities would diminish (Jeong & Davidson-Shivers, 2006). Others contend that online social interactions exist in a context dominated by racial, gender, age, and class dynamics (Mann & Stewart, 2000; Kramarae, 1995) where individuals can glean information about discussants in subtle ways. Discussants may react to one another based on presumptions about gender because gender information is revealed through interactions, politeness markers in messages, and/or communication style (Herring, 1993, 1996a, 2000, 2003). Moreover, during social interactions, people of lower-status groups often self-monitor their language use and non-verbal communication in ways that underscore predominant stereotypes about role relationships (Arnold & Miller, 2001). It is also likely that discussants bring preexistent notions, learned early in life, about hierarchy and control to CMC environments wherein males are often perceived to fill the dominant role in social relations (Pedersen & Macafee, 2007). Thus, electronic discourse reveals much about one's gender, notwithstanding prior claims about CMC being gender-neutral and democratic. It is possible that discussants' ability to glean gender information from electronic text, their preexistent ideas about gender and social relations, and the lack of familiar visual cues contribute to the arousal of asocial behavior in CMC. While the online environment may be physically safe, relative anonymity in the virtual world creates potential for distressing interaction (Mann & Stewart, 2000) that can be exacerbated when students manage conferences with minimal instructor interaction. Thus, instead of defusing gender disparities the online world may intensify them.

GENDER DIFFERENCES IN CMC

Huffaker and Calvert (2005) reported that compared to women, men use more active and resolute language, but that the language of women was not inevitably passive or compliant. Women are more concerned with politeness (Herring 1996b, 2000) and they "...tend to hedge, qualify, and justify their assertions (using such words as maybe, possibly, and perhaps), express support of others, make apologies, and in general, manifest a more consensus-making orientation and epistolary style" (Jeong & Davidson-Shivers, 2006, p. 544).

Herring (1996a) reported that women prefer epistolary communication characterized by interpersonal interaction, and alignment with others and that the epistolary (conversation/interactive) schema consists of: (a) opening convention, (b) link to previous discourse, (c) content message, d) link to following discourse, and (e) closing convention. Men prefer expository communication characterized by intention to convey information and to challenge others (Herring, 2003). The expository schema consists of: (a) identification of problem, (b) proposal of solution, (c) evidence in support of solution, and (d) evaluation of solution (Herring, 1996a). Fahy (2002) found that in all epistolary categories, women surpassed men and men were more expository and opposed.

Gender differences affect how men and women interact (Herring, 2000; Fahy, 2002). Studies report disparities in male-female interactions with women contributing fewer messages and their messages receiving fewer replies (Herring, 2000; Panyametheekul & Herring, 2003; Jeong, 2003). At the same time, women have been shown to be more responsive than men to messages addressed to them (Fahy, 2002). In another form of CMC (blogging), women were found to persist longer and write more but their postings often received fewer comments than male posts. Moreover, their style of writing in blogs was diary-like whereas men tended to be opinion oriented (Herring & Paolillo, 2006; Pedersen & Macafee, 2007).

The aforementioned gender differences may accentuate or impede communication. Awareness of gender communication disparities is especially important when educators employ innovative pedagogical methods that afford students greater autonomy as with peer-directed discussions. Ignorance of these differences in text-based CMC can stifle learning as well as evoke frustration and animosity among discussants.

SOCIO-EMOTIONAL CONTENT

Non-standard orthographic forms (NSOF) pervade CMC and they include abbreviations (e.g., "IMHO"), emoticons (e.g., "smiley faces"), deliberate misspellings, and variations in punctuation (Baron, 2004; Hancock, 2004; Herring, 2001). In a medium void of traditional nonverbal communication, discussants formulate messages to convey socio-emotional content in order to achieve their relational aims. They become accustomed to the lack of nonverbal cues and compensate with different types of NSOF such as emoticons and repeated punctuation. As purported by social information processing theory, discussants communicate socio-emotional content (Nastri, Peña, &

Hancock, 2006; Walther, 1992) to attain relational goals, and they form perceptions of conversational partners based on how they use text and orthographic forms (Jaffe, Huang, & Oshagan, 1995). Discussants structure messages to communicate information as well as to be expressive, which may help them regulate dialogue, sustain contacts, and convey identity (Nastri, Peña, & Hancock, 2006). NSOF allow discussants to inform others about their emotional state as well as their feelings on issues (Nastri, Peña, & Hancock, 2006).

Some researchers (e.g., Quina et al., 1987) contend that compared to the language of men, female discourse has a greater degree of social warmth, is more expressive (Ivy & Backlund, 1994), and it may possess aesthetic qualities (Mulac, Bradac, & Mann, 1985; Mulac & Lundell, 1986). Witmer and Katzman (1997) found that women use NSOF in electronic discourse more often than men. They purported that these communication forms may be a means by which women express emotion, hedge, and/or possibly infuse aesthetics in communication.

It is plausible that NSOF, indicative of social expression and relational intent, may offer valuable information about the nature of educationally-oriented dialogue. For instance, do expressive forms occur randomly in messages or when discussants engage in expository or epistolary communication? Are discussants more expressive in terms of NSOF when they align with and support others (epistolary) or when they engage in expository communication? At the same time, can one anticipate less socio-emotional communication among men than women in peer-conferences, because, as suggested by previous research (Tannen, 1991; Herring, 1993; Fahy, 2002), men are less likely to engage in this kind of communication (Jaffe, Huang, & Oshagan, 1995)? These are important issues because fundamentally peer-directed online discussions exist for students to partake in social dialogue, learn, foster social relations, and, in the process, align with and support their peers. Understanding the factors that contribute to these aims is therefore of much importance.

PURPOSE OF STUDY

The study investigated gender in text-based asynchronous educational discussions by examining how men and women communicate online. Specifically, it examined the type of messages and interactional exchanges that occurred to more fully understand the influence of gender in peer-directed discussions, discussions run primarily by students. The researchers were also interested in how students used non-standard orthography in online communication.

The discussion conferences examined in the study were distinctive for several reasons: (a) the instructor established them for students who were taking part in a new and challenging teaching practicum; (b) they served to help students support and mentor peers; and (c) they were administered by students with minimal instructor involvement. The practicum afforded students a shared experience that exposed them to the challenges of beginning teaching and the conferences provided a venue for communicating and engaging with peers about those experiences. Researchers have noted that the social context and shared understanding among discussants are important factors that affect communications. The context in which a discussion takes place helps shape the structure of communication and it provides information that discussants use to interpret situations accurately (Riva & Galimberti, 1998). A shared understanding among participants that has evolved through prior communication and/or common experience (such as teachers' professional socialization) can influence, positively or negatively, messages and their interpretation (Dickey, Wasko, Chudoba, & Thatcher, 2006). The researchers reasoned that the common teaching experience would likely influence students to adopt an epistolary style of communication where they aligned with and supported one another. Moreover, it would induce expressiveness among both genders as well as empathy for peers who were undergoing similar experiences. Thus, the researchers expected male-female interactions and use of NSOF to be comparable.

The study examined the following research questions:

1. In peer-directed conferences, are there gender differences in the type of messages that comprise communication?
2. In peer-directed conferences what, if any, gender differences exist in interactional exchanges. Specifically, the following three questions were examined: (a) are men and women comparable in the extent to which they persist in the message chain; (b) do men and women respond equally to one another; (c) do men and women receive equal numbers of isolated messages?
3. In peer-directed conferences, to what extent do men and women use socioemotional content in messages and what, if anything, do these forms indicate about communication?

METHOD

Participants

The study used a sample population comprised of 46 undergraduate students enrolled in a required instructional methods course at a mid-sized university in the central region of the United States. The sample consisted of 23 females and 23 males, who ranged in age from 18 to 22 years old. They were competent users of online media and had familiarity with posting and reading messages in online discussion conferences. During participation, all students were engaged in a teaching practicum. They used the discussions conferences because the instructor established them as a peer-directed support network for the practicum. After the discussions occurred, the researchers, in consultation with the instructor, identified the corpus of data to be used for analysis and so all communication occurred in the natural setting of the discussion activity.

Procedure

Discussions

Students participated in 12 discussion conferences about various topics ranging from their initial reactions to teaching, technology issues at host schools, assignments, and interacting with students and teachers. They posted 277 messages across all discussions. Over the six-week practicum period, students posted questions about and descriptions of their experiences. The instructor monitored discussions but contributed only when necessary.

The researchers analyzed the discussions in several different ways to address the research questions presented above. Using the Transcript Analysis Tool - TAT (Fahy, Crawford, & Ally, 2001), an adaptation of Zhu's (1996, 1998) discussion content categorization, they performed a content analysis on the discussion transcripts to examine research question 1. To investigate research question 2, three measures regarding interaction exchanges were obtained from the discussions: (a) male-female persistence in the message chain, (b) male-female response patterns, and (c) isolated messages. Finally, the researchers made three observations to investigate research questions 3, (a) number of NSOF in all discussions by gender; (b) number of NSOF in proximity to other statement types; (c) amount of slang used in discussions by gender. Each approach is discussed more fully in the following sections.

Content Analysis Procedure

The researchers analyzed the content of the discussion transcripts using the Transcript Analysis Tool

(TAT), a tool for examining the content and social processes of online interactions (Fahy, 2005) that consist of eight categories (see Table 1). Using TAT, one researcher coded each sentence of the transcript while another individual coded portions of it. The coders compared their coding decisions and reconciled disagreements. The researcher re-coded the entire transcript one month later.

The agreement rate between two different coders was 68%. A Cohen's kappa of.57 suggests 'moderate' inter-rater agreement that is better than chance, $p <.001$. Intra-rater procedures (i.e., code-recode by one coder) after the 30-day interval resulted in a 76% agreement rate. The obtained Cohen's kappa value was.67 indicating a 'good' level of intra-rater agreement that was significantly better than chance, $p <.001$, given that Kappa values of.40 to.60 are considered fair,.60 to.75 as good, and over.75 as excellent (Bakeman & Gottman, 1997, p. 66).

Interactional Exchanges Procedure

In public discussion conferences, women post fewer messages, receive fewer responses, and often will not persist in discussions because other discussants frequently do not respond to their messages (Herring, 2000). To examine these factors in the peer-directed conferences, the researchers obtained three measures:

a. **Male-female persistence in the message chain:** Hierarchical arrangement of messages in discussions allows one to observe the extent to which dialogue persists. Deeper hierarchies suggest persistence and imply intensity in communication. If one gender is censored, then that group's persistence level will be shallow. In this study, when a discussant participated, either he/she initiated a new thread or responded to an existing message. The researchers use the term *initial post* to denote the first message of a thread. They refer to all messages that are direct responses to initial posts as *subtopic 1*. All responses to *subtopic 1* messages are denoted as *subtopic 2* and responses to *subtopic 2* as *subtopic 3* and so on.
b. **Male-female response patterns:** The researchers examined response sequences to identify whether men and women responded to one another equally. For each message and its direct response, the researchers identified the sex of the poster and respondent. They counted only direct responses. Suppose message A is an initial post sent by a female, message B a response to A (subtopic 1) sent by a male, and message C a response to B (subtopic 2) sent by a male. In this scenario, B is the direct response to A and C the direct response to B. Thus, the male-female

Table 1. Abridged transcript analysis tool categories as presented by Fahy (2001; 2005)

Categories indicative of epistolary communication	
1A - Vertical question	Assume a "correct" answer exists
1B - Horizontal question	Recognizes there may not be one right answer
2B - Referential statements	Comprise direct answers to questions
3 - Reflections	Show speaker expressing thoughts, judgments, opinions
4 – Scaffolding	Initiate, continue, acknowledge interpersonal interaction
Categories indicative of expository communication	
2A - Non-referential statements	Little self-revelation; do not invite dialogue; impart facts or information.
5A - Quotations	Quotations or paraphrases of others' words
5B - Citations	Citations or attributions of quotations or paraphrases

response sequence between A and B would be counted as *female post –male response* (FM), and then B and C counted as *male post – male response* (MM). The researchers calculated transitional probabilities of response sequences for males and females. A transitional probability "…is the probability with which a particular target event occurred, relative to another given event" (Bakeman & Gottman, 1997, p. 95).

c. **Isolated messages:** Disregarding a person's comments is a type of social censure in face-to-face communication (Donath, Karahalios, & Viegas, 1999). In text-based CMC, silence is often misinterpreted and it may increase dissatisfaction and enmity among users (Kalman & Rafaeli, 2005). The researchers tallied the number of messages that did not receive replies for men and women.

Fahy (2003, Attachment A) provided the following examples of TAT message categories:

- **1A-Vertical questions:** "What are the categories in Bloom's taxonomy?"
- **1B-Horizontal questions:** "What is good teaching?"
- **2A-Non-Referential statements:** "Although our office has been in the business of providing program in-service and training workshops since its inception, it is new to the area of computer-mediated communications."
- **2B-Referential statements:** "I want to add to Lauren's point about the importance of context in assessing technologies."
- **3-reflections:** "I felt, as a teacher, that I had failed the most needy students – it's the reason I left teaching after ten years and lots of private tears."
- **4-Scaffolding and engaging:** "Thanks for your brilliant description of the problems new teachers face – you could have been describing any one of us, I think."
- **5A-Quotations and paraphrases:** "Every tool carries with it the spirit by which it has been created."
- **5B-Citations:** "Werner Karl Heisenberg, Physics and Philosophy, 1958."

Non-Standard Orthographic Forms in Messages

Following the approach of Nastri and Hancock (2006, Content Analysis ¶ 3), the researchers reviewed the discussion transcripts and coded speech elements as NSOF each time a message included a "…non-standard orthography such as emoticons, repeated punctuation (e.g., 'Woo hoo Friday!!!!!,' or 'Is it really raining again?!?!?!'), ellipses, intentional misspellings (e.g., 'sleeeeeping', or 'riiiight'), or abbreviations (e.g., 'lol' for laughing out loud, or 'brb' for be right back)." The researchers first recorded the number of NSOF in all discussions across topic levels (topic levels refers to the *initial post, subtopic1, subtopic2* and so on) by gender, as an indication of expressive speech acts. Secondly, they observed the number of NSOF in proximity to other statements types, such as referential, scaffolding, and non-referential. This observation examined the extent to which NSOF were present in the context of other message statements. For example, will students be inclined to make a smiley face on the same line as a non-referential statement versus a scaffolding statement? The researchers counted each NSOF and its proximity, embedded within or adjacent to, a TAT statement. Thirdly, the researchers observed the amount of slang used in discussions across topic levels by gender, to ascertain the extent to which dialogue became less formal over time. It is likely that as students connected socially and discussion progressed, dialogue became less formal and, at the same time, students aligned with and supported one another. For this measure, the researcher tallied all instances of words such as "Hey", "Dunno", "Kus", "Yea", "Ya", "Yeh", and "Gosh".

RESULTS

Gender Differences in Message Types

To address the first research question concerning gender and message types, the overall number of statements generated by each gender was used as the base of the percentages. A series of chi-square tests were performed to assess whether men and women differed in their usage of each type of statement. The results of the analyses are summarized in Table 2. For both men and women, non-referential statements were the most common followed by reflections, scaffoldings, and then referential statements. When gender differences were examined more closely, 5% of statements from women and about 3% of statements from men consisted of signatures. This gender difference was found to be statistically significant. As shown in Table 2, among the epistolary types of statements, women had a significantly larger proportion of scaffoldings in their messages (17%) than the men (about 14%). On the expository types of statements, men had a significantly larger proportion of non-referential sentences in their messages (43%) than the women (37%).

The researchers ranked the proportions of statements generated within each gender. As shown in Table 3, men and women were similar in ranking for all statement types except horizontal and vertical questions, signatures, and introductions. However, horizontal questions ranked higher than signatures for men whereas signatures ranked higher for women. Similarly, vertical questions ranked higher than introductions for men whereas

Table 2. Proportions of each TAT statement type generated within Gender

Statement Type	Men		Women		Total		χ^2 *	p
	Count	Percent	Count	Percent	Count	Percent		
Introduction	11	1.3%	28	2.5%	39	2.0%	3.26	.07
Signature	23	2.7%	57	5.1%	80	4.1%	6.94	.008***
Epistolary Types								
1A: Vertical Questions	12	1.4%	9	.8%	21	1.1%	1.06	.30
1B: Horizontal Questions	33	4.1%	28	2.5%	61	3.2%	3.25	.07
2B: Referential Statements	90	10.5%	134	12.1%	224	11.4%	1.11	.29
3: Reflections	206	23.9%	251	22.6%	457	23.2%	.40	.53
4: Scaffolding, engaging	116	13.5%	190	17.1%	306	15.5%	4.64	.03**
Expository Types								
2A: Non-referential Statements	366	42.5%	408	36.8%	774	39.3%	6.49	.01**
5A: Quotations, paraphrases	2	.2%	5	.5%	7	.4%	.18	.67
5B: Citations	0	0%	0	0%	0	0%		
Total	861	100%	1110	100%	1971	100%		

* $df = 1$ for each test performed
** $p \leq .05$
*** $p \leq .01$

introductions ranked higher than vertical questions for women.

Gender Differences in Interactional Exchanges

Persistence of the Message Chain

Table 4 shows the persistence of messages by gender. There were 86 (31%) initial postings and 191 (69%) subtopic postings (subtopic 1 through 7). As shown in Table 4, male posts were somewhat dispersed over levels one and two, whereas women made the highest amount of postings (22.7%) in level two and showed greater persistence beyond level 3. To examine if there were gender differences in persistence, a chi-square test was performed at each level (see Table 5). There were no statistically significant gender differences in persistence at levels 1 to 3. However, at level 4, significantly more of the postings came from the women (71%) than from the men (29%), $\chi^2(1) = 3.86$, p =.05. Statistical analyses could not be performed on levels 5 to 7 given the small total number of postings made at each of those levels.

Table 6 presents a transitional frequency matrix for the response sequence data and table 7 presents the transitional probabilities. Each cell indicates the number of times a specific event occurred. Males responded to messages posted by other males 49 times and females responded to messages posted by males 52 times. The initial

Table 3. Ranking of most common TAT statements generated by men and women

Statement Type	Men	Statement Type	Women
Non-referential	42.5%	Non-referential	36.8%
Reflections	23.9%	Reflections	22.6%
Scaffolding, engaging	13.5%	Scaffolding, engaging	17.1%
Referential	10.5%	Referential	12.1%
Horizontal Questions	4.1%	Signature	5.1%
Signature	2.7%	Horizontal Questions	2.5%
Vertical Questions	1.4%	Introduction	2.5%
Introduction	1.3%	Vertical Questions	.8%
Quotations	.2%	Quotations	.5%
Citations	0%	Citations	0%

Table 4.Gender differences in persistence

Level	Men		Women		Total	
	Count	Percent	Count	Percent	Count	Percent
Level 1: Initial Post	46	16.61	40	14.44	86	31.05
Level 2: Subtopic 1	45	16.25	63	22.74	108	38.99
Level 3: Subtopic 2	28	10.11	24	8.66	52	18.77
Level 4: Subtopic 3	6	2.17	15	5.42	21	7.58
Level 5: Subtopic 4	4	1.44	1	0.36	5	1.81
Level 6: Subtopic 5	1	0.36	1	0.36	2	0.72
Level 7: Subtopic 5+	2	0.72	1	0.36	3	1.08

events, such as a female posting a message, are in the Initial column and the target events or the events occurring later in time, such as a male responding to a message sent by a female, are in the Target columns. The were fours possible event sequences: 1) male posted message, male responded; 2) male posted message, female responded; 3) female posted message, male responded; 4) female posted message, female responded. To compute the transitional probabilities, the frequency for a particular cell is divided by the total frequency for the row (Bakeman & Gottman, 1997, p. 98). A .49 probability was found for a male response, given a preceding male post. The highest probability (.59) was for a female response, given a preceding female post and the lowest probability (.41) was for male response, given a preceding female post (see Table 7). However, the probability of a male responding to a preceding male post was not found to be significantly different from the probability of a female responding, $\chi^2(1) = .09$, $p = .77$. Likewise, the probability of a male response to a female post was not significantly different from the probability of a female response, $\chi^2(1) = 2.84$, $p = .09$.

Isolated Messages

There were 24 total isolated messages across all conferences, 9% of total messages. There was no significant differences in the amount of isolated messages for men and women; men posted 11 initial messages to which no one responded and women posted 13 messages, $\chi^2(1) = .17$, $p = .68$. The researchers identified the themes of isolated messages to ascertain if their content was distinct from messages that received responses. A prevalent theme occurring in most (83%) of the isolated messages related to students describing a teaching experience. An example of one such message is presented below:

Hi everyone, Today was my first experience teaching. It was wonderful. I taught PE and the kids

Table 5. Gender differences in persistence at each level

Level	Men		Women		Total Count
	Count	Percent	Count	Percent	
Level 1: Initial Post	46	53	40	47	86
Level 2: Subtopic 1	45	42	63	58	108
Level 3: Subtopic 2	28	54	24	46	52
Level 4: Subtopic 3	6	29	15	71	21
Level 5: Subtopic 4	4	80	1	20	5
Level 6: Subtopic 5	1	50	1	50	2
Level 7: Subtopic 5+	2	67	1	33	3

Male-Female Response Sequences

Table 6. Observed frequencies in two-event response sequences by male and female posters

Initial	**Target**		
	Male	Female	Total
Male	49	52	101
Female	37	53	90

were great. I was a really nervous when I started but it was fine once I got going. I made a list of the student names and it really helped that I knew them all and call them by name. I gave the students a guide on how to take notes and they really liked it. Overall, it was really good.

Another common theme occurring in 29% of the messages related to issues of disciplining or managing students. However, these themes were prevalent in all messages, not only those that were isolated. Of all isolated message, 42% were either the last or second to last message in the discussion. Additionally, the highest volume discussion conference has the most isolated messages.

Table 7. Transitional probabilities in two-event response sequences by male and female posters

Initial	Target	
	Male	Female
Male	0.49	0.51
Female	0.41	0.59

Non-Standard Orthographic Forms in Messages

There were 277 posts of which 141 (52%) contained NSOF. In 141 unique messages, there were 201 NSOF elements, most (41%) occurring in initial postings and 29% in subtopic 1 (see Figure 1). Females made the majority (65%) of NSOF and males made 35% of them. The overall amount of NSOF decreased steadily after level 1, as did the amount of messages in each level. However, Figure 2 shows the proportion of messages in each topic level that contained NSOF relative to the number of messages in that level.

The percent of NSOF in close proximity to other statements type is shown in Table 8. Of all the NSOF, 28% were positioned within or adjacent to a scaffolding statement. Seventeen percent were positioned near non-referential statements and 12% were positioned near reflections. No NSOF were positioned near vertical questions, quotations, or citations.

Out of 277 total messages, 34 had slang. In those 34 messages, there were 51 instances of slang use. Much (47%) of the slang occurred in topic level 1. Over all topic levels, women made 76% of the slang and men made 24%. Figure 3

Figure 1. Non-standard Orthographic Forms use by gender across topic levels

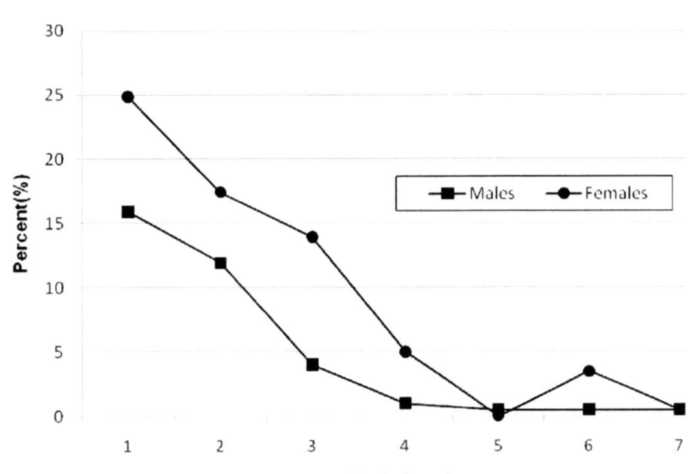

Figure 2. Percent of messages containing NSOF relative to the number of messages for each topic level

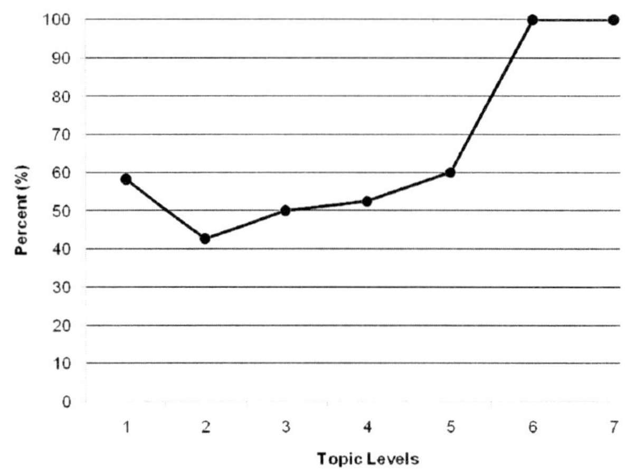

Figure 3. Slang use by gender across topic levels

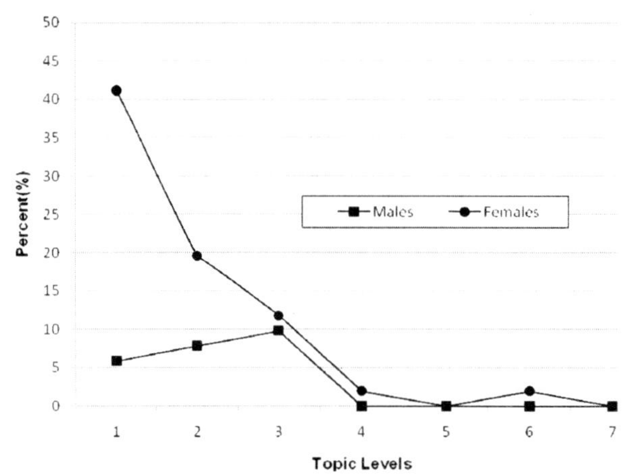

shows the use of slang by topic level for men and women.

DISCUSSION

This research set out to examine gender differences in communication and interactional processes in peer-directed conferences. In the following section, the researchers examine the findings in terms of the research questions.

Gender Differences in Message Types

Question 1: In peer-directed conferences, are there gender differences in the type of messages that comprise communication?

Despite the supportive nature of the conferences and students sharing a new teaching experience, there were gender disparities in messages types. This suggests that the shared (teaching) experience did not influence message types and the observed gender differences would be evident regardless of the nature of the conferences.

Table 8. Non-standard orthographic forms in proximity to other statements

Statement Type	NSOF %
1A-Vertical	0
1B-Horizontal	2
2A-Non-referential	17
2B-Referential	4
3-Reflections	12
4-Scaffolding	28
5A-Quotations	0
5B-Citations	0

Messages posted by women were more of an epistolary nature relative to those posted by men, which is consistent with other research (Herring, 1996a, 1996b, 2000; Fahy, 2002) but not what the researchers expected. Communication is shaped by the social context in which discussion occurs as well as shared experiences among discussants (Dickey, Wasko, Chudoba, & Thatcher, 2006; Riva & Galimberti, 1998). Consequently, the researchers anticipated that the common experience of beginning teaching and the nature of the peer-directed conferences would engender epistolary-type messages (reflecting alignment and support) equally among genders. However, several indicators show that this was not the case. First, the epistolary (conversation/interactive) message schema is characterized by opening and closing conventions. Women used introductions (openings) and signatures (closings) or similar rules in messages more than men. In fact, women used signatures significantly more than men. Second, women exceeded men in all epistolary categories except vertical and horizontal questions. Third, the messages of women had significantly higher proportions of scaffolding statements, an indicator of epistolary discourse. Fourth, compared to women, men used significantly more non-referential statements, indicators of expository discourse. The findings coincide with Fahy's (2002) research, even though his conference was of a different nature, instructor moderated, and related to a specific course topic.

Factors Contributing to the High Use of Expository Discourse

As mentioned, the researchers anticipated greater use of epistolary-type statements because of the nature of the conferences and the common (new) teaching experience, which was quite personal for students. In level 1, many students of both genders made postings that informed about their experiences. Below is an example of one such post:

This was my first day and it was a unique sort of experience. My third class only had 7 students so that was a different kind of experience because the group was so small. I had many more students in my first class and several of them had special needs. I start to teach my own lessons on Monday. I thought it was suppose to be today but I guess I was wrong. Oh well, now I'm prepared for Monday.

Possibly because of their intent to inform others, men and women used non-referential statements (expository) more than any other statement type. While speculative, the structure of messages may have influenced communication. Epistolary discourse has a structure characterized by opening and closing conventions (Herring, 1996a) that is an important communicative form in text-based CMC, especially in discussions of the type examined here. Of all the messages posted, only 2% used openings and 4% used closings. In the aforementioned post, for example, there is no indication of the person to whom the message is addressed. One assumes that the sender is addressing the entire group. In addition, there is no indictor of who sent the message other than an impersonal name stamp provided by the conferencing system. In a face-to-face conversation, it is probable that if person A makes a statement such as, "*I feel very uneasy about my ability to control the students in my large unwieldy class.*", person

B, when responding, would address the person by name or he/she may engage in some form of non-verbal communication to signal interest and support such as altering his/her tone of voice, or leaning toward person A. Because many familiar non-verbal cues are unavailable in text-based CMC, discussants must rely on other forms to foster alignment and support. Opening and closings can help promulgate epistolary messages (support and alignment) and serve as an important communicative function in several ways. First, unlike face-to-face conversations multiple people "speak" simultaneously in CMC and thus rules of turn-taking become less obvious. For instance, suppose Liam posts a new message (initial post - level 1) that relates an experience he had in class. Two people respond (level 2 – subtopic 1 postings) to him using openings and closings. A third person, intending to respond to Liam, uses one of the level 2 messages for her reply and she does not include an opening. As a result, it is not immediately clear to whom the third person addressed the message, to Liam or the other two posters. Thus, openings help identify the addressee and let him/her know that someone is waiting for a response. Second, openings help personalize messages and establish relational connections with the addressee and/or to a previous posting. Addressing a message to a person or specific group will, in all likelihood, encourage recipients to read and respond. Third, openings signify the message beginning. As messages get deeper in the message chain and discussants include previous postings in them, it becomes difficult to ascertain where messages begin.

Like openings, closings are useful for the several reasons. First, they identify the end of the current message. It is not always obvious where a message ends because discussants often embed multiple messages in a single post. Second, closings identify the message poster. While a name stamp is provided by the conferencing system, it is not personalized or initiated by the poster. Moreover, the name stamp typically does not follow the end of the message and so the reader's eyes must scan for it in the message header. Third, closings (and openings) are politeness markers (Herring, 1994).

Initiating Conferences with Expository Statements

The researchers observed that discussants used expository-type statements (non-referential statements) the most in level 1. Their use of epistolary-type statements was low in level 1 but it increased in level 2. This intimates that initially discussants showed a tendency to inform and then in level 2 they strove to support and align. The propensity to inform at the onset of the conferences is noteworthy because it may have impacted recipients' ability to adequately attend to messages. In face-to-face group communication, multiple people will yield a turn so that only one person speaks at a time. In CMC, discussants "speak" simultaneously, often about divergent topics. This is particularly pertinent at level 1 in the message hierarchy as numerous simultaneous postings compete for participants' attention. As everyone "speaks" about his/her own topic, there is more information discussants must attend to and correspondingly an increased probability of missed information. At the same time, message order becomes important, with messages appearing higher in the list likely to receive more attention than those lower in the list. Unlike postings in level 1, messages in levels 2 and beyond have relational connections to previous postings, which may help discussants filter information and/or attend to a particular message thread. Due to a potential onslaught of expository-type messages in level 1, it could be useful to employ some form of message filtering to help aid discussants (and instructors) discern message content, especially in high volume conferences. For example, Jeong and Joung (2007) had students insert labels into message subject headings to identify message content. Instructors could instruct students to label postings with descriptors such as general information, action needed, interesting to know, suggested strategy-teaching, or suggested strategy-classroom management, among others. Assuming the labels accurately depict message content, the technique could help discussants focus on the information they need and thus it may engender richer dialogue within specific conferences or threads. While it may be impossible to know specific categories of message labels at the start of a conference, this information could be garnered over time and be used in subsequence discussion activities.

Gender Differences in Interactional Exchanges

Question 2: In peer-directed conferences what gender differences exist in interactional exchanges?

Persistence in the Message Chain

In CMC men tend to open and close discussions in mixed-sex groups (Herring, 2000). In this study, male and female persistence in the message hierarchy was comparable. Although the majority of men ended participation at level subtopic 2 and most women ended participation at subtopic 3, slightly more men persisted past subtopic 3, which may reflect Herring's observation of a male tendency to close discussions. The relatively high degree of female persistence to subtopic 3 may correspond to an epistolary communication style and with the overall finding that women exhibited a greater (although non significant) tendency than men to respond to both sexes. Possibly in an effort to support and align with others, women persisted to subtopic 3 with a higher number of posts.

Overall there was not a great deal of persistence for either men or women. Given that some of the topics were personal and contentious with potentially significant implications (e.g., classroom discipline, problems with cooperating teachers, inappropriate behavior), the researchers expected more in-depth discussion. In these conferences, even though a topic was of considerable importance, students communicated relatively briefly about it and then moved on. What is germane to this observation is that in educational discussions situations may arise that are problematic and/or controversial in nature. When an instructor or moderator is engaged, he/she can follow up on key points to foster greater discourse and ultimately help students work toward resolving issues. This is an area of additional research since this study only investigated male-female persistence and not factors that enhance or impede in-depth discourse. However, while it appears that students can effectively manage peer-directed conferences without gender disparities in persistence, the role of an instructor or moderator is still important.

Male-Female Response Sequences and Isolated Messages

The amount of initial posts or the topics started by men and women were comparable, although men had slightly more (2%) than women. While not significant, women gave 6.5% more replies to initial posts than men, of which more than half (55%) were replies to messages posted by men. Conversely, men made 75% of their subtopic 1 replies to other men and 24% to women.

Scholars have noted that during CMC women post fewer messages than men and they receive fewer responses (Herring, 2000; Panyametheekul & Herring, 2003; Jeong, 2003). In this study, women posted more messages than men but received fewer replies. Differences in how men and women responded to one another were not significant, although men were less likely to respond to women than they were to other men. Women responded equally to men and other women. The least likely response sequence was men responding to women.

The volume of postings by women and the fact that women and men had equal numbers of isolated messages suggests that women were not prohibited from participating nor were they socially censored. Herring (1993) reports that in some CMC discussions women are discouraged from participation based on the reactions they received from their postings. The nature of the conferences in this study may have fostered interactions in which women felt comfortable posting messages. Students were likely looking for support and advice about issues pertaining to their student teaching and thus there was no censorship, or asocial behavior.

The number of isolated messages in the conferences was relatively small. Their themes were similar to messages that receive responses. Many isolated messages occurred at the end of discussions and they were most prevalent in the highest volume conference, possibly because of the increased amount of information that competed for discussants' attention. To address isolated messages, it would be useful for instructors to appoint a moderator to review and/or close discussions to ensure, when necessary, that all postings receive a reply.

Unlike other studies (e.g., Jeong, 2003) women exhibited a tendency to respond to other women as well as men, while men responded more to other men. It is possible that the overall tenor of conferences enabled these gender differences to emerge. The new teaching experience and the conferences may have engendered a discourse style typically associated with women characterized by support and alignment with others (Panyametheekul & Herring, 2003) and thus, women made more posts and replies. On the other hand, many men are socialized to be reserved in terms of receiving and giving social support or expressing emotions and thus they may have been disinclined to respond to the posts of women. Herring (2000) contends that the socialization of men (and women) is the fundamental root of discordant behaviors in CMC.

Non-Standard Orthographic Forms in Messages

Question 3: In peer-directed conferences, to what extent do men and women use socio-emotional content in messages and what, if anything, do these forms indicate about communication?

More than half of all messages used NSOF and women used them more than men. The researchers anticipated that as discussion progressed students would become more socially connected and communication would reflect this characteristic. Because NSOF indicate social expression and relational intent, one might expect them to be more prevalent in subtopic levels as students gain familiarity with each other. It is plausible that with increased social relations, students would exhibit greater tendency to align and support others and thus epistolary communication would emerge. Moreover, over time one might expect increased usage of NSOF and less formal language (slang).

Interestingly, the highest amount of NSOF and slang occurred in level 1 and then use dropped in level 2, which is the opposite of what the researchers expected. When NSOF were examined relative to the number of postings at each level, use declined after level 1 but then increased steadily after level 2 (see Figure 2). It is noteworthy that NSOF and slang decreased in level 2 while epistolary statement increased. These observations may be attributed to the several factors. First, because discussants knew one another, they felt comfortable using NSOF and slang in level 1. Secondly, they could have written posts informally despite the weightiness of the matter. For example, a student might post a message such as the following in level 1,

AHHHHHHHHHH!!! I'm at a lossssssss! I have three students who just will not listen to me & they talk NON-STOPPPPP during my class. Da.... I'm clueless. My CT [cooperating teacher] seems 2b

getting impatient with my inability to manage them. Does anyone have suggestions? Please help me ☺

While the message has NSOF and slang, the underlying issue concerns the poster, which is readily apparent to the reader. Possibly as discussants moved to level 2 they recognized that although many of their peers wrote expressively or informally about issues, the issues were nonetheless of some gravity. As a result, they responded more formally in effort to empathized with or support the poster. Third, discussants' expressiveness in level 1 could have been rooted in their sentiments toward the teaching practicum. Thus, level 1 provided discussants an opportunity to relate their new teaching experiences (expository discourse), while in level 2 they began addressing (epistolary discourse) issues presented by other discussants. The fact that expository discourse (non-referential statements) was highest in level 1 while epistolary discourse (scaffolding) was low in level 1 and increased in level 2 seems to support this contention.

Women used more NSOF and less formal language than men, which is consistent with research indicating that women are more inclined to use socio-emotional communication (Tannen, 1991; Herring, 1993; Fahy, 2002; Jaffe, Huang, & Oshagan, 1995). Conceivably, NSOF may coincide with a tendency to align and support peers. While research is needed to examine the relationship between NSOF and epistolary communication (specifically scaffolding) in peer-directed discussions, discussants showed an inclination to use NSOF when making scaffolding statements. However, of all NSOF, 28% were positioned within or adjacent to scaffoldings, whereas 17% and 12% were near non-referential and reflections, respectively. In addition, NSOF and slang decreased in level 2 while epistolary discourse increased, which was unexpected. This observation suggests that as discussants responded to the issues of their peers, they were less expressive. Thus, the relationship between NSOF, slang, and epistolary (scaffolding) discourse is unclear, if a relationship exists at all.

CONCLUSION

It is important to point out the findings presented here are not conclusive due to the limitations and scope of this study. The study looked at a specific type of discussion conference with a unique population. Additional research is required to examine communication types and interaction across larger groups engaged in discussions on varying topics.

In discussions of this nature, students can engage in positive discourse with minimal instructor involvement. There will be gender differences in the type of messages that comprise communication and in the use of socio-emotional content. However, overall men and women can participate equitably. They will persist comparably, respond equally to one another, and receive equal numbers of isolated messages.

The study findings bring to light important implications regarding communication processes in online asynchronous conferences and they offer additional insight into how gender affects communication. First, they suggest that regardless of the shared (teaching) experience and the nature of the conferences gender differences will exist in terms of epistolary and expository discourse. Second, instructors need to be aware that gender differences will likely occur in online conferences and, as a result, they should actively monitor conferences. The discussions in the study were fairly innocuous. Equal numbers of men and women engaged in non-graded dialogue about a teaching practicum in which they were generally experiencing similar issues and challenges. It is probable that gender disparities would be even more pronounced as competition for grades increased, discussion content became adversarial, and the distribution of males and females became uneven. Third, students should be educated about gender differences in text-based CMC so they are cognizant of their own communication and its impact on dialogue. A student who uses non-referential statements pervasively throughout messages may inhibit discourse and be unable to fully engage in key communication processes. In addition, if an expository style of communication is warranted, discussants should be instructed to structure messages accordingly with openings and closings. Therefore, strategies that recognize and account for gender are needed to help students facilitate dialogue and engagement. It is plausible that group performance could be enhanced by assigning specific roles to discussants based on gender and communication preferences (Jeong & Davidson-Shiver, 2006).

The finding suggests that even though differences in male-female communication may exist (as found by research question 1) interaction is not prohibited. Given the nature of the conferences described, students can self-govern discussions with members having equal opportunity to engage in communication. This is important because women often feel censored or inhibited from contributing in conferences that are not moderated. Herring (2000) reports that women are inclined to do better in moderated conferences. In this study, students governed conferences with little instructor involvement and yet the contributions across genders were comparable; in fact, women had more messages of longer length. Such findings are valuable because enabling student autonomy may foster learner-centeredness and ultimately self-reliant learners. However, it is important to point out that men received more replies to their messages and, while not significant, they were less inclined to respond to women while women responded equally to men and women. To ensure equitable exchanges among men and women, instructors or moderators should monitor discussions because the differences observed in this study may become more pronounced when discussions are graded or as they grow competitive.

The use of socio-emotional content among men and women indicates gender differences in online communication. Women were more expressive than man and they used NSOF and slang to a greater extent. Over time, their use of socio-emotional content did not steadily increase as expected. Discussants used socio-emotional content when opening the conferences but use decreased as they began to address the issues of their peers, particularly in level 2. While additional research is needed to further explore the relationship between NSOF, slang, and epistolary (scaffolding) discourse, discussants showed a tendency to use socio-emotional content when making scaffolding statements.

REFERENCES

Arnold, J., & Miller, H. (2001). Academic masters, mistresses, and apprentices: Gender and power in the real world of the web. *Mots Pluriels, 19*. Retrieved March 10, 2009, from http://www.arts.uwa.edu.au/MotsPluriels/MP1901jahm.html

Bakeman, R., & Gottman, J. (1997). *Observing Interaction: An introduction to sequential analysis*. Cambridge, UK: Cambridge University Press. doi:10.1017/CBO9780511527685

Baron, N. S. (2004). See you online: Gender issues in American college student use of instant messaging. *Journal of Language and Social Psychology, 23*(4), 397–423. doi:10.1177/0261927X04269585

Dickey, M. H., Wasko, M. M., Chudoba, K. M., & Thatcher, J. B. (2006). Do you know what I know?: A shared understandings perspective on text-based communication. *Journal of Computer-Mediated Communication, 12*(1). Retrieved March 16, 2009, from http://jcmc.indiana.edu/vol12/issue1/dickey.html

Donath, J., Karahalios, K., & Viegas, F. (1999). Visualizing conversation. *Journal of Computer-Mediated Communication, 4*(4). Retrieved March 3, 2009, from http://jcmc.indiana.edu/vol4/issue4/donath.html

Fahy, P. (2002). Epistolary and Expository Interaction Patterns in a Computer Conference Transcript. *Journal of Distance Education, 17*(1), 20–35.

Fahy, P. (2003). Indicators of support in online interaction. *International Review of Research in Open and Distance Learning, 4*(1), 1-16. Retrieved April 28, 2008, from http://www.irrodl.org/index.php/irrodl/article/view/129

Fahy, P., Crawford, G., & Ally, M. (2001). Patterns of interaction in a computer conference transcript. *The International Review of Research in Open and Distance Learning, 2*(1). Retrieved September 30, 2008, from http://www.irrodl.org/index.php/irrodl/article/view/36

Fahy, P. J. (2005). Two methods for assessing critical thinking in computer-mediated communications (CMC) transcripts. *International Journal of Instructional Technology and Distance Learning, 2*(3). Retrieved June 5, 2008, from http://www.itdl.org/Journal/Mar_05/article02.htm

Hancock, J. T. (2004). Verbal irony use in face-to-face and computer-mediated communication. *Journal of Language and Social Psychology, 23*(4), 447–463. doi:10.1177/0261927X04269587

Herring, S. C. (1993). Gender and democracy in computer-mediated communication. *EJC/REC, 3*(20). Retrieved May 18, 2008, from http://www.internetstudies.pe.kr/txt/Herring.txt

Herring, S. C. (1994). Politeness in computer culture: Why women thank and men flame. In M. Bucholtz, A. Liang, & L. Sutton (Eds.), *Cultural Performances: Proceedings of the Third Berkeley Women and Language Conference* (pp. 278-94). Berkeley, CA: Berkeley Women and Language Group.

Herring, S. C. (1996a). Two variants of an electronic message schema. In Herring, S. C. (Ed.), *Computer-mediated communication: Linguistic, social, and cross-cultural perspectives* (pp. 81–106). Philadelphia, PA: John Benjamins.

Herring, S. C. (1996b). Posting in a different voice: Gender and ethics in computer-mediated communication. In Ess, C. (Ed.), *Philosophical Perspectives on Computer-Mediated Communication* (pp. 115–145). Albany, NY: SUNY Press.

Herring, S. C. (2000). Gender Differences in CMC: Findings and Implications. *CPSR Newsletter, 18*(1). Retrieved May 30, 2008, from http://www.cpsr.org/issues/womenintech/herring

Herring, S. C. (2001). Computer-mediated discourse. In Schiffrin, D., Tannen, D., & Hamilton, H. E. (Eds.), *The Handbook of Discourse Analysis* (pp. 612–634). Malden, MA: Blackwell Publishers.

Herring, S. C. (2003). Gender and power in online communication. In Holmes, J., & Meyerhoff, M. (Eds.), *The Handbook of Language and Gender* (pp. 202–228). Oxford: Blackwell Publishers. doi:10.1002/9780470756942.ch9

Herring, S. C., & Paolillo, J. C. (2006). Gender and genre variation in weblogs. *Journal of Sociolinguistics, 10*(4), 439–459. doi:10.1111/j.1467-9841.2006.00287.x

Huffaker, D. A., & Calvert, S. L. (2005). Gender, identity, and language use in teenage blogs. *Journal of Computer-Mediated Communication, 10*(2). Retrieved May 3, 2008, from http://jcmc.indiana.edu/vol10/issue2/huffaker.html

Ivy, D. K., & Backlund, P. (1994). *Exploring GenderSpeak: Personal effectiveness in gender communication*. New York: McGraw-Hill.

Jaffe, J. M., Lee, Y., Huang, L., & Oshagan, H. (1995). *Gender, Pseudonyms, and CMC: Masking Identities and Baring Souls*. Presented at the 45th Annual Conference of the International Communication Association (ICA), Albuquerque, New Mexico, USA.

Jeong, A. (2003). *Gender interactions in online debates: Look who's arguing with whom.* Paper presented at the Annual Meeting of the American Educational Research Association, Chicago, Ill, April. Retrieved January, 2009, from http://mailer.fsu.edu/~ajeong/GenderInteraction2.doc

Jeong, A., & Davidson-Shivers, G. V. (2006). The effects of gender interaction patterns on student participation in computer-supported collaboration argumentation. *ETR&D, 54*(1), 543–569. doi:10.1007/s11423-006-0636-4

Jeong, A., & Joung, S. (2007). Scaffolding collaborative argumentation in asynchronous discussions with message constraints and message labels. *Computers & Education, 48*, 427–445. doi:10.1016/j.compedu.2005.02.002

Juler, P. (1990). Promoting Interaction, Maintaining Independence: Swallowing the mixture. *Open Learning, 5*(2), 24–33. doi:10.1080/0268051900050205

Kalman, Y. M., & Rafaeli, S. (2005). Email chronemics: Unobtrusive profiling on response time. In *Proceedings of HICSS-38: Hawaii International Conference on System Sciences* (pp. 108b). Los Alamitos, CA: IEEE Computer Society Press.

Kramarae, C. (1995). A backstage critique of virtual reality. In Jones, S. (Ed.), *Cybersociety: Computer-mediated communication and community* (pp. 35–56). Thousand Oaks, CA: Sage.

Lee, G. B. (1996). Addressing anonymous messages in cyberspace. *Journal of Computer-Mediated Communication, 2*(1), Retrieved May 6, 2008, from http://jcmc.indiana.edu/vol2/issue1/anon.html

Mann, C., & Stewart, F. (2000). *Internet communication and qualitative research: A handbook for researching online.* London: Sage Publications.

Mulac, A., Bradac, J. J., & Mann, S. K. (1985). Male/female language differences and attributional consequences in children's television. *Human Communication Research, 11*(4), 481–506. doi:10.1111/j.1468-2958.1985.tb00057.x

Mulac, A., & Lundell, T. L. (1986). Linguistic contributors to the gender-linked language effect. *Journal of Language and Social Psychology, 5*(2), 91–101. doi:10.1177/0261927X8652001

Murphy, K. L., Harvell, T. J., Sanders, B., & Lu Epps, M. (1999). *Students as designers and teachers of their courses via computer-mediated communication.* Paper presented at the Annual Convention of the Association for Educational Communications and Technology, Houston, TX, February. Retrieved, December 14, 2008, from http://www.coe.tamu.edu/~kmurphy/writings/aect99webdesign.html

Nastri, J., Peña, J., & Hancock, J. T. (2006). The construction of away messages: A speech act analysis. *Journal of Computer-Mediated Communication, 11*(4). Retrieved June 6, 2008, from http://jcmc.indiana.edu/vol11/issue4/nastri.html

Panyametheekul, P., & Herring, S. (2003). Gender and turn allocation in a Thai chat room. *Journal of Computer-Mediated Communication, 9*(1). Retrieved June 6, 2008, from http://jcmc.indiana.edu/vol12/issue2/waldvogel.html

Pedersen, S., & Macafee, C. (2007). Gender differences in British blogging. *Journal of Computer-Mediated Communication, 12*(4). Retrieved December 23, 2009, from http://jcmc.indiana.edu/vol12/issue4/pedersen.html

Quina, K., Wingard, J. A., & Bates, H. G. (1987). Language style and gender stereotypes in person perception. *Psychology of Women Quarterly, 11*(1), 111–122. doi:10.1111/j.1471-6402.1987.tb00778.x

Riva, G., & Galimberti, C. (1998). Computer-mediated communication: Identity and social interaction in an electronic environment. *Genetic, Social, and General Psychology Monographs, 124*(4), 434–464.

Tannen, D. (1991). *You Just Don't Understand: Men and Women in Conversation*. New York: Ballantine Books.

Walther, J. B. (1992). Interpersonal effects in computer-mediated interaction: A relational perspective. *Communication Research, 19*(1), 52–90. doi:10.1177/009365092019001003

Witmer, D. F., & Katzman, S. L. (1997). On-Line smiles: Does gender make a difference in the use of graphic accents? *Journal of Computer-Mediated Communication, 2*(4). Retrieved March 6, 2009, from http://jcmc.indiana.edu/vol2/issue4/witmer1.html

Zhu, E. (1996). Meaning negotiation, knowledge construction, and mentoring in a distance learning course. In *Proceedings of Selected Research and Development Presentations at the 1996* (pp. 821–844). Indianapolis, IN: National Convention of the Association for Educational Communications and Technology.

Zhu, E. (1998). Learning and mentoring: Electronic discussions in a distance learning course. In Bonk, C. J., & King, K. S. (Eds.), *Electronic collaborators: Learner-centered technologies for literacy, apprenticeship, and discourse* (pp. 233–259). Mahwah, NJ: Lawrence Erlbaum Associates.

Section 2

Multimedia Learning Tools

Chapter 5
Video Analysis as a Reflective Tool:
Providing Pre-Service Teachers a Gradual-Replay Lens on their Developing Practice

Pru Cuper
Keene State College, USA

Yi Gong
Keene State College, USA

ABSTRACT

The purpose of this chapter is to present and explain the effects of a videotaping assessment instrument designed to help pre-service teachers hone specific aspects of their developing practice. In an educational era marked by emphasis on both quantitative assessment and reflective practice (sometimes considered conflicting targets), this instrument is particularly effective in providing quantitative data while simultaneously evoking gradual and productive self analysis in pre-service teachers. The authors begin with a discussion of the use of videotaping in pre-service teacher education over the years (the benefits and the drawbacks), before proceeding to discuss the merits of this particular assessment instrument as well as their thoughts on future revisions and research.

INTRODUCTION

We live in an era that is both ripe and rife with new technologies. At times, the unending flow of technological innovations and improvements is exciting, but at other times it is overwhelming. For teacher educators, whose primary work is to develop pre-service teachers into the next generation of effective classroom teachers, the draw of new technologies is strong. Certainly, they offer instantaneous communication and a wealth of materials to enhance learning—at all levels. Additionally, today's pre-service teachers are, in most cases, extremely comfortable with these new technologies. Many use video and audio files as part of their daily communication practices—through cell phones and Blackberries, Facebook and MySpace accounts, to name a few.

Today's pre-service teachers are used to technologies that offer fast and easy means of sharing pictures, thoughts and plans. But how does their comfort with technology translate into what they

DOI: 10.4018/978-1-61520-899-9.ch005

will be required to know and do in the classroom setting? Most importantly, how will it lead to the deep, reflective practice that is necessary (but oftentimes disregarded) in the fast-paced world that is so familiar to them? This question challenges teacher educators today. It is the question that led us to develop a means for harnessing a useful-but-constantly-evolving technological tool, videotaping, in a way that would also encourage reflective practice amongst our pre-service teachers.

In this chapter, we discuss the steps we went through as we developed the Student Teaching Performance Checklist (STPC), an assessment tool designed to guide pre-service teachers' pedagogical progress while simultaneously triggering self analysis and reflection. To accomplish these tasks, we begin by viewing and discussing videotapes of their classroom practice with them, using the STPC to focus the conversation. Next, we encourage them to revisit the videotapes and the STPC categories on their own and at a pace that is comfortable for them—to, in effect, use a guided, gradual-replay lens on their practice vs. the instant-replay lens that seems endemic to many 21st Century endeavors.

Like many teacher preparation programs, we have used videotapes of our pre-service teachers' work in the past, but we have found that, without the specific assessment guidelines that the STPC provides, we sometimes overlook key aspects of what is essential to becoming an effective classroom teacher. More importantly, prior to using the STPC we did not consistently encourage our students to take a second (or third), deeper look at their own work while keeping the necessary components of good teaching practice in mind—to gradually replay their interactions with students in order to hone their teaching skills.

Our chapter begins with a review of the use of videotaping in teacher education. We share success stories as well as challenges from the field using Bandura's (1977) theories of self-efficacy and various research studies on reflective practice in teacher education as a foundation. We follow with a brief discussion of the issues, controversies and problems inherent in videotaping pre-service teachers. Next, we offer an in-depth explanation of our experiences in this realm—our solutions and recommendations, including an explanation of the assessment tool we developed to guide our pre-service teachers' practice. We close the chapter with our thoughts on next steps; the research that is still needed in this area based on what we have discovered as we ventured into using an "old" (but constantly evolving) technology in a carefully designed way.

BACKGROUND

Teaching is arguably the most "human" of all professions. As such, it is riddled with the inevitable complexities that underlie human interactions and human growth. Because of this, mentoring and supervision of pre-service teachers has offered an invigorating challenge to teacher educators since public schooling became a governmental requirement in America close to a century ago. Teacher educator considerations include (but are not limited to): 1) the great range of natural abilities within the pre-service teacher ranks; 2) the array of areas and topics that perspective teachers need to know about and be able to teach; 3) the theory-to-practice debate... how much of a theoretical base is necessary and how do we (teacher educators) balance theory and practice? 4) the wide array of student needs that pre-service teachers will be required to accommodate and address. Needless to say, these are only the first round of considerations.

Ultimately teacher educators must find ways, within a relatively short span of time, to help their pre-service teachers become successful classroom professionals. One of the most powerful means of promoting this growth is to *show* future teachers what they look like in the classroom setting, to videotape and discuss their teaching performances with them. Over time this strategy has proven extremely successful. In fact, video evidence has been used as a catalyst to promote rich dialogue, which supports multiple perspectives, meanings and interpretations of classroom events (Jones & McNamara, 2004) for many years. Fortunately, the technologies related to this work have become exponentially more powerful over the years and easier to use as well. And as the technologies have become more facile, researchers have had time to consider other effects of videotaping in teacher education, such as the development of self-efficacy and reflective practice in pre-service teachers.

VIDEOTAPING IN PRE-SERVICE SUPERVISION

Case-based teaching and learning in teacher education, which oftentimes involves videotapes of pre-service teaching performance, has intuitive appeal as an instructional practice and definite advantages over the traditional lectures and textbooks that have been used in teacher education for many years (Beck, King, & Marshall, 2002). For starters, it represents a more realistic view of the dynamic complexities and ambiguities of classroom teaching and subsequent student learning. It also enables pre-service teachers to detect specific issues and problems within a complex and authentic context; foster critical analysis of such issues and problems; and, develop habits of reflection that are essential to honing effective teaching practice. Studies show that case-based, videotaped instruction improves pre-service teachers' ability to teach effectively in a variety of ways: 1) to identify instructional problems within the classroom setting; 2) to consider alternative perspectives and use evidence of multiple sources to develop solutions; 3) to consider the consequences of their solutions, and; 4) to generate final solutions and conclusions from cases (Beck et al, 2002). But while case-based instruction shares these outcomes, the form that it takes varies greatly from one site to the next—depending as much on learning targets as instructional technology infrastructures and support. Fortunately, there has been steady positive progress in this area since videotaping became more widely used in teacher education close to twenty years ago.

Early on, McIntyre and Paper (1993) described the development of an interactive videodisk project in an introduction to education course at Southern Illinois University at Carbondale. The project was based on three constructs of learning: situated cognition, anchored instruction, and reflective judgment. Their video protocols consisted of: 1) video recordings of original and unrehearsed classroom events; 2) organized collections of relevant theoretical knowledge, such as concepts, definitions, and facts, and; 3) recorded interviews of teachers' elaboration on their actions, thoughts, and decisions during classroom events.

In a somewhat similar vein, Dymond and Bentz (2006) developed a digital video library for their full-time special education teachers who enrolled in a graduate special education course to update their special education teaching certification. These teachers were required to videotape their use of specific instructional strategies with individuals with mild disabilities. Their process of building a digital video library began with identifying who, what, and where to videotape. They then obtained permission before collecting the actual digital video, then editing and storing their digital movies as a teaching tool for their pre-service teachers.

Cennamo, Abell, George and Chung (1996) at Purdue University developed a series of case-based interactive videodiscs to facilitate reflective thinking about science teaching among pre-service elementary teachers. Their approach of using videodiscs as an instructional tool is distinctive in the following aspects. First, they used realistic cases that recorded the actual teachers' reaction to things that worked well and things did not work well, which allowed pre-service teachers to experience the complexity of the real classroom experience.

Second, they used continuous cases that presented the classroom events over a two-week period, which offered the pre-service teachers an opportunity to see the interrelationship of classroom events. Third, they provided multiple modes of representation so that pre-service teachers could explore the cases through lesson plans, classroom teaching videos, teacher reflections, student products and student notes. Last and most important, the videodiscs were used not only for individual pre-service teacher's reflection and knowledge construction, but also for small and large-group discussion that facilitated the exchange of ideas among pre-service teachers.

Using the most current technologies, Wu and Kao (2008) integrate video streaming technology with a web-based peer assessment system in their teacher education program. In this example, pre-service teachers' performance is recorded into online streaming video. The streaming video, online peer assessment form and comment text boxes are all shown on the same page. The peer assessment form includes ten clear objectives ranging from correct content, appropriate examples, inspiring learning, organized lectures, provoking thinking, being aware of students, proper wording and handling of student "incidents" to considerations of time management. Comment text boxes allow peers to enter qualitative data. Beside each comment text box, there is a text box for inputting where, in the video clip, the commented action occurred. Pre-service teachers can reply to their peers' comments using a "reply" text box. In addition, they are able to play the comment-associated video segment. The comments are given by peers in an anonymous way so peers are comfortable providing professional feedback. The whole streaming video, peer assessment system requires two computer servers, one for storage of student data and the other for streaming video applications. While this is technologically demanding, the system offers opportunities for rich, collaborative feedback.

VIDEOTAPING AND SELF EFFICACY

Long before videotaping became a common practice, teacher educators were drawn to the concept of self efficacy as a possible determinant of teaching success. Bandura (1977) defined efficacy expectations as "the conviction that one can successfully execute the behavior required to produce desired outcomes" (p.193). He posited that the amount of effort and the duration of persistence of people dealing with obstacles and adverse experiences are determined by efficacy expectations. The stronger people perceive their self-efficacy to be, the more active effort they will put forward (Bandura).

Bandura (1977) identified four sources of efficacy expectations. These included *performance accomplishment, vicarious experience, verbal persuasion,* and *emotional arousal*. Among these, *performance accomplishment* is especially applicable to teacher education as development of the sense of self efficacy, according to Bandura, is based on mastery experiences. These are precisely the types of experiences pre-service teachers (and their supervisors) seek during their methods and student teaching experiences. Derived from Bandura's description of self-efficacy, teachers' self-efficacy is defined as teachers' beliefs in their capability to "perform" in a manner that will bring about student learning. Understandably, teachers' self-efficacy is thus considered a key factor in the process of initiating and sustaining positive change in teaching practices (Gabriele & Joram, 2007).

Brand and Wilkins (2007), in their empirical study of pre-service teachers' self-efficacy development during their methods course experiences, confirmed that, although all four sources of efficacy expectation influenced pre-service teachers' self-efficacy beliefs, mastery experiences are the most influential source. They concluded that the pre-service teachers "[repeatedly] alluded to these [mastery] experiences as being instrumental in enhancing their understanding of ideas that they perceived as very difficult or providing them with strategies that would improve their beliefs about their teaching competencies" (p. 313.).

However, Gabriele and Joram (2007) argued that Bandura considered the interpretation of performance, rather than performance itself, primary in developing self-efficacy and they emphasized that teachers' reflections on their teaching performance and the criteria used in evaluating success are the critical sources of teacher self-efficacy.

The question then becomes, how do pre-service teachers get the best portrait of their own teaching performances, the performances that will enhance their self efficacy? A likely answer lies in the effective use of videotaping during pre-service teaching performances. As developing teachers are given the opportunity to view themselves taking on the complex role of the classroom teacher, they must carefully consider what is occurring beneath the surface of the videotaped story. They must be guided by their supervisors in the use of reflective practice that will help illuminate what they are viewing in terms of human interactions and human growth and their part in the student learning process.

VIDEOTAPING AND REFLECTIVE PRACTICE

When reviewing the history and current use of case-based learning and its potential for developing self efficacy in pre-service teachers, the concept of reflective practice surfaces repeatedly. Reflection was defined by Dewey (1933) as "active, persistent, and careful consideration of any belief or supposed form of knowledge in light of the grounds that support it and the future conclusions to which it tends" (p.7). Since Dewey's early definition, many others have offered their own definitions for reflective practice. Oftentimes, these definitions involve a continuum, or tiered levels of reflection.

Larrivee's (2008) 3-tiered work in this area is particularly pertinent to the teacher education discussion. Larrivee's first level of reflection is described as *surface reflection*, focusing on strategies and methods to reach predetermined goals. At the second level, *pedagogical reflection,* teachers shift their reflection focus to educational goals, the theories underlying approaches, and the connections between theories and practice of teaching. At the third level, *critical reflection,* teachers reflect on the moral and ethical implications as well as the consequences of their teaching on students. Keeping Larrivee's reflective levels in mind, much of the literature on the use of videotape indicates that using video helps master teachers become more reflective in their teaching; facilitate the change of reflection from personal idiosyncrasies to thinking about growth in teaching and student learning; and, focus more on whether or not teachers' behaviors met students' learning needs (Welsch & Devlin, 2007).

Similar in some respects to Larrivee's work, Stockero (2008) used a quasi-experimental design to study the effect of video case curriculum on pre-service teachers' reflective abilities. She found that, through a pre-service teachers' mathematics methods course, pre-service teachers who were exposed to a videotaped, case-based curriculum differed from others in terms of their reflective abilities. They focused more on individual student thinking and tended to ground their reflection in evidence from classroom transcripts and student work. The videotapes facilitated their ability to revisit what had actually transpired in the classroom, versus relying on a memory of what had occurred. Cognitive emphasis was then turned toward what caused certain events to occur, rather than the typical "how did I do?" (rather than a "how did *they* do?") attitude that is not uncommon in early teaching situations.

Rosaen and her colleagues (2008) also documented the effectiveness of using video records in promoting pre-service teachers' reflective practice. In this case, interns were required to teach, videotape and reflect on two lessons per semester in a year-long internship in a post-baccalaureate program. Using a cross-case analysis technique, this research team found that, when using video-based reflection, interns tended to make more specific observations, discuss more instructional elements than behavior management, and pay more attention to the students with respect to instruction and achievement.

In a somewhat different vein, but with reflective practice still at the forefront, Yung and her colleagues (Yung, Wong & Cheng, 2007) adopted a different approach to using videos in their post-graduate education program. The same videos of two science lessons taught by exemplary teachers were used to elicit *progressive* reflections from pre-service teachers. They found that, at the beginning of the exercise, videos served as a stimulus to provoke pre-service teachers' thinking and help them to find a reflection focus. As the same videos were played at several different times during the course, the videos facilitated pre-service teachers' reflection on their changing conceptions of good science teaching from different perspectives and with a primary focus on different elements of solid teaching practice.

ISSUES, CONTROVERSIES, PROBLEMS

With constant improvement in video technologies and clear definition of the theoretical rationale for video-based approaches, teacher education programs are likely to be drawn to this powerful learning tool. The potential for fostering self-efficacy and reflective practice is clear. However, when implementing video-based supervision in student teaching field experiences, several issues persist.

First, there is the problem of confidentiality when videotaping in public school settings. Video-taping will inevitably include students' images and their live movements as well. College instructors and classroom cooperating teachers need to be aware of the confidentiality issue when using students' images. Permission from parents or legal guardians is a necessity and a detailed plan for subsequent video use must be clearly communicated with all parties involved. Many public schools have developed standard parental/guardian agreement forms for the controlled use of photo and video images that can be also used by college and university teacher education faculty. However, it is important to note that even when using pre-service teachers' video cases for group reflection or discussion in the college classroom, proper permission must be obtained. To cover all eventualities, we strongly advise teacher educators to be cognizant of federal regulations regarding the use of student images and to consult with their cooperating school districts before beginning video work in the classroom.

A second effect of videotaping involves pre-service teachers' performance and the fact that videotaping may escalate anxiety levels, thereby lowering performance levels and causing bias in the performance appraisal. Using various strategies to make pre-service teachers comfortable while being video-taped is the instructor's responsibility. By the same token, students in the classroom also need to be reassured about being videotaped to avoid interruptions in their learning potential. While students tend to get used to this practice over time, the first session or two must be carefully planned to lower the impact on student learning.

Although emerging technologies make videotaping and editing much easier than ever before, it still takes considerable time for college instructors and/or pre-service teachers to produce meaningful video segments for various purposes. Ideally, an Information Technology (IT) support group should be in place to relieve instructors of heavy technology-related duties that can interfere with their instructional duties. Such support is not always easy to come by and requires a commitment on the part of Teacher Education programs hoping to use videotaping as a meaningful learning opportunity for pre-service teachers.

As we have stressed previously in this chapter, technology alone does not automatically improve the preparation of pre-service teachers. A thorough understanding and deep investigation of the underlying pedagogical theories is necessary if video-based supervision is to be both effective and productive. Video-based supervision can definitely improve pre-service teachers' reflection at the technical level, as most of the research has shown; however, to help pre-service teachers develop the habit of in-depth reflection curriculum and instruction design must also be taught and carefully implemented.

SOLUTIONS AND RECOMMENDATIONS

The authors of this chapter teach at a public, liberal arts college that began as a Normal School in 1909 and now offers 12 certification options. After successful completion of their foundation courses, students in our Teacher Education programs begin their field experience in one of two Methods courses. A growing number of our Methods instructors use video in the field supervision process – primarily to develop pre-service teachers' teaching skills, but also to hone their ability to engage in self-directed reflection.

For our Methods faculty using video in their field practice, the approach is similar to the Objective Knowledge Growth Framework, a reflective-deduction model of professional development (Chitpin, Simon, & Galipeau, 2008). While carefully reviewing videotape of their teaching performance, Teacher Education faculty and pre-service teachers use a locally-developed assessment checklist (see Table 1) designed by the authors to identify strengths and weaknesses. Through discussion and self-guided reflection, pre-service teachers then develop tentative solutions to address the issues they have identified. A second video session gives them an opportunity to determine how their tentative solutions are working. After viewing both video clips, they write an in-depth reflection of the entire process, sharing their analysis with their college supervisors and cooperating field professionals as well.

The authors started using videotaping in their supervision of pre-service teaching in the fall of 2006. At the time, this initiative was new to the college's Teacher Education program and was generously supported by a college-level technology grant. The grant covered the cost of the video-recording equipment, video-editing software, and even included a small faculty stipend for the extra work the initiative entailed.

The idea of incorporating videotaping in pre-service teaching is not new, but it was not broadly practiced within our Teacher Education program prior to 2006. Before this time, college and field supervisors used very traditional, paper-based supervision methods. Pre-service teachers submitted their lesson plans for supervisory feedback and approval before they were allowed to teach their lessons. College supervisors observed the teaching of their pre-service teachers and then filled out an observation form. Afterwards, pre-service teachers and their supervisors spent time going over the categories and notes on the observation form. Suggestions and an improvement plan were co-constructed during the post-observation meeting. While this was accepted practice for many years, we found that it was not particularly effective toward developing a reflective-deductive model of pre-service instruction.

First, the post-teaching discussion and follow-up self reflection were totally memory-based. When teaching, pre-service teachers (especially at the beginning of their field experience) tend to follow strictly the steps prescribed in their lesson plan and do their best to "act out" their lesson. Memory of their teaching behavior, their interaction with students, and the response from their students tends to be very limited. This directly affects their ability to reflect realistically on what took place in the classroom. College supervisors are likely to face the same problem. It is extremely difficult to describe the details of their pre-service teacher's performance in a vivid way. Oftentimes, the comments on the observation forms are abstract and theoretical, which is hard for pre-service teachers to use in a productive fashion. Our experience tells us that this memory-based approach may lead to lofty discussions and somewhat far-fetched, ungrounded reflection. It serves little purpose in helping pre-service teachers reinforce their strengths and improve on areas that need further development. On some occasions, pre-service teachers' instruction becomes a random effect. For example, a pre-service teacher may have done very well in questioning during his/her first lesson but did not continue this good (questioning) work in the second lesson because it was not highlighted and/or discussed in the follow-up session.

Another problem with a memory-based, post-teaching discussion is that some students tend to be defensive at this fragile point in their teaching development. Although the college supervisor may try very hard to assure the pre-service teachers that the comments on the observation form will be used for improvement in a formative way, pre-service teachers are more likely to connect such comments with their final grades in the course; thus they will try to justify their behaviors. Without "evidence" to show pre-service teachers their actions and the learning consequences for the students, supervisors may find it difficult to convince their pre-service teachers of what needs to be addressed. This is especially true of those pre-service teachers with negative attitudes stemming from poor performance.

Finally, a memory-based approach limits the potential expansiveness of a follow-up discussion. Teaching is a complex phenomenon, including not only the teacher, but also the students and other contextual factors such as the subject area being addressed, classroom setting, student grouping, and cultural differences within the class, to name a few. Teaching is the interaction between the teacher and all of these elements. It is extraordinarily difficult to retrieve such interaction purely from memory. Discussion and reflection on pre-service teaching without the interaction of all of these elements lacks the depth and meaning that could be garnered if these elements were brought into focus.

When we first implemented videotaping in our supervision, we simply videotaped the whole teaching session. We then re-played the tape with our pre-service teachers, providing feedback during viewing and post-teaching discussion in what we refer to as an "add on" approach. This approach certainly improved communication between college supervisors and pre-service teachers and the video sometimes helped pre-service teachers identify teaching challenges on their own. Videotaping in this way also increased pre-service teachers' ability to identify contextual issues in their teaching—such as student grouping, interaction among students, and classroom setup. The simple use of videotaping as an add-on supervision tool did overcome some weaknesses in the traditional, memory-based supervision approach. We saw it increased our pre-service teachers' ability to make connections between their teaching practice and the underlying theoretical aspects of instruction. It also made it easier for them to internalize supervisors' comments and suggestions. However, we found some inherent weaknesses within the video add-on approach.

For starters, the add-on approach tends to be more reactive than proactive. In many cases, the expectations for effective teaching skills were not explicitly stated to pre-service teachers. Indeed, some good teaching behaviors proved to be more random behaviors rather than intentional, built-in habits. For example, some pre-service teachers demonstrated effective disciplinary strategies by using proximity, but they did not always realize what they were doing at the time and were therefore only likely to repeat the natural strategy if it was brought to their attention during the shared video viewing.

Additionally, the add-on approach proved to be more evaluative than reflective. Pre-service teachers proved able to identify the strengths and weaknesses of their teaching by viewing a videotape with their college supervisors; however, simply reviewing such a videotape did not encourage pre-service teachers to reflect on their actions and further investigate the effect of these actions on student learning. One pre-service teacher, for example, demonstrated good questioning skills by redirecting questions to engage more students in critical thinking and conversation. Even though such a sound teaching behavior was recognized by both the pre-service teacher and the supervisor, the pre-service teacher was not able to conceptualize questioning skills as only one element of good teaching.

Based on our marginally positive experience using videotaping as an add-on, we decided to try a different approach. Inspired by the professional framework developed by Danielson (1996), we created the Student Teaching Performance Checklist (STPC), an assessment tool to accompany and enhance the videotaping of pre-service field experience. The checklist went through several revisions and included critical feedback from our cooperating field professionals as well as our pre-service teachers. The checklist focuses on the performance aspect of classroom teaching, but it is only a performance that can be successful if the pre-service teacher understands sound curriculum and instruction design and is working from a supervisor-approved lesson that is grounded in knowledge of developmental/cognitive and social theory.

The checklist has two broad categories, each with numerous, related subcategories. The first is *Instruction and Classroom Management,* which focuses primarily on the academic/content portion of the experience with particular attention to student engagement. The second is *Presence and Delivery Style* which focuses more on the physical nature of the teaching experience, including voice, movement around the classroom and amongst the students, and general body language. In designing the checklist, we were mindful of length and the "overload" factor facing pre-service teachers new to the classroom teaching experience. The Comments column to the right of the checklist items gives the Teacher Educator and/or field supervisor space to explain the assessments offered in each category.

STUDENT TEACHING PERFORMANCE CHECKLIST

After one semester's practice with the newly-developed performance assessment tool, we determined and formalized how it should be used. (While there are clear cut steps in the process we, of course, allow for individual differences depending on pre-service teachers' level of maturity and ability to use critical feedback productively.)

1. **Explain in detail the STPC.** This is important to ensure pre-service teachers are cognizant of the expectations of them and at the same time understand the theoretical tenets underlying those expectations.
2. **Videotape the teaching.** The videotaping should be done selectively. Videotaping an entire teaching session will not help pre-service teachers and supervisors to identify the most important areas for improvement. Instead, it tends to make the video viewing tedious and lacking in real focus.
3. **Fill out the checklist with check marks and comments.** The checklist should be filled out by both the supervisor and pre-service teacher separately, but while they review the videotape together. This approach can empower pre-service teachers to actively

Table 1. Student teaching performance checklist

Performance Categories		**Comments**
I. Instruction and Cognitive Classroom Management A. Questioning		**I. Instruction and Classroom Management**
Determines students' prior or related knowledge		
Asks open-ended questions		
Clarifies and/or rephrases questions when students do not understand		
Allows appropriate wait time		
Re-directs questions to increase student involvement		
Uses prompting and probing to facilitate student thinking		
Uses questions to summarize/provide closure		
B. Presentation of Materials		
Uses visual aids that meet all learners' needs		
Writes on board (chart paper, etc.) clearly/correctly		
Positions self so students can see and be seen		
Provides adequate/necessary modeling for learning		
Stays on topic but allows for spontaneous learning		
C. "With-it-ness" and Timing		
Is aware of and responds to all students		
Shows no gender/ethnicity bias and/or favoritism		
Offers a learning agenda with clear transitions		
Timing/tempo/pace is appropriate to age group		
II. Presence and Delivery Style E. Responsiveness		**II. Presence and Delivery Style**
Handles unexpected questions appropriately		
Handles unexpected interruptions appropriately		
Handles behavior issues appropriately		
Models behavior that is expected of students		
F. Movement and Body Language		
Maintains good posture (head up, hands out of pockets, proper eye contact with students)		
Moves about room/uses proximity to students appropriately		
Stays on task and attentive to the needs of students		
Uses affirming and specific responses		
G. Prosody/Voice		
Speaks with a tone, pitch and speed that is context appropriate		
Articulates words/sentences clearly		
Uses inflection when reading aloud and speaking		
H. Professionalism		
Dresses appropriately for the activity and school setting		
Uses mature and appropriate language		
Displays a positive attitude that invites engagement		

Key: (√) Observed at appropriate level; (No √) Not observed/minimally observe Copyright 2007, Pru Cuper & Yi Gong©

reflect on their own teaching. It also allows space for registering different perspectives on the videotaped lesson.

4. **Edit and make a copy of videotape.** Pre-service teachers are given a copy of the edited video. They can thus review it for reinforcement and reflective purposes over time. Of course, the videotapes can also become part of the pre-service teacher's professional e-portfolio (where available).
5. **Encourage reflection.** The edited video and the finished STPC provide pre-service teachers with rich content to reflect upon. Compared with the traditional approach, the STPC-enhanced approach allows pre-service teachers to reflect on their teaching more specifically and in a more target-oriented fashion. Our students spoke of using the "gradual-replay lens" described at the beginning of our chapter as a real benefit to reflective self analysis and growth. They explained how they would repeatedly replay those aspects of their teaching tapes that demonstrated areas that needed attention and improvement, taking notes and planning ways to amplify their current practice.
6. **Revisit the videotapes and STPC comments.** The ultimate goal of using video-based reflection is to help pre-service teachers improve their teaching. Immediately before teaching their next lesson, we require our pre-service teachers to review their edited video and their written reflections. This can help refresh their memory and help them to visualize both the positive and developing aspects of their teaching. Used in this way, the videotapes serve as the beginning of a new and improved cycle of practice.

We found using video-based supervision and reflection to be very effective in improving our pre-service teachers' skills in various areas, particularly in questioning skills, providing directions, modeling new activities, and classroom management. The most valuable advantage of the new approach is that pre-service teachers became able to do in-depth reflection of their teaching as a habitual practice.

Revisiting research on videotaping and reflective practice, scaffolding has proven to be of great importance in helping pre-service teachers develop the disposition and habit of reflection (Yung et al., 2007). Scaffolding also enables pre-service teachers to reach the level of reflection that is beyond their current ability level (Harford & MacRuairc, 2008). Our work with pre-service teachers attests to the fact that using a combination of focused videotapes, self-assessment, and supervisory feedback to scaffold learning is sound and successful practice. In most instances, our pre-service teachers' reflections extended beyond the surface level. They were able to enjoy pedagogical reflection (Larrivee, 2008) and to reflect on the causes of classroom events and to appreciate the levels of their students' cognitive processing. They also become capable to make connections between learning theories and their teaching behaviors. While we did not witness instances of critical reflection, we look toward this as a possible target for the future as we refine our work in this area.

The above mentioned Steps 2 through 6 compose the gradual replay lens through which pre-service teachers develop their teaching via visualizing, scaffolding, reflecting, internalizing, reinforcing, and improving. This up-going spiral cycle of practice is not only applicable in student teaching, but can also prove instrumental in improving the practice of in-service teachers. We believe the gradual replay lens model has two-fold benefits. Teaching, like dancing and acting, is a performance. Teachers can become cognizant of how well they "performed" through viewing their teaching practice in light of the guidelines offered in the STPC. By viewing their performances gradually and in multiple sittings, with focus on differing actions and subsequent student responses, pre-service teachers can improve their teaching in a more intentional and conscious way. Another key benefit of this model of teacher preparation is that teacher educators (with permission) can use the videos and relevant data of the performance of their pre-service teachers to re-design curriculum and adjust instruction.

FUTURE RESEARCH DIRECTIONS

While there has been considerable success to date, there is still much research and practical work to do if we are to use videotaping technologies to their maximum potential in teacher education. Taking into account what has been accomplished over the years and in light of our own experience, we joined with our cooperating field professionals in creating the following list of critical considerations.

1. **Videotaping Equipment Selection.** There is a wide variety of videotaping equipment currently available. Camcorders that use DVDs or miniDVs are very convenient in exporting video signals to computers for editing. Camcorders, which are portable and handy and can run for relatively long periods of time, are popularly used in field supervision. In addition, most of the newer digital cameras have videotaping functions that can record short video segments. This functionality allows supervisors to focus on brief teaching moments that target areas of concern without needing to spend considerable time "editing down" to what is essential. Finally, Webcams offer a strong alternative option, especially in circumstances that require long distance supervision.
2. **Video Editing Software.** There are a number of programs available that can help convert video between a variety of formats, such as AVI, MP4, WMV, MPEG. These programs can also be used to select video segments from an entire video clip. Once video is transferred to a computer in any acceptable format, iMovie™ or Movie Maker™ can be used to edit the video for diagnostic purposes. After that, notes, questions, and short reflections can be added to the video through products such as iMovie™ or Movie Maker™.
3. **Assessment Tool Development.** Assessment tools for student teaching performance in the classroom are of critical importance if videotaping is to be helpful. Assessment tools, whether in a checklist format or any other format, help to explicitly convey expectations to pre-service teachers. If carefully and thoughtfully designed (with curriculum and developmental considerations in place), they can provide an opportunity for pre-service teachers to conduct self-assessment and to identify their strengths and areas-in-need-of-development based on clearly-defined criteria. The most effective assessment tools are constructed locally by individual teacher education program faculty to reflect the learning outcomes in that specific program.
4. **Videotaping – the Action.** Selective videotaping of pre-service teachers' classroom performance is strongly recommended. Selective videotaping of targeted areas reduces the time needed for editing afterwards and the raw footage can immediately be used for post-teaching discussion. In addition, videotaping should not just zoom in on the pre-service teacher but also span the interaction between teacher and students; students' reaction to directions; students' movement; and other elements of the overall teaching experience.
5. **Video-Based Discussion**. Post-teaching discussion between the college supervisor and the pre-service teacher should take place as soon as possible after teaching. Any lag will diminish the effect of this method. An assessment tool (such as the SPTC) should be filled out by both the supervisor and the pre-service teacher to engage him/her in

active reflection after reviewing the teaching video.

6. **Video-Based Reflection**. Video can be edited by the supervisor or the pre-service teacher. Edited video should be gradually replayed (as per our description) when the pre-service teacher is working on his/her reflection. To ensure pre-service teachers conduct in-depth reflection, guidelines for reflection should be provided beforehand by the supervisor.
7. **Longitudinal Use of Edited Video.** Pre-service teachers are able to continue to improve their teaching when they are provided with edited video series of their teaching across semesters or academic years. Such video also provides supervisors a tool to assess pre-service teachers' progress over time.
8. **Peer Assessment.** Edited video of pre-service teachers' performance can also be used in the college classroom for peer assessment. Best practices can be showcased and common mistakes (with permission, of course) can be analyzed collectively.
9. **E-Portfolio.** The power of electronic portfolio storage is that it allows pre-service teachers to archive their teaching videos in an assessment management system. There are numerous versions currently on the market–each offering some unique features that may be particularly useful, depending on programmatic needs. A collection of pre-service teachers' video "stories" can be used as a direct and visible measure of the performance and learning outcomes of a teacher education program, particularly when they are considered with regards to pre-defined criteria such as those we included in the STPC.

Working with our cooperating professionals from the field, we offer these ideas and suggestions as a helpful guide for using video as a supervision tool. Certainly, as technology advances, there will be easier ways to use technology to fulfill our collective mission. Working together, our target is to help pre-service teachers reach the highest level of performance and critical reflection possible. Their target, in turn, must be to enhance student learning. With scaffolding and careful use of technology over time, we believe this can happen. We also realize that it may require turning the gradual-replay lens on ourselves, to develop an assessment tool that explores what is needed of teacher educators and field supervisors as we provide feedback to our pre-service teachers. We too must take a look at our own practice to determine if we are being adequately self-analytic and reflective in what we do.

Aside from the above-listed considerations, two lines of further research can enhance our gradual replay lens practice. One line of research would involve investigating how this model actually impacts pre-service teachers' self-efficacy and their perception of teaching over time. Such research could help ensure the use of the model in its most productive direction, to offer a means of gradually implementing improved teaching practices. The other line of research would focus on investigating the effect of various teaching behaviors on student learning. This could help us identify effective teaching behaviors necessary to pre-service teachers' inventory of teaching practices. While there is already a wealth of research in this area, the focus has not been on reviewing and discussing videotapes of pre-service teachers over time, and (with their permission) sharing their work and their critical/targeted responses with subsequent cohorts of teacher candidates.

CONCLUSION

Video-based supervision can improve pre-service teachers' reflection at the technical level, as most of the research has demonstrated. But, as we have stressed throughout this chapter, the use of any technology alone will not automatically improve the preparation of pre-service teachers. When we consider what teacher educators need *to think about* and *do* as they implement new technologies, we believe it is essential to ensure, first and foremost, a thorough understanding and deep investigation of the underlying developmental and pedagogical theories that lead to effective teaching practice. The next area for teacher educators to explore with their students involves the many facets of effective curriculum design—from determining meaningful learning objectives to creating the most appropriate ways to assess how well students have met those objectives. With this knowledge in place, video-based supervision that features a commitment to the gradual-replay/reflective approach we offer in this chapter can be both motivational and highly effective. Under the guidance of their field supervisors, watching themselves "perform" successfully, in the sense of engaging their students in rich and valuable learning experiences, is one vital step in the complex process of becoming effective teachers.

The gradual replay lens model of video-based supervision, in a broader sense, can be implemented not only in teacher preparation, but also at any level of teacher development. Once the professional development school relationship is constructed, this model can be used for in-service teachers' instructional improvement as well. The technology leadership role, in this sense, is not limited to building the technology infrastructure; rather, it is expected to cultivate a rich culture for teachers, pre-service teachers, and college professors to model best teaching practices, exchange reflective responses, and maintain continuous improvement as its ultimate goal.

REFERENCES

Bandura, A. (1977). Self-efficacy: Toward a unifying theory of behavioral change. *Psychological Review*, *84*(2), 191–215. doi:10.1037/0033-295X.84.2.191

Beck, R. J., King, A., & Marshall, S. K. (2002). Effects of videocase construction on pre-service teachers' observation of teaching. *Journal of Experimental Education*, *70*(4), 345–361. doi:10.1080/00220970209599512

Brand, B. R., & Wilkins, J. L. M. (2007). Using self-efficacy as a construct for evaluating science and mathematics methods courses. *Journal of Science Teacher Education*, *18*(2), 297–317. doi:10.1007/s10972-007-9038-7

Cennamo, K. S., Abell, S. K., George, E. J., & Chung, M. L. (1996). The development of integrated media cases for use in elementary science teacher education. *Journal of Technology and Teacher Education*, *4*(1), 19–36.

Chitpin, S., Simon, M., & Galipeau, J. (2008). Pre-service teachers' use of the Objective Knowledge Framework for Reflection during practicum. *Teaching and Teacher Education: An International Journal of Research and Studies*, *24*(8), 2049–2058. doi:10.1016/j.tate.2008.04.001

Danielson, C. (1996). *Enhancing professional practice: A framework for teaching*. Alexandria, VA: ASCD.

Dewey, J. (1933). *How we think: A restatement of the relation of reflective thinking to the educative process*. Boston: Heath and Company.

Dymond, S. K., & Bentz, J. L. (2006). Using digital videos to enhance teacher preparation. *Teacher Education and Special Education*, *29*(2), 98–112. doi:10.1177/088840640602900202

Gabriele, A. J., & Joram, E. (2007). Teachers' reflections on their reform-based teaching in mathematics: Implications for the development of teacher self-efficacy. *Action in Teacher Education*, *29*(3), 60–74.

Harford, J., & MacRuairc, G. (2008). Engaging student teaches in meaningful reflective practice. *Teaching and Teacher Education: An International Journal of Research and Studies*, *24*(7), 1884–1892. doi:10.1016/j.tate.2008.02.010

Larrivee, B. (2008). Meeting the challenge of preparing reflective practitioners. *New Educator*, *4*(2), 87–106. doi:10.1080/15476880802014132

McIntyre, J. D., & Paper, S. (1993). Using video protocols to enhance teacher reflective thinking. *Teacher Educator*, *28*(3), 2–10. doi:10.1080/08878739309555031

Rosaen, C. L., Lundeberg, M., Cooper, M., Fritzen, A., & Terpstra, M. (2008). Noticing noticing: How does investigation of video records change how teachers reflect on their experiences? *Journal of Teacher Education*, *59*(4), 347–360. doi:10.1177/0022487108322128

Stockero, S. (2008). Differences in pre-service mathematics teachers' reflective abilities attributable to use of a video case curriculum. *Journal of Technology and Teacher Education*, *16*(4), 433–458.

Welsch, R. G., & Devlin, P. A. (2007). Developing pre-service teachers' reflection: Examining the use of video. *Action in Teacher Education*, *28*(4), 53–61.

Wu, C. C., & Kao, H. C. (2008). Streaming video in peer assessment to support training pre-service teachers. *Educational Technology & Society*, *11*(1), 45–55.

Yung, B. H. W., Wong, S. L., & Cheng, M. W. (2007). Tracking pre-service teachers' changing conceptions of good science teaching: The role of progressive reflection with the same video. *Research in Science Education*, *37*(3), 239–259. doi:10.1007/s11165-006-9024-7

ADDITIONAL RESOURCES

Jones, L., & McNamara, O. (2004). The possibilities and constraints of multimedia as a basis for critical reflection. *Cambridge Journal of Education*, *34*(3), 279–296. doi:10.1080/0305764042000289929

Romano, M. E. (2006). "Bumpy moments" in teaching: Reflections from practicing teachers. *Teaching and Teacher Education*, *22*, 973–985. doi:10.1016/j.tate.2006.04.019

SchÖn. D.A. (1987). Educating the Reflective Practitioner: Toward a New Design for Teaching and Learning in the Professions. San Francisco, CA: Jossey-Bass Inc.

Sherin, M. G. (2004). New perspectives on the role of video in teacher education. In *Using Video in Teacher Education: Advances in Research on Teaching* (pp. 1–27). Elsevier Ltd.

Star, J. R., & Strickland, S. K. (2008). Learning to observe: Using video to improve pre-service mathematics teachers' ability to notice. *Journal of Mathematics Teacher Education*, *11*(2), 107–125. doi:10.1007/s10857-007-9063-7

KEY TERMS AND DEFINITIONS

Case-Based Teaching: The use of real-world cases to illustrate both theoretical and pedagogical points in teacher education. Videotapes from classroom settings are a common form of case-based teaching.

Cooperating Field Professionals: Employees of public schools who are partnering with Teacher Education college faculty in the educational development of pre-service teachers. This includes principals as well as field supervisors and other staff members who interact directly with pre-service teachers.

Field Supervisors: Professional educators teaching in public and/or private school settings who have been hired to evaluate pre-service teachers' progress in conjunction with college faculty serving in this role.

Methods Courses: Courses in the teacher education sequence that involve extended field practice in the "methods" of instruction in various subject areas.

Normal School: An institute of higher education devoted solely to teacher preparation.

Pre-Service Teachers: Students enrolled in a teacher preparation program.

Chapter 6
A Multimedia Learning Tool that Allows High School Teachers and their Students to Engage in Scientific Research

Jacqueline S. McLaughlin
The Pennsylvania State University - Lehigh Valley, USA

ABSTRACT

This chapter presents a new and different type of multimedia learning tool, the so-called "research module." This unique, learner-centered, multimedia tool aims to create a learning environment wherein high school teachers and their students engage in higher-order, inquiry-based activities that allow them to "do" actual scientific research in the classroom. This chapter also describes the design and implementation of these computer-based resources, as well as assessment data on student learning, and perceptions of both textbooks and computer-based learning tools. It also reveals high school teachers' attitudes toward the use of both computer-based resources and textbooks.

Scientific inquiry refers to the diverse ways in which "scientists" study the natural world and propose explanations based on the evidence derived from their work. Inquiry also refers to the activities of "students" in which they develop knowledge and understanding of scientific ideas, as well as an understanding of how scientists study the natural world. (National Science Education Standards, p. 23.)

DOI: 10.4018/978-1-61520-899-9.ch006

INTRODUCTION

Can technology change the way science is taught? The answer is yes. Strategically designed interactive technology is allowing us to link skilled educators and research scientists from around the world with high school teachers for professional development, and with their students for high impact, or higher-end inquiry learning. In short, technology is allowing us to build new and effective multimedia learning tools and strategies for the 21st Century classroom, which bring real-world research experiences to life for teachers and students.

Technology is helping biology instructors redefine their "pedagogical toolboxes" for the 21st Century classroom. Indeed, new, technology-centered, *multimedia learning* tools are evolving, and through their evolution, are allowing instructors to re-imagine the endless possibilities for teaching in innovative and exciting ways. Moreover, they are creating interactive classrooms, empowering instructors to be facilitators of learning, and helping to excite the next generation of researchers and scientifically aware citizens.

Definitions

According to Mayer (2001), the term *multimedia* means the presentation of material using both words and pictures. The words can be printed (e.g., on-screen text) or spoken (e.g., narration). The pictures can be static (e.g., illustrations, graphs, charts, photos, or maps) or dynamic (e.g., animation, video, or interactive illustrations). This definition is broad enough to cover a textbook, a computer-based narrated animation, and a "research module" – which you will read about herein.

Mayer and his associates have been carrying out research for years to figure out how to best use words and pictures to foster meaningful learning. In fact, they have proposed a "Cognitive Theory of Multimedia Learning" to explain how the mind works in multimedia learning (Mayer and Moreno, 1999). According to Mayer, *multimedia learning* refers to learning elicited by words and pictures, and *multimedia instruction* is the presentation of words and pictures that are intended to foster learning. Importantly, there are two contrasting views of multimedia learning – *multimedia learning as information acquisition* and *multimedia learning as knowledge construction.*

Basically, if you view multimedia learning as information acquisition, then multimedia is merely an information delivery system. According to this viewpoint, learning simply involves adding information to a student's memory bank. Not surprisingly, the information acquisition view is sometimes called the "empty vessel" view because the learner's mind is seen as an empty container that needs to be filled by the teacher pouring in the information.

In contrast, if you view multimedia learning as knowledge construction, then multimedia is a cognitive aid (think of yourself as an architect). According to this view, multimedia learning is a sense-making activity in which the learner seeks to build a coherent mental representation from the presented material. Unlike information, which is an objective commodity that can be moved from one mind to another, knowledge is personally constructed by the learner and cannot be delivered in exact form from one mind to another. In this view, the teacher functions as a facilitator who provides guidance to frame and support the learner's cognitive processing. The responsibility for learning shifts to the student, and the teacher becomes the guide who highlights what to pay attention to, how to mentally organize the information, and how to make it relate to prior knowledge. As Mayer's states, the teacher here is "an aid to knowledge construction."

Mayer, like myself, favors the knowledge-construction viewpoint because it is more aligned with the research base of how people learn (Bradsford et al., 1999). The knowledge-construction view of multimedia learning is consistent with our mutual goal of using multimedia in the classroom – to help students develop an "understanding" of the presented material rather than exposing students to, and overloading them to, vast quantities of information. Importantly, Mayer, also supports, as I do, "*learner-centered*" rather than "*technology-centered*" *multimedia approaches* when it comes to multimedia design for student learning (Mayer, 2009). Learner-centered approaches begin with an understanding of how the human mind works and ask, "How can we adapt multimedia technology as an aid to human cognition?" In contrast, technology-centered multimedia approaches begin with the functional capabilities of multimedia and ask, "How can we use these capabilities in designing multimedia tools?" The bottom line is this: The former focuses on using multimedia technology as an aid to human cognition, while the latter aims only to incorporate man-kind's cutting-edge multimedia technology into pre-existing lesson plans. As Mayer states, simply providing "access to technology" is an approach with a 100-year history of failure. Norman (1993, p. xi) eloquently makes a similar point about technology-centered approaches: "We need to reverse the machine-centered point of view and turn it into a person-centered point of view. Technology should serve us."

Inquiry exists on a continuum from a pure verification experience in a classroom or laboratory (textbook/lab manual) to a full-fledged research immersion in a real-world laboratory (Weaver et al, 2008). The levels of." intellectual ownership and responsibility increase along this gradient, in that students transition from simple confirmation of details to engaging in full-fledged professional science practice itself. So propelled to move inquiry into K-12 classrooms was the US National Research Council (NRC) that in 2000, after providing a set of standards that "outline what students need to know, understand, and be able to do to be scientifically literate at different grade levels" (NRC, 1996), it published a book devoted entirely to defining the term inquiry and showcasing how teachers *and* students can use this modality to learn how to do science, about the nature of science, and science content.

The reality of large-class sizes, scarce resources and/or overscheduled teachers is such, however, that until this day, education at the secondary level predominantly focuses on lower levels of inquiry–memorization of textbook content and packaged laboratory activities, with only an occasional outdoor activity. Moreover, the science that underlies this curriculum in general remains watered-down, in the form of vocabulary words and definitions, for example, and color-coded diagrams, graphs, and tables. By the time pre-service science teachers come to their supervised field experiences, they face the daunting tasks of preparing lessons for students with sub-optimal materials and methods in an age where understanding of science is crucial.

A well-known approach to undergraduate education involves direct mentoring by a scientist, such that an undergraduate works in the lab of a scientist to perform hands-on research. Using this approach, students engage in many of the activities and critical-thinking processes as scientists—such as making observations, formulating questions, gathering evidence, interpreting reproducible data, and communicating results. Moreover, they come to appreciate that science is not a linear process; it's the "application" of conceptual knowledge in a particular field(s) to the intellectual task of asking "questions" in an attempt to answer the why's, how's, and if's of our natural world. These apprenticeship-based and authentic research experiences, however, generally only take place outside the normal course time and rarely, if ever, exists with regard to high school curricula. The latter are lucky if they get to partake in a science fair project with adequate research guidance. Indeed, as pointed out in the National Science Education Standards (National Research Council, 1996), the activities and thinking processes used by scientists are not always familiar to the K-12 educator seeking to introduce inquiry into the classroom or laboratory. A survey completed in 2007 found that K-12 math and science teachers reported spending an average of 39% of their time on inquiry-based instruction (Marshall et al., in press). Further observations suggested that the inquiry being implemented was often of poor quality.

Science teaching at the secondary level can involve research-level inquiry, if teachers are trained to do scientific research and have the proper tools. By taking part in "scientific research experiences themselves, teachers can better understand basic research techniques (Pasley, 1998), procure an increased understanding of science as a research endeavor (Dotterer & Pasley, 2000), and establish a greater sense of authority when describing the research process with students. As a result, such teachers become more proficient in doing actual scientific research alongside their students; in fact, it becomes a priority. The *Highlights Report: Inside the Classroom (2003)* indicates that if teachers experience basic research and believe that it is important for their students to engage in research, the content of their courses will shift towards students uncovering concepts through inquiry.

Yet, in an age where the costs of complying with unfunded mandates such as the No Child Left Behind Act of 2001 (or NCLB, US Public Law 107-110, which requires states to develop assessments in basic skills to be given to all students in certain grades in return for receiving federal funding for schools) fall to already over-burdened school budgets, in-service teachers find themselves without resources and/or the time for professional development—greatly limiting available time and resources for developing teaching approaches that harness the critical thinking skills, rigor, creativity, and spirit of basic research that will simultaneously help their students master science content standards. It is no wonder then that, even though the NRC called for inquiry to be a greater force in our science classrooms, in the past 13 years inquiry has still not become prevalent in our science classrooms at any grade/ability level.

Without training and the right pedagogical tools, teachers fall back on, lean on, and are further removed from being weaned-off the old textbook and cookbook laboratory activities. The reality: While science is a practice that must be engaged in, most textbooks teach instead the history of science. Science is currently taught as a series of facts (National Science Council, 2003). Complicating matters more are the facts that most students in high school are not reading their science textbooks, nor understanding the content (American Association for the Advancement of Science, 2000).

Today's high school science classrooms must, therefore, take bold steps to engage students in the high end of Bloom's taxonomy (analyze, evaluate and create). To do this, they need to re-define the pedagogical tools for the 21st Century classroom. Indeed, technology can be used to create new, "learner-centered" (again, focus here is on the nature of the human cognitive system, not on the capabilities of technology itself, Mayer, 2009) multimedia learning tools and multimedia-learning strategies that shift students away from mere textbook-learning modalities so as science becomes real. Such multimedia learning tools can bridge the gap between teaching and research by bringing real-world research scientists, and their experiences and actual scientific data directly into high school (and undergraduate) classrooms to educate teachers and students about the science behind numerous, pressing global biological issues.

BACKGROUND

According to the authors of the National Science Education Standards (National Research Council, 1996), students need "access to skilled professional teachers, adequate classroom time, a rich array of learning materials, accommodating work spaces, and the resources of the communities surrounding their schools." Although national, state, and local budget cuts continue to constrain students' access to all of these resources, curriculum developers nationwide have been collaborating with skilled teachers and scientists to create effective, integrated learning strategies that strengthen teachers' professional skills, make optimal use of classroom time, and broaden student access to learning materials via the Internet. Guidelines have been proposed by leading national science education organizations for the integration of technology into science classrooms and for the preparation of science teachers (Flick & Bell, 2000). These guidelines include the following:

1. Technology should be introduced in the context of science content.
2. Technology should address worthwhile science with appropriate pedagogy.
3. Technology instruction in science should take advantage of the unique features of technology.
4. Technology should make scientific views more accessible.
5. Technology instruction should develop understanding of the relationship between technology and science.

Although textbook publishers have produced rich arrays of highly interactive CD-ROM materials for several decades, they often are priced outside the reach of many public school district budgets. Science teachers need more affordable options for accessing highly interactive science materials. Federal attempts over the last decade to close the digital divide through an estimated $3 billion annual e-rate Internet funding (Universal Services Administrative Company, 2007) and the concurrent "Moore's Law" (Moore, 2003) of halving prices while doubling computing power have rendered the Internet a far more accessible medium for many public school science teachers and students. The project that is discussed in this chapter takes advantage of the increasingly more affordable Internet to deliver high quality, multimedia-learning materials for enhanced scientific inquiry instruction in high school.

ISSUES, CONTROVERSIES, PROBLEMS

In response to increased public school access to the Internet, the Office of Science Education (OSE) at the National Institutes of Health (NIH) recently launched a Curriculum Supplement Series of web-based materials that continues to grow as funding and expertise are allocated to this project (OSE, 2006). The major advantages of these materials for teachers are:

1. Access to the materials in print or multimedia formats is free via the Internet.
2. Practicing science teachers and NIH scientists co-author the materials.
3. Each learning module is aligned to national and state science standards.
4. Teacher guides and complete lesson plans are also included at no charge.

The modules already available from the growing collection at the NIH Web site follow an adaptation of the classic Atkin-Karplus (and later Lawson) model of sequenced instruction, applying a Piagetian learning cycle. Recent cognitive research on how people learn and, particularly, on how children learn science has refined the earlier Piagetian cycles to occur much earlier and more iteratively in young learners' brains (Bransford, Brown, & Cocking, 1999; Donovan & Bransford, 2005; Duschl, Schweingruber, & Shouse, 2007).

Observing the integration of conceptual frameworks to existing semantic maps and conceptual frameworks recommended in this updated work on learning science, the authors of the NIH-sponsored curriculum have utilized the "5E" instructional model (Bybee, 1993) that encourages learners to Engage, Explore, Explain, Extend, and Evaluate (BSCS, 2006). Teacher education programs should have access to these materials via the Internet, which is increasingly available in schools at lower costs than many packaged textbook ancillaries. Furthermore, faculty members who design curriculum for the NIH curriculum should consider incorporating these resources into their required curricula.

Even as the NIH materials have begun to meet the national needs for multimedia science education tools that integrate authentic research, a similarly engaging internet-based project that is the subject of regional interest to the mid-

Atlantic has simultaneously been reaching these same consistently high standards by integrating authentic scientific research from local, national, and international field sites into sequenced multimedia learning materials. And, just as the NIH modules have been co-authored and field tested by science teachers, so too, have the CHANCE research modules been co-authored and field-tested (McLaughlin, 2006; McLaughlin and Arbeider, 2008; McLaughlin, 2010). Moreover, these research modules expand on the 5E model in use on the NIH web site to incorporate the most current knowledge of how students learn science. Notably, McLaughlin and Arbeider (2008) have shown how these new environmental science and ecology multimedia learning tools are carefully aligned with the four perspectives of learning environments: learner-centered, knowledge-centered, assessment centered and community centered (Donovan & Bransford, 2005).

SOLUTIONS AND RECOMMENDATIONS

Even as the NIH materials have begun to meet the national needs for multimedia science education tools integrating authentic research, a similarly engaging Internet-based project has been created to address these same standards for the students of Pennsylvania—by integrating authentic scientific research from Pennsylvania communities into sequenced learning materials. Just as the NIH modules are free, have been co-authored by science teachers and scientists, aligned with national and state standards, and supply teacher guides and lesson plans, so too, do these CHANCE research modules, as this article will demonstrate.

Launched in 2004, the CHANCE professional development program is partnership between The Pennsylvania State University (PSU) and the Pennsylvania Department of Education (PDE), along with several funders. It was developed to (a) engage Pennsylvania in-service and pre-service high school teachers in environmental and conservation science through the excitement of hands-on field research in selected ecosystems in Costa Rica, and to (b) enhance the way Pennsylvania teachers teach and the way Pennsylvania students learn by using real-world scientific data in the classroom.

These goals are achieved by participation in a field course and through the development, training, and implementation of the CHANCE research modules. The CHANCE modules, which are the focus of this chapter, are a set of seven internet-based, environmentally themed, multimedia-learning tools (htpp://www.CHANCE.psu.edu). Targeted toward high school science students, each module features a student-as-researcher approach through student manipulation of a data set contributed by scientists who are currently investigating the same topic. The CHANCE modules provide opportunities to work with real scientists, and research data helps students transition from learning via a textbook or cookbook lab to professional science practice.

These interactive multimedia learning tools support standards-based teaching (Pennsylvania Environmental Science and Ecology Standards, http://www.pa3e.ws/resources/academic-standards.html), enforce complex thinking and problem solving, embrace research skills, include appropriate assessments to measure student performance, and portray real-world environmental issues. Yet, what makes the CHANCE modules so extremely unique is their ability to provide the balance of "whole science."

Using multimedia technology, the modules transport the students to a virtual research location. The format is similar to the idea of a virtual field trip, but instead of being guided by a teacher, students are guided by a renowned research scientist. After completing several interactive and challenging assignments that cover essential core concepts, the students are taken to a research location where they engage in the same process of scientific inquiry used by the researcher who has co-authored the module. Students then manipulate authentic data in order to draw conclusions about an environmental issue. For example, in the most recently developed module on global warming, students first examine the major layers of the earth, and the unique layer that sustains life, the biosphere. They then learn about the carbon cycle, and how humans are shifting carbon from the lithosphere to the atmosphere. Then, after visiting the Scripps Institute of Oceanography in Hawaii, they plot the late Dr. Charles Keelings' data on atmospheric CO_2 levels and average global temperature taken since 1960 to verify the evidence that atmospheric CO_2 has been rising since the industrial revolution. Finally, students are transported to Costa Rica to work with Dr. Deborah Clark, an ecologist at the Organization of Tropical Studies, Costa Rica, known for her research on carbon stores and fluxes in tropical forests. Students take actual measurements of canopy tree annual growth over a sixteen-year period, gathering data published by Clark in 2003 in the journal, Proceedings of the National Academy of Sciences (PNAS), to demonstrate how increased canopy temperature affects rainforest productivity.

The following is a more in-depth description of how multimedia instructional technology is used to simulate Dr. Clark's actual field research:

After locating Costa Rica and Puerto Viejo on an interactive map, users are welcomed to the LaSelva Research Station—taking in the sights and sounds of the rain forest as they learn more about this private biological reserve, one of the most important research sites in the world for studying the rainforest. Students then get to meet Dr. Clark, learn about her "Trees Project" on the affect of temperature on tree productivity, her research methods, and how she and her staff monitor over 2000 canopy trees in old-growth lowland rainforest. After being shown how to use a virtual diameter tape measure, they begin the research activity by virtually measuring the diameter and growth change of trees over a span of 15 years, and recording measurements in a table. Finally, they plot the table data on a graph, calculate a growth median, and compare it to the actual graph data set that Dr. Clark has published in her research paper. From interpreting this data, students discover that while canopy temperature has been increasing in the La Selva rainforest, tree growth (girth) has been decreasing.

Clark's research is adapted in one of seven CHANCE modules that have been developed and are in use by high schools and educational organizations throughout the world (see list of CHANCE "sponsors" on its web site). These modules focus on the following global topics: invasive plant species; raptor migration; amphibians as indicators of environmental change; sea turtle nesting behaviors and survival; deciduous forest biodiversity; species extinction; and, global climate change (Figure 1). Modules in the planning stages include topics on watershed restoration, waste disposal, water pollution, and the newest technology in electricity production—burning 'culm'—the main waste product of coal incineration.

Each module maximizes classroom or laboratory functionality. In addition to an animated research scenario, the modules' template includes links to teacher guidelines; state and national standards; suggested websites; and ideas for alternative creative, collaborative, and experiential classroom activities. Exclusive to these interactive modules is the CHANCE "Progressive Notebook," which allows students to continually record their experimental research findings as they progress through the module—observing and carrying out a virtual experiment—in the manner of a "real-life" researcher collecting data.

Once a module is completed, the "Progressive Notebook" component can be printed for teacher review. While answer keys are available for each module (teachers can e-mail the appropriate authors --high school teacher, selected scientist, and the director), a teacher using a module should first complete it in its entirety to become familiar with the content and the scientific methodology employed, then set up a rubric of their own to grade students' answers. Also, teachers who have

Figure 1. CHANCE modules table of contents

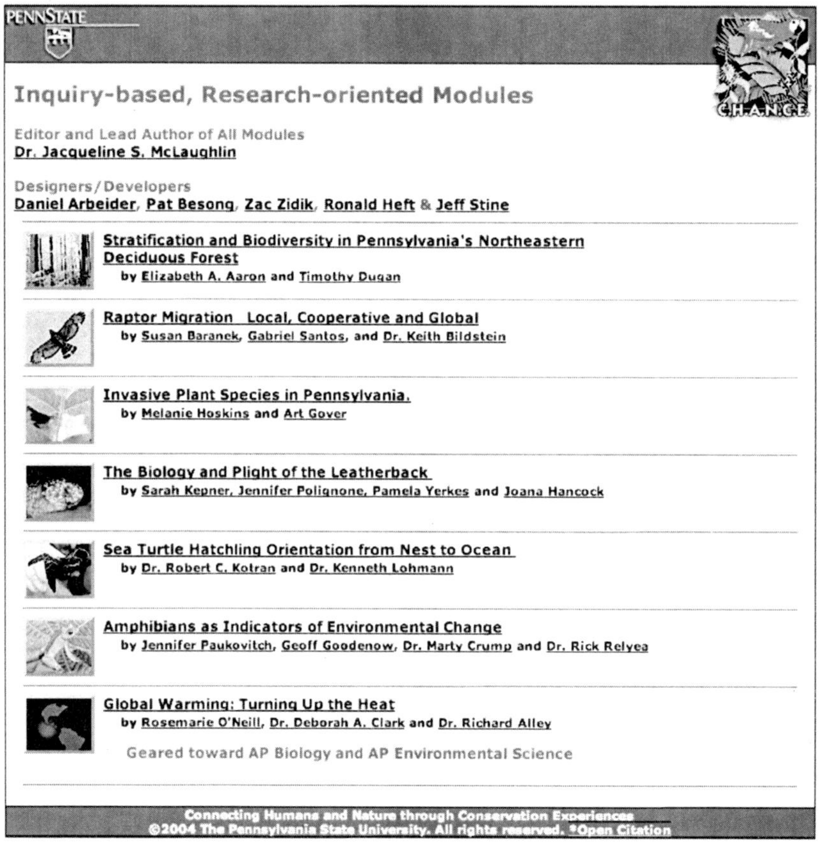
PENNSTATE
C.H.A.N.C.E.
Inquiry-based, Research-oriented Modules
Editor and Lead Author of All Modules
Dr. Jacqueline S. McLaughlin
Designers/Developers
Daniel Arbeider, Pat Besong, Zac Zidik, Ronald Heft & Jeff Stine
Stratification and Biodiversity in Pennsylvania's Northeastern Deciduous Forest
by Elizabeth A. Aaron and Timothy Dugan
Raptor Migration Local, Cooperative and Global
by Susan Baranek, Gabriel Santos, and Dr. Keith Bildstein
Invasive Plant Species in Pennsylvania.
by Melanie Hoskins and Art Gover
The Biology and Plight of the Leatherback
by Sarah Kepner, Jennifer Polignone, Pamela Yerkes and Joana Hancock
Sea Turtle Hatchling Orientation from Nest to Ocean
by Dr. Robert C. Kotran and Dr. Kenneth Lohmann
Amphibians as Indicators of Environmental Change
by Jennifer Paukovitch, Geoff Goodenow, Dr. Marty Crump and Dr. Rick Relyea
Global Warming: Turning Up the Heat
by Rosemarie O'Neill, Dr. Deborah A. Clark and Dr. Richard Alley
Geared toward AP Biology and AP Environmental Science
Connecting Humans and Nature through Conservation Experiences
©2004 The Pennsylvania State University. All rights reserved. *Open Citation

their students complete the suggested additional "Classroom Activities" that are provided for each module on a side link, may choose to grade these as well.

The CHANCE modules are also unique due to the way in which each module is developed through an intricate collaboration between teachers, a prominent scientist(s), program director, a research institution, governmental organization, or non-governmental organization, and instructional technology experts. This partnership has ensured that the final products are a valid representation of cutting edge scientific research, address the most recent pedagogical practices in science education, and utilize effective and engaging multimedia instructional technology from animations, videos, and virtual explorations to allow students to explore, critically think about, and understand key environmental science issues and biological concepts.

Importantly, the CHANCE modules adhere to Pennsylvania state standards, and provide embedded assessments. Similar to many state science assessments, a large portion (50%) of the Pennsylvania System of School Assessment (PSSA) focuses on the nature of science. At all grade levels, students must demonstrate proficiency in not only content-based knowledge, but also in their understanding of scientific processes. The Nature of Science portion of the Pennsylvania state-exam addresses the following specific areas: (a) unifying themes of science; (b) inquiry and design; (c) technology education; (d) technological devices; and (e) science, technology, and human endeavors. The CHANCE modules offer students experience in all of these areas while at the same time, addresses specific content. For example, one of the specific assessment anchors requires that students "apply knowledge of scientific investigation or technological design in different contexts to make inferences to solve problems." Each of the CHANCE modules does just this in its own unique context. Students analyze evidence in order to describe relationships – this is exactly what the state tests are requiring students to be able to accomplish.

Throughout all CHANCE modules, students are required to answer increasingly difficult questions. These lower-to higher-level thinking questions further their understanding and are the key to inquiry-based learning. For example, after working through an animation of a roadside disturbance in the module on invasive species, students learn about the Tree of Heaven (*Ailanthus altissima*), also known as Ailanthus, an invasive tree species originally from Asia, which is having a devastating impact on many of the natural-plant communities in Pennsylvania. Students are asked to make a hypothesis as to what will happen if one Ailanthus tree seed germinates, takes root, and is allowed to grow for a period of 10 years in the pond/meadow plant community they studied in the required activity. Thus, students must consider not only what they now know about the population density and biology (life cycle) of the native species in this ecosystem, but also the biology of Ailanthus (life cycle) and the negative influences of invasive species, in general, to predict and explain how this plant will affect the survival of the native plant species already in existence.

These modules are freely available to anyone in the nation teaching high school biology or environmental science or to anyone who is looking for an engaging alternative to teaching basic biological and ecological principles and environmental issues while advocating environmental stewardship (http://www.CHANCE.psu.edu). Of significance is the fact that dialogue among educators is encouraged, and teachers and their students can contact the module authors, their research mentors, and the director via direct links.

It is essential to note that CHANCE modules are meant to be authentic learning tools for both teacher and student; they are not meant to be "online" textbooks or test banks. They should be considered just one pedagogical tool in a teacher's toolbox and never meant to totally replace textbooks or an entire curriculum. To cover all the academic standards for environmental science and ecology and to cater learning to meet all types of learning modalities, the modules can and should be used in conjunction with textbooks, classroom discussions, laboratories, fieldwork, and other inquiry-based technology tools.

The CHANCE modules allow scientists, from all over the world, to virtually work beside our youth sitting in classrooms and to share their experiences and to think about and "do" their research. Indeed, Robert DeHaan reports in his exemplary review on the state science education in the United States that, "using real-research strategies to teach has profound effects on student learning, and could have profound effects in promoting a scientifically literate society and a reinvigorated research enterprise (DeHaan, 2005)."

THE CHANCE MODULE PASSES THE TEST

Using the tools of science to teach science, the goal of these learning objects is to produce levels of understanding, knowledge retention and transfer that are greater than those resulting from traditional lecture classes by blending teaching and basic research through technology. Thus, a point that is worthy to consider is the actual degree to which the CHANCE modules exceed text-based instruction. In order to assess if the use of research modules enhance student learning of core biological concepts and required Pennsylvania Environmental and Ecological Standards set forth by the Pennsylvania Department of Education (www.pde.state.pa.us/k12/lib/k12/envec.pdf), research was conducted to assess learning before and after module use in selected Pennsylvania high school classrooms. Comparisons were made on similar groups of students who were taught the same concepts using a textbook only.

Methods

Participants

These modules were used in several tenth grade classrooms in the Pennsylvania Pocono Mountain (suburban), Allentown (urban), and Salisbury Township School Districts (suburban) in the spring of 2008. Twelve classes of 20-30 tenth grade students per teacher for a total of 212 students were asked to take part in this study (Table 1). The tenth-grade students who participated in this study were enrolled in either Gifted High Potential (GHP), College Prep (CP), or Applied levels of biology study.

Five tenth grade teachers were selected for this study. Four acted in the classroom as Research Assistants who carried out teaching and assessment duties and also assisted with the collection of the informed consent documents, and with recruitment, consenting, and data collection from the students. The fifth teacher acted as the Research Coordinator whose job was to coordinate teacher involvement with student participants and to ensure blind scoring of assessments and surveys. A senior instructional designer at The Pennsylvania State University, Ann Taylor, helped the Director and teachers develop the assessment tools: Concept Assessments (tests) and Attitude Surveys. The Director and her undergraduate research students, Stephen Seaquist and Foram Dave, blindly scored assessments and surveys, carried out statistical analysis, and interpreted data.

All teachers had worked with the principal investigator, CHANCE Director, to complete a day-long CHANCE module training workshop, and agreed to participate in this study, and also completed a separate two-hour workshop on the use of the chosen textbook product, Biology, by Rob DeSalle and Michael Heithaus (2008).The latter workshop was held on August 27, 2007 at the Penn State Lehigh Valley campus and presented by David Bray, Sales Representative, Holt, Rinehart and Winston.

Experimental Design

The 10th grade students in the chosen biology classrooms completed three selected CHANCE modules in conjunction with related chapter readings of the above mentioned textbook, or these same textbook chapters alone. To assess the impact of the modules on student learning, the following null hypothesis was tested:

There will be no significant difference in achievement (assessment performance) between high school students who experience science using on-line CHANCE research modules in conjunction with related chapters of a standard high school biology textbook (treatment group) versus students using these chapters alone (comparison group).

Table 1. Comparison of textbook and module groups pre and post scores

	Number of Students	Mean Score	t-value
Textbook Group Pre-Test	115	55.792	0.896
Module Group Pre-Test	97	57.708	
Textbook Group Post-Test	115	63.107	3.114*
Module Group Post-Test	97	69.937	
$p<0.001$; N Total =212			

All students in the comparison group were evaluated with a pre-study Concept Assessment (test) and Attitude Survey before completing Unit 2 on ecology (chapter 4--Ecosystems, chapter 5--Populations and Communities, and chapter 6--The Environment) of the Holt textbook. As the teachers progressed through the unit, the students in the comparison group completed questions from the Holt testbank and did all activities that were provided for each of the designated chapters of Unit 2. Additionally, all students were assessed with Concept Assessments (tests) after completing each of the designated chapters of Unit 2. After finishing the three designated textbook chapters, all students completed the same Attitude Survey that was administered pre-instruction. Three months after the completion of the assigned text chapters all students were re-assessed using the same Concept Assessment tool that was administered pre-study to determine the impact of the treatment on the students' long-term memory.

After completing the same pre-study instruments described above, all students in the experimental group completed each of three selected CHANCE modules (the treatment of the study) in conjunction with selected readings and assignments from Unit 2 on ecology (chapters 4--Ecosystems, chapter 5--Populations and Communities and 6--The Environment) of the Holt textbook. The three CHANCE modules used with the experimental group covered material similar to the overarching themes/concepts of each selected book chapter. The students carried out all of the activities embedded within the CHANCE modules and answered questions that are provided in each module using the CHANCE on-line "Progressive Notebook." All students were assessed with identical Concept Assessments (tests) that were used for the comparison group after completing each of the three CHANCE modules. Again, the latter included completing all the module activities while using the CHANCE on-line "Progressive Notebook" and completing selected chapter readings and assignments of the Holt textbook. After finishing the designated modules and textbook chapter content of Unit 2, all students completed the same Attitude Survey that was administered pre-instruction. Three months after the completion of the assigned modules and text content, all students were re-assessed using the same Concept Assessment tool that was adminitered pre-study to determine the impact of the treatment on the students' long-term memory. Selected results are briefly described below as this study and all its data is being prepared for another manuscript.

Curriculum

Teaching Methodology

Both groups covered the same essential themes and, for the most part, unless otherwise indicated, covered the same key concepts. The teachers and Director met and developed a protocol to handle incidents when, in the experimental group, a chosen CHANCE module did not address one or more of the key concepts that were included in the selected chapters used by the textbook group. The devised plan of action included using the textbook as a supplement to the modules so that both groups still were taught identical material. Each teacher/researcher strictly adhered to this agreed upon procedure to ensure reliability. (Example, deciduous forest module only covers this particular biome; and, in much more detail than the textbook. To ascertain that module students learned about the other biomes, such as the rainforest and the desert, textbook content describing the other biomes in the world was required.)

The implementation of the content for each group varied such that the control group was taught in a traditional manner with the teachers utilizing the lower-end inquiry teaching modality of "questioning" through text and the use of diagrammatic representations. In contrast, the experimental group was taught the material in the higher-end inquiry teaching modality of multimedia interaction using real-world experimental simulations and research data.

Curriculum Content

The broad curriculum theme for the unit covered by both groups in this study was Ecology. Again, the textbook used in this study was the Holt, Biology (DeSalle & Heithaus, 2008). All teachers in the study were provided with new classroom sets of the textbooks and teaching ancillaries. The Ecology Units included chapters 4, 5, and 6.

3.1 Each textbook chapter covered by the teachers embraced the following core content:

Chapter 4: Ecosystems

Text and the use of diagrammatic representations allow students to answer major questions:

- What is an ecosystem? How does energy flow in ecosystems? What are the major terrestrial biomes and how does temperature and sunlight affect the biodiversity in each of them?
- Key Concepts Covered: ecosystems, abiotic factors, biotic factors, succession, terrestrial biomes, aquatic ecosystems, food chains, food webs, producers, consumers, biodiversity, climatograph.

Chapter 5: Populations and communities

Text and the use of diagrammatic representations allow students to answer major questions:

- What is a population? How do populations grow? What are the factors that affect population size? How does competition for resources affect species in an ecosystem? What are the factors that contribute to the resiliency of an ecosystem?
- Key Concepts Covered: population, community, species, exponential growth, logistic growth, carrying capacity, population density, invasive species, competition, fundamental niche, realized niche, keystone species.

Chapter 6: The environment

Text and the use of diagrammatic representations allow students to answer major questions:

- How are humans and the environment connected? How does ecosystem disruption affect biodiversity? How are humans affecting the biosphere? How do conservation and restoration solve environmental issues?
- Key Concepts Covered: fossil fuels, greenhouse effect, global warming, deforestation, water pollution, air pollution, biodiversity, extinction, habitat disruption, overharvesting, water and air pollution, sustainability.

3.2 Each CHANCE module covered by the teachers embraced the following core content through the specific modalities described below:

Module used to cover overarching content in Chapter 4 – Stratification and Biodiversity of the Northeastern Deciduous Forest

Web-based multimedia activities allow students to:

1. Explore the distribution of temperate deciduous forests around the world and analyze the abiotic factors that define them (Figure 2);
2. Identify the vertical layers found in Pennsylvania's northeastern deciduous forest;
3. Analyze data on the total area of Pennsylvania's deciduous forestland from 1630 to 2002 obtained from Pennsylvania Department of Conservation and Natural Resources (DCNR);
4. Examine the re-growth (ecological succession) of an area of Pennsylvania's deciduous forest since 1907 to the present;
5. Analyze the distribution of tree species in Pennsylvania's northeastern deciduous forest;

Figure 2. In the module "Stratification and Biodiversity in Pennsylvania's Northeastern Deciduous Forest," students examine the climatic zones and the location of deciduous forests around the world, then plot a climatograph from a northeastern deciduous forest to understand how the abiotic factors, temperature and precipitation, define the climate of this biome

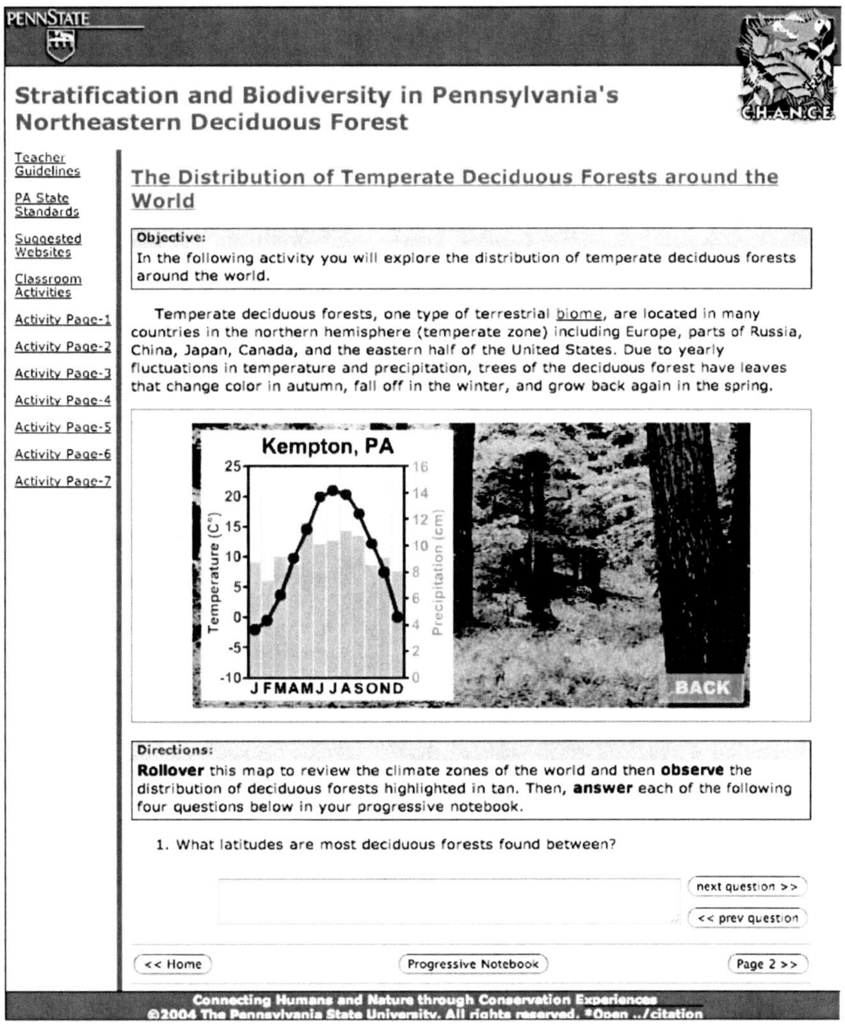

6. Interpret real data from the Pennsylvania Regeneration Study on the effect of the population increase of white-tailed deer and their over-browsing on Pennsylvania's northeastern deciduous forest; and
7. Observe the biodiversity found along the forest floor of one Maple tree in the deciduous forest, then explain why not just one species of tree, but the overall "tree species diversity" is essential to the continued success of a healthy forest.

Key Concepts Covered: ecosystems, abiotic factors, biotic factors, succession, terrestrial biomes, food chains, food webs, producers, consumers, biodiversity, climatograph.

Module used to cover overarching content in Chapter 5 – Invasive Plant Species in Pennsylvania

Web-based multimedia activities allow students to:

1. Observe and read about "native" plant species of Pennsylvania by viewing a slide show of real images taken throughout the state;
2. Observe and read about, using a virtual slide projector, the negative impacts of "invasive" plant species of Pennsylvania (Figure 3);
3. Collect, calculate, record, and analyze data on the population densities of native species like the Eastern Hemlock, Winterberry and Indian Grass in a Pennsylvania pond/meadow plant community—simulated here to help them learn about this common biological measurement that is often used by ecologists, foresters and conservationists to predict species survival;
4. Examine information on the Tree of Heaven (Ailanthus altissima), aka Ailanthus, an invasive trees species, originally from Asia, which is having a devastating impact on many of the natural plant communities in Pennsylvania;
5. Investigate the effects Ailanthus has on the population densities of selected native plant species found in the given Pennsylvania pond/meadow plant community over a ten year period.

Key Concepts Covered: population, community, species (native versus invasive), exponential growth, logistic growth, carrying capacity, population density, invasive species, competition, fundamental niche, realized niche, keystone species.

Module used to cover overarching content in Chapter 6 – Amphibians as Indicators of Environmental Change

Web-based multimedia activities allow students to:

1. Learn what an amphibian is and how it fits into the modern classification of living things;
2. Explore the unique biology and habitat of Costa Rica's Golden toad;
3. Visit an educational site created by the United States Environmental Protection Agency (EPA) to learn about the greenhouse effect and global warming (the most supported theory behind the golden toads' disappearance in 1989), and why global warming continues to be a threat to amphibian species;
4. Investigate the negative effects of pesticides in aquatic communities by carrying out an experimental simulation that repeats Dr. Relyea's experiment concerning the impact of common pesticides on amphibian populations in aquatic communities in Pennsylvania (Figure 4); and
5. Explore data from the International Union for the Conservation of Nature (IUCN) Redlist of Threatened Species, the IUCN Redlist categories and their criteria, and data from the 2006 Global Amphibian Assessment (GAA), to understand the reality amphibian global decline.

Key Concepts Covered: fossil fuels, carbon cycle, global warming, deforestation, water pollution, air pollution, biodiversity, extinction, habitat disruption, overharvesting, water and air pollution, sustainability.

4. Assessment Tools

In order to assess students' content knowledge each teacher/researcher, in either the textbook or module group, utilized four different Concept Assessments (tests). The teachers and Director created these end-of-chapter or module tests to assess students' understanding. These tests were titled according to the three chapters utilized from the Holt textbook. The Chapter 4 test included nine multiple-choice, four true-or-false, fourteen open-ended (requiring analysis of graphs, data, and figures), and one essay item. The Chapter 5

Figure 3. In the module "Invasive Plant Species of Pennsylvania," students use a virtual animated slide projector to observe and read about the negative impacts of invasive plant species of Pennsylvania

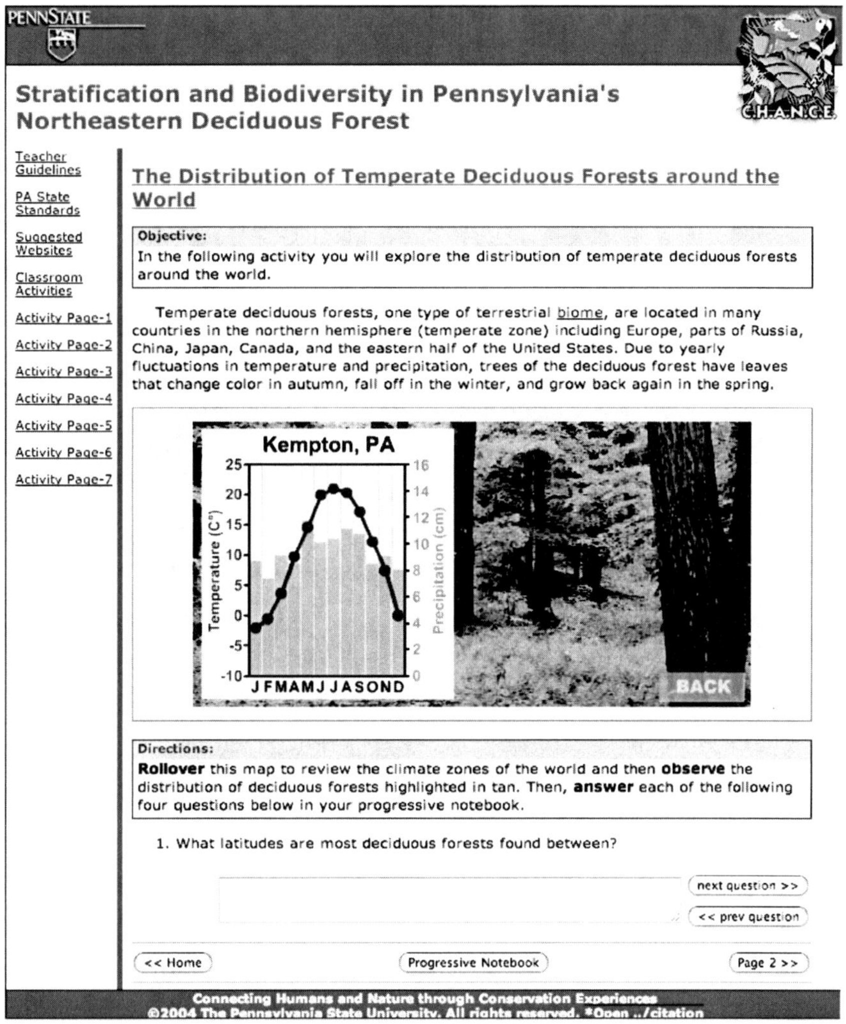

test included nine multiple-choice, four true-or-false, twelve open-ended (requiring analysis of graphs, data, and figures), and one essay item. The Chapter 6 test included nine multiple-choice, four true-or-false, fourteen open-ended (requiring analysis of graphs, data, and figures), and one essay item. In terms of Webb's Depth of Knowledge Levels (http://dese.mo.gov/divimprove/sia/msip/DOK_Chart.pdf) the multiple-choice and true-or-false items were aligned with level one (recall) or level two (skill/concept). The open-ended items were at levels two and three (strategic thinking). The essay items aimed for levels three and four (extended thinking). Sample questions from the Chapter 4 test are provided in Figure 5.

The pre- and post Concept assessment tools consisted of a compilation of the same multiple-choice items found on the three chapter assessments described above.

Additionally, Attitude Surveys were administered to both teachers and students. The items consisted of Likert scale questions (strongly agree; disagree; neither agree or disagree; agree; strongly agree) and open-ended evaluation questions and

Figure 4. In the module "Amphibians as Indictors of Environmental Change," students investigate the negative effects of pesticides in aquatic communities by carrying out an experimental simulation concerning the negative impact of common pesticides on amphibian populations in aquatic communities in Pennsylvania

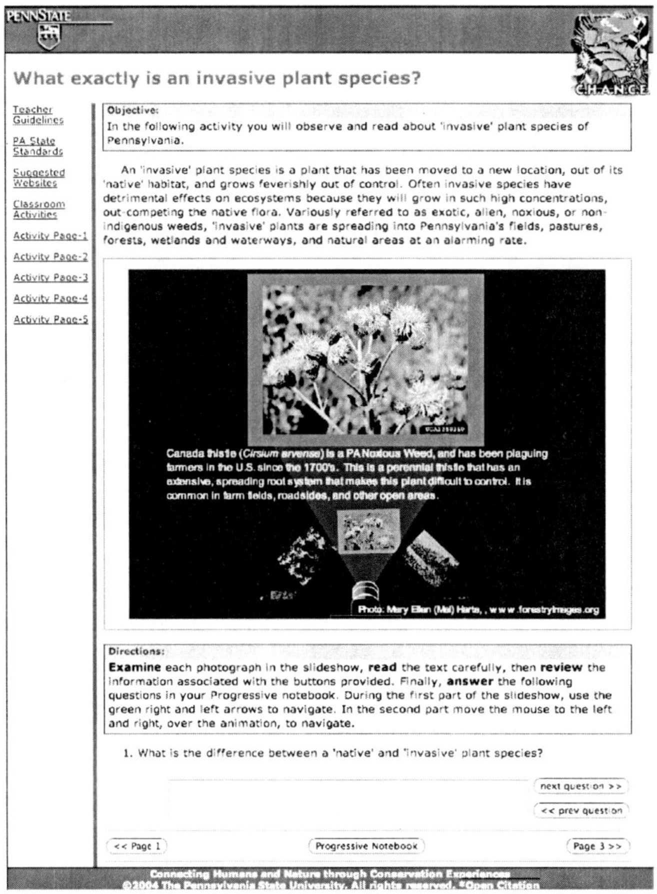

were given pre- and post study. Teachers completed 20 items. Students completed 17 items.

All pre-assessments were administered in the winter 2008 and post-assessments occurred at the end of the academic year.

5. Data Analysis

The Research Coordinator ensured blind scoring of assessments and surveys. All instruments were sent to the Coordinator by the teachers/researchers then categorized by group and academic level. Assessments and surveys were then sent to the Director without knowledge of the high school, and teacher or student participants. All Concept Assessments multiple-choice, true-or-false, and open-ended items were graded using a key and the essays were graded based on a rubric addressing expected learning outcomes.

To determine whether there was a difference in student performance on the pre- and post-tests that were administered before and three months after the completion of the assigned text chapters or modules, T-statistics and means were obtained for both groups. Significant differences were determined based on the.005 p level scale.

Figure 5. Sample questions from chapter 4 showing multiple choice, open-ended, and essay examples. Webb Taxonomy Levels are also indicated. The theme for this assessment was ecosystems.

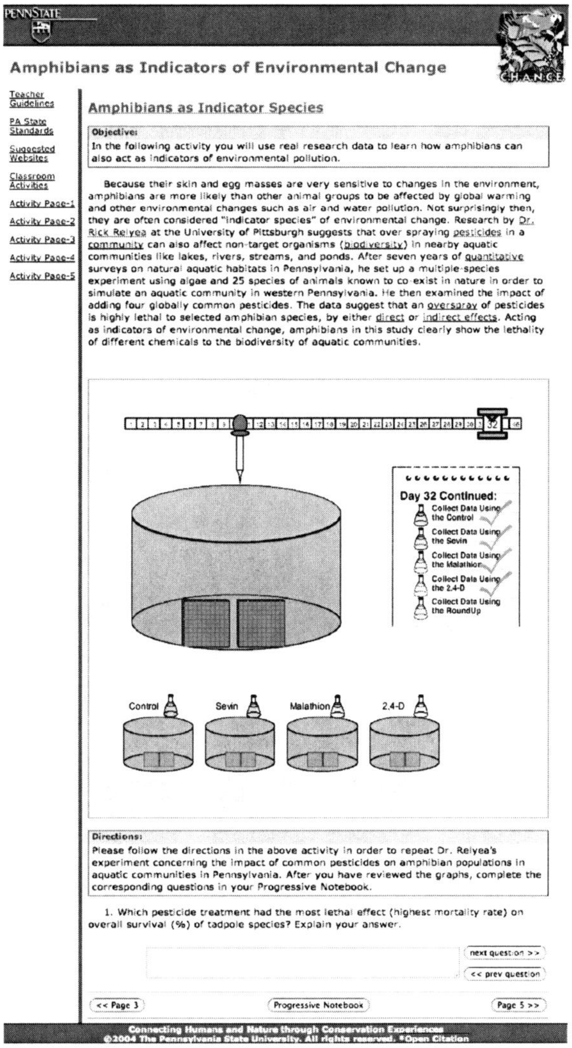

RESULTS

Data analysis revealed that between the pre-and post-tests, the student participants who used the CHANCE modules to enhance their studies scored higher on Concept Assessments given for each chapter/module. Moreover, post-test scores for the module group showed a gain of 12.99 percentage points while the textbook group showed a gain of only 5.91 percentage points. A t-test evaluating the difference in the final post-test scores between the textbook and module groups indicate statistical significance at the p=0.001 level (Table 1 and Figure 6). Interestingly, both student populations showed no significant difference at the pre-assessment stage. The groups varied by only 1.91 percentage points.

Data published elsewhere, revealed that the Gifted High Potential and College Prep groups of students who utilized the CHANCE research modules scored higher on the three chapter Concept Assessments than the students using only their textbook, and that the Applied Group faired lower (McLaughlin and Fadigan, 2010).

Figure 6. Line graph plotting the average test scores for all student participants in either the textbook or module group, demonstrating an average 12.99% increase in long-term retention among students using both modules and textbooks vs. textbook-only instruction.

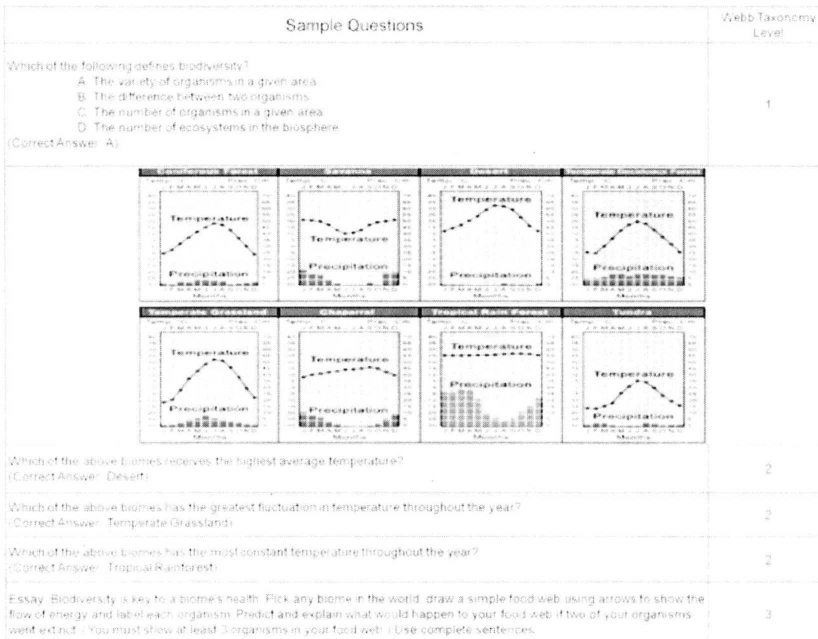

Sample Questions	Webb Taxonomy Level
Which of the following defines biodiversity? A. The variety of organisms in a given area B. The difference between two organisms C. The number of organisms in a given area D. The number of ecosystems in the biosphere (Correct Answer: A)	1
Which of the above biomes receives the highest average temperature? (Correct Answer: Desert)	2
Which of the above biomes has the greatest fluctuation in temperature throughout the year? (Correct Answer: Temperate Grassland)	2
Which of the above biomes has the most constant temperature throughout the year? (Correct Answer: Tropical Rainforest)	2
Essay: Biodiversity is key to a biome's health. Pick any biome in the world, draw a simple food web using arrows to show the flow of energy and label each organism. Predict and explain what would happen to your food web if two of your organisms went extinct. (You must show at least 3 organisms in your food web.) Use complete sentences.	3

Of major interest was the qualitative data from the post-assessment student Attitude Surveys, which indicated that more than 50 percent of the respondents (n=188) disagreed with the statement, "I found my biology textbook interesting," while over 81 percent of the same group of students agreed with the statement, "I feel comfortable using computer-based resources as learning tools." Even more important, teacher attitude assessment revealed a host of qualitative advantages of using the computer-based modules.

The four teachers participating in this study taught both textbook-based and module-based courses and, in post-study surveys, their attitudes about the two approaches were unanimous. All four said that they use textbooks but consider them just one of the many tools that they can use for teaching and learning, and stated that, currently, they do not have sufficient supplementary teaching materials to draw upon. In addition, all of the teachers:

- "strongly agreed" they value their ability to understand the scientific research behind the biological concepts that they teach. --"strongly agreed" that their students will learn the scientific content better if allowed to engage in scientific research. --"disagreed" that their students understand what is meant by scientific research and can see research in science as a career opportunity. (WHEW...no wonder they are ALL pre-med!!)
- "agreed" or "strongly agreed" that they want their students to appreciate that science is built on data from the cumulative efforts of real-world research scientists who perform basic research experiments.

The teachers also described exactly how using the CHANCE research modules helped their students discover the scientific ideas and concepts for themselves, better understand what a researcher does, apply science ideas to everyday situations, learn to analyze real data and draw conclusions, understand how science contributes to society, and become better advocates for the environment. When asked about their use of technology in the classroom, teachers said the technology made it easier to teach about the environment, to do more hands-on experiments in the classroom, to use the CHANCE modules again, use other computer-based resources in their classroom, and to engage in professional development programs that allow them to learn about the research behind the scenes of the concepts they teach. With regard to CHANCE modules in particular, two teachers commented:

I appreciated everything being in one place, since a major drawback of using technology is the time it takes to find all the materials that are out there. And, many times what is out there, is either too boring, simplistic, or way too complicated. It's nice to know that tools are being developed that engage both teacher and student. How awesome that famous scientist can come to your classroom.

FUTURE RESEARCH DIRECTIONS

In order to reach the largest number of secondary students, completed CHANCE modules (or the larger program itself) are showcased on a wide variety of education and science web sites, including PDE, PSU, National Association of Biology Teachers (NABT), National Science Teachers Association (NSTA), Caribbean Conservation Corporation (CCC), Widecast, LaSelva Biological Field Station of the Organization of Tropical Studies (OTS), and Hawk Mountain Sanctuary (see complete list on the CHANCE web site). As stated previously, these modules are freely available to anyone in the nation teaching high school biology or environmental science, or to anyone who is looking for an engaging alternative to teaching basic biological and ecological principles and environmental issues while advocating environmental stewardship.

Nearly 100 high school teachers from around the United States have been trained in the field, through the CHANCE field course, to be more like scientists. As part of the long-term plan to bring the modules into as many classrooms as possible, CHANCE has been featured in more than 30 workshops and presentations, reaching more than 600 teachers. The CHANCE program continues to evolve, however, based on ongoing research and evaluation findings. We are developing new CHANCE modules specifically for undergraduate students majoring in biology. These new modules will use the existing structure and format to bring real-world research directly into the college classroom, but coverage will include the key concepts needed at the collegiate level in evolution, biodiversity, cell biology, developmental biology, molecular biology, ecology, and so on.

In a recent field test of CHANCE materials by both veteran (in-service) and pre-service teachers, the newer teachers showed more interest and likelihood to implement digital technology than their more experienced counterparts, demonstrating a clear generational preference (McLaughlin and Arbieter, 2008). Sixty-eight teachers (ten of whom were pre-service and 58 in-service) evaluated one module using both the "cyberguide" for Web Site Design, and the "cyberguide" for Content Evaluation (MacLachlan, 1996). A subset of 46 teachers (10 of them pre-service) also completed a brief "Implementation Survey." The teachers' responses to the "Invasive Plant Species in Pennsylvania" module served as a feedback mechanism for the module design team. Although responses to the cyberguide modules were equally strong among both pre-service and in-service teachers, the pre-service teachers were far more likely to select CHANCE materials for definite future implementation than were the in-service teachers. Additionally, in free response comments collected after the evaluation workshop, pre-service teachers in particular noted that they expected to use the CHANCE modules during their upcoming student teaching practicum experiences–suggesting that they will be more likely to incorporate the CHANCE materials into their classrooms in the future.

Many research challenges lie ahead. For example, we must better understand the differences in implementation methods of pre-service and in-service teachers, as well as how best to meet the needs of both. We know that it is not possible to provide intensive training to all teachers, so we must also find ways to ensure that teachers who do not receive formal professional development on the implementation of the CHANCE modules (or multimedia tools in general) are able to use them to their full capacity. We must also conduct further research to determine how integrating inquiry-based multimedia learning tools, like the CHANCE modules, into the curriculum can improve science education for students in all grades. We must also develop assessments that measure how effectively students use scientific inquiry and how thoroughly they understand the scientific subjects they have been taught.

Important findings of the research presented in this chapter, and that of additional data being published elsewhere, included the positive effects upon students' learning demonstrated via both short-term (immediate assessment) and long-term (three months post assessment) after using the research modules. Indeed, the premise behind the design of the CHANCE research modules was to create new, "learner-centered" multimedia tools that aid students in the higher inquiry-based learning of science (application, integration, and understanding), or to expand their cognitive abilities. Mayer (2009, p. 20-21) defines three types of learning outcomes: no-learning; rote learning, and *meaningful learning*. "Meaningful learning is distinguished by good transfer performance as well as good retention performance." Future research will therefore examine the design features of the CHANCE modules that appear to be fostering meaningful learning so as to augment these features in future modules. Additionally, we have only measured learning outcomes data for the CHANCE modules for a short time, so our next research project will involve a longitudinal study to determine whether the stronger learning outcomes among high school students are attributable to the CHANCE modules and not to the novelty effect.

Another finding, which was only briefly discussed herein, that is especially interesting to me is the fact that the "Applied Students" using textbooks fared better than their module-using counterparts in all Concept Assessments immediately after, as well as three months later. (Importantly, these average scores were still lower than similar grade sets obtained for the "College Prep" and "Gifted High Potential" groups.) Moreover, feedback from this group suggests that these students are uninterested in learning about science in general, and uninterested in the idea of using real-research data or indeed any assignments beyond those associated with their textbooks. Several of these students noted that the CHANCE modules were "too hard." This lack of student motivation and/or intimidation by real-research simulations to enhance higher order inquiry by this group of students, typically classified as the "lower" group, is worthy of further exploration. These results also stress an urgent need for relevant technology-based curriculum materials for non-college bound students as well as those with an academic career path.

CONCLUSION

CHANCE research modules evolved from this bleak reality: On average, K-12 teachers use computers or engage in lab experiences with their students less than one time per week for little more than word processing, e-mail, or game and drill software (Becker, 2000; Singer, Hilton, & Schweingruber, 2005; Smith, Banilower, McMahon, & Weiss, 2002; Wetzel, 1993). Yet, today's youth spend an average of 6 ½ hours a week using various forms of media—about a quarter of that time juggling more than one form of media at a time. The amount of time spent on computers has more than doubled over the last 5 years (Kaiser Family Foundation, 2005). Thus, using digital technology is second nature to the Millennial generation, students born between 1980 and 1994, and research shows that they prefer video, audio, and interactive media, and they prefer to learn by doing (Carlson, 2005). Indeed, the results of the student surveys listed in this paper augment this argument.

Moreover, in a recent field test of CHANCE materials by both veteran (in-service) and pre-service teachers, the newer teachers showed more interest and likelihood to implement digital technology than their more experienced counterparts, demonstrating a generational preference in teaching with multi-media (McLaughlin and Arbeider, 2008). Complicating matters more are the facts that most students in high school are not reading their science textbooks, nor understanding the content (American Association for the Advancement of Science, 2000). Moreover, most pre-service science teachers are taught to teach technology as a separate component of high school education rather than as a topic integrated into the curriculum (Willis & Mehlinger, 1996; The Milken Exchange & the International Society for Technology in Education, 1999; Thomas & Livingston, 2004), while over the past decade spending on technology in the United States tripled, now totaling more than $6 billion (WestEd Policy Brief, 2002).

Thus, it has become obvious that new types of interactive multimedia learning tools need to be developed for both high school science teachers and students that supports standards-based teaching, enforces complex thinking and problem solving, embraces research skills, includes appropriate assessments to measure student performance, best utilizes the content provided in traditional textbooks that fill today's market, and shows real-world uses. The CHANCE modules accomplish all of these goals in a way that balances what we know about how students learn science (Bransford et al., 1999; Duschl et al., 2007), support "meaningful learning" (Mayer and Wittrock, 1996) through multimedia that avoids cognitive overload (Mayer and Moreno, 2003), and delivers these modules to teachers via the increasingly more affordable and student-favored medium of the Internet.

The CHANCE modules take full advantage of the digital propensity of students and new teachers alike and promote inquiry-based learning by allowing students to explore, observe, question, hypothesize, manipulate, analyze, and think critically about real science data and information from accredited research programs in Pennsylvania and around the world. Experienced teachers embrace the authentic science that forms the basis for CHANCE modules and pick up easily on the interactive nature of the materials. This computer-based interactive approach is particularly attractive to secondary students, most of whom enjoy the virtual experiences today's technology affords. Best of all, CHANCE modules promote active learning by providing opportunities for students to participate as individuals directing their own learning process.

The CHANCE modules are purposefully designed to be more engaging and interactive than a textbook by allowing students to learn how the world works. These modules cover key biological and environmental science concepts using higher-end, inquiry activities that provide compelling animations, video, factual information, and research-based exploration that necessitate students working with real research data. Using the tools of science to teach science, the goal of these learning objects is to produce levels of understanding, knowledge retention, and transfer that are greater than those resulting from traditional lecture classes by blending teaching and basic research through technology.

At the core of the CHANCE modules and the larger professional program they represent is the underpinning objective to enhance environmental awareness in U.S. high-school and undergraduate student populations. Our environment faces serious threats resulting from human activity – water pollution, air pollution, loss of biodiversity, depletion of natural resources, and watershed depletion – all of which must be understood in the context of basic biological principles and solid research. Thus, in order to help students understand the real world environmental issues that confront them and to become informed citizens, it is time for teachers to understand research and how science works (higher order inquiry), not just by textbook content (lower order inquiry). Think: teachers as researchers! CHANCE's field component trains teachers in environmental science, ecology, and conservation practices on an international, eye-opening level via hands-on field work in Costa Rica. CHANCE's research modules equip teachers with multimedia learning tools that provide inquiry-based activities in areas that foster their students' competencies in biological concepts and real world environmental issues like climate change, species extinction, water pollution, loss of wetlands, etc., while at the same time instilling an inclination toward environmental advocacy.

The Pennsylvania Department of Education recommends the CHANCE field course and research modules as ways of helping high school teachers and their students meet the nine state standards in environmental science and ecology. Because most states must meet similar standards, the CHANCE program provides a viable framework for improving or reforming high school biology education nationwide.

The impact of the CHANCE field course and its modules on teachers and their students has been overwhelmingly positive. Put simply, hundreds of teachers from all over Pennsylvania and the nation are embracing these resources. Free response comments by Pennsylvania high school teachers after completing the CHANCE field course and module training included the following:

I am a high school Biology and AP Environmental Science teacher. The CHANCE program was the BEST professional development program that I have participated in, during 20 years of teaching. The interactive approach to Conservation Biology, integrating research was invaluable. I learned the importance of providing my high school students with this skill, and the modules make this task truly possible. In addition, seeing, feeling, touching, participating in programs in Costa Rica was absolutely a life- changing experience that I bring to my classroom every day. Paula Wang, CHANCE 2007.

First, the experience of field work in Costa Rica has helped invigorate me in the classroom; second, the wealth of experiences, pictures, knowledge and research picked up during the trip (and in the accompanying assignments) has provided me with tons of new material for my classroom; and third, the available modules are helping me integrate interactive technology into my classes as well as being valuable curricular material in their own right. Rick Bloom, CHANCE 2007.

The CHANCE program is grounded in the belief that only a well-informed citizenry will be qualified to create policies and develop programs that will help stem the extensive alteration of our natural world. Publishing data in a peer-review article is important; yet, only a select few can actually read and can understand targeted and complex data. Conveying complex data at a level that allows high school students to think and ponder real world questions is one of the most worthwhile endeavors that scientists can undertake, for it is in the imperative of the messages, delivered to those who will build on what they learn in their classrooms, that our very futures depend.

I also believe that technology can help us bridge this gap. Technology is allowing us re-imagine new pedagogical tools for the 21st century classroom. With technology, we can create new learner-centered environments that allow high school teachers and their students to engage in real-world scientific research--and essentially conquer higher-order inquiry in their classrooms. Moreover, by doing actual science through this tool, both teacher and student gain a stronger understanding of the process, the methods, the struggles, the triumphs, time commitment, and the social impact of the enterprise known as science itself.

ACKNOWLEDGMENT

For belief in CHANCE and its impact, I thank Dr. Patricia Vathis (PDE), Mrs. Ellyn Schindler (sanofi pasteur), and Mr. James Bus (ATAS International, Inc.), and all other partners, sponsors, and collaborators for their endorsement and backing (complete list on our web site). I am also especially grateful to the following NGO's for their devotion to the CHANCE field course and allowing this program to blend real-world research with science education: The Organization of Tropical Studies (OTS) in La Selva, Costa Rica; The Smithsonian Tropical Research Institute in Bocas del Toro, Panama; Widecast (Duke University) in Gandoca, Costa Rica; and, The Caribbean Conservation Corporation (CCC), Costa Rica. For amazing assistance with module development and design, I am beholden to all the CHANCE high school teacher authors, research scientist mentors, and multimedia design specialists who used their talents to help create a different type of pedagogical tool. For support in the jungles and the beaches of Costa Rica and now Panama, I thank Dr. Kathleen Fadigan for her expertise and devotion to field-based experiential teaching and learning. For the research assessment team who worked to build assessment tools and to carry-out the research presented herein, especially Jennifer Paukovitch, gratitude is also extended. And last, but not least, I thank Ronald Heft for preparing the figures and tables showcased herein.

REFERENCES

American Association for the Advancement of Science. (2005). *High school biology Textbooks: A benchmark-based evaluation.* Retrieved from the AAAS Project 2061 Textbook Evaluations Web site: http://www.project2061.org/publications/textbook/hsbio/report/default.htm

Anderson, L., & Krathwohl, D. (Eds.). (2001). *A Taxonomy for Learning, Teaching, and Assessing: A Revision of Blooms Taxonomy of Educational Objectives.* New York: Addison Wesley Longman, Inc.

Beatty, A. (1997). *Learning from TIMSS: Results of the Third International Mathematics and Science Study, Summary of a Symposium.* Committee on Science Education K-12, National Research Council. Washington, DC: The National Academies Press. Retrieved from http://www.nap.edu/catalog.php?record_id=5937

Becker, H. (2000). *Findings from the teaching, learning, and computing survey: Is Larry Cuban right?* Paper presented for the Council of Chief State School Officers' Annual Technology Leadership Conference, Washington, DC.

Bloom, B. S. (Ed.). Engelhart, M.D. Furst, E.J., Hill, W.H., & Krathwohl, D.R. (1956). Taxonomy of Educational Objectives: Handbook 1: Cognitive Domain. New York: David McKay.

Bransford, J., Brown, A., & Cocking, R. (1999). *How People Learn: Brain, Mind, Experience and School.* National Research Council.

BSCS. (2006). *The BSCS 5E instructional model: origins and effectiveness: a report prepared for the Office of Science Education, National Institutes of Health.* Retrieved from http://www.bscs.org/library/BSCS_5E_Model_Full_Report2006.pdf

Bybee, R. (1993). An instructional model for science education. In Developing biological literacy. Colorado Springs, CO: Biological Science Curriculum Study.

Carlson, S. (2005). The net generation goes to college. *The Chronicle of Higher Education, 52*(7), A34. Retrieved from http://chronicle.com/free/v52/i07/07a03401.htm.

Center for Science, Mathematics, and Engineering Education. (1996). *National Science Education Standards.* Washington, DC: The National Academies Press. Retrieved from http://books.nap.edu/openbook.php?record_id=4962&page=1

Clark, D. A., Piper, S. C., Keeling, C. D., & Clark, D. B. (2003). Tropical rain forest tree growth and atmospheric carbon dynamics linked to interannual temperature variation during 1984-2000. *Proceedings of the National Academy of Sciences of the United States of America, 100*(10), 5852–5857. doi:10.1073/pnas.0935903100

Council of Chief State School Officers. (2005). State indicators of science and mathematics education 2005, Washington, DC.

DeHaan, R. (2005). The impending revolution in undergraduate science education. *Journal of Science Education and Technology, 14*(2), 253–269. doi:10.1007/s10956-005-4425-3

DeSalle, R., & Heithaus, M. (2008). *Biology*. New York: Holt, Rinehart and Winston.

Donovan, M., & Bransford, J. (2005). *How Students Learn: Science in the Classroom.* Washington, DC: The National Academies of Science Press. Retrieved from http://books.nap.edu/openbook.php?record_id=11102&page=1

Donovan, M. S., Bransford, J. D., & Pellegrino, J. W. (Eds.). (1999). *How people learn: Bridging research and practice*. Washington, DC: National Academy Press.

Dotterer, R. E., & Pasley, J. D. (2000). *New Frontiers in Physiology/ Physiology Insights and Final Evaluation Report.* Chapel Hill, NC: Horizon Research Inc.

Duschl, R., Schweingruber, H., & Shouse, A. (2007). *Taking Science to School: Learning and Teaching Science in Grades K-8*. Washington, DC: The National Academies of Science Press. Retrieved from http://books.nap.edu/openbook.php?record_id=11625&page=R1

Flick, L., & Bell, R. (2000). Preparing tomorrow's science teachers to use technology: Guidelines for Science educators. *Contemporary Issues in Technology & Teacher Education, 1*(1). Retrieved from http://www.citejournal.org/vol1/iss1/currentissues/science/article1.htm.

International Society for Technology in Education. (1999). *Will new teachers be prepared to teach in a digital age? A national survey on information technology in teacher education.* Santa Monica, CA: Milken Exchange on Education Technology. Retrieved October 29, 2006 from http://www.milkenexchange.org/research/iste_results.html

Kaiser Family Foundation. (2005). Generation M: media in the lives of 8-18 year-olds. *Kaiser Family Foundation Web Site.* Retrieved from http://www.kff.org/entmedia/entmedia030905pkg.cfm

MacLachlan, K. (1996). Web Evaluation. *WWW Cyberguides web site.* Retrieved from http://www.cyberbee.com/guides.html

Marshall, J. C., Horton, B., Igo, B. L., & Switzer, D. M. (in press). K-12 science and mathematics teachers' beliefs about and use of inquiry in the classroom. *International Journal of Science and Mathematics Education.*

Mayer, R. E. (2001). *Multimedia Learning* (1st ed.). New York: Cambridge University Press.

Mayer, R. E. (2009). *Multimedia Learning* (2nd ed.). New York: Cambridge University Press.

Mayer, R. E., & Moreno, R. (2003). Nine ways to reduce cognitive load in multimedia learning. In Bruning, R., Horn, C. A., & Pytlik Zillig, L. M. (Eds.), *Web-based learning: What do we know? Where do we go?* (pp. 23–44). Greenwich, CT: Information Age Publishing.

Mayer, R. E., & Wittrock, M. C. (1996). Problem-solving transfer. In Calfee, R., & Berliner, R. (Eds.), *Handbook of educational psychology* (pp. 47–62). New York: Macmillan.

McLaughlin, J. (2006a). The CHANCE program: Promoting learning for teachers and students through experiences and inquiry. *The American Biology Teacher*, *68*(4), 17–24. Retrieved from https://royercenter.cwc.psu.edu/CHANCE/press/NABT-CHANCE-04-2006.pdf. doi:10.1662/0002-7685(2006)68[e17:TCPPLF]2.0.CO;2

McLaughlin, J., & Arbeider, D. A. (2008b). Evaluating multimedia-learning tools based on authentic research data that teach biology concepts and environmental stewardship. *Contemporary Issues in Technology & Teacher Education*, *8*(1), 1–19. Retrieved from http://www.citejournal.org/tempcite/vol8/iss1/science/article1.cfm.

McLaughlin, J. S. (2006b). Using technology to blend teaching and basic research. *Science Teacher (Normal, Ill.)*, *73*(8), 48–53.

McLaughlin, J. S. (2010) Re-imagining Science Education and New Pedagogical Tools: Blending Research with Teaching. *Educause Quarterly*, 33 (1). Online at http://www.educause.edu/eq.

McLaughlin, J. S., Arbeider, D. A., Stine, J. L., Dugan, T. R., & Besong, P. J. (2008a). *CHANCE* (*Online*). Retrieved from http://chance.psu.edu/

McLaughlin, J. S., & Fadigan, K. A. (2010). The CHANCE (Connecting Humans and Nature Through Conservation Experiences) Program: Transitioning from Simple Inquiry-based Learning to Professional Science Practice. In Yager, R. (Ed.), *Exemplary Science Programs: Science for Resolving Issues/Problems*. Arlington, VA: NSTA Press.

Moore, G. E. (2003). *No exponential is forever... but we can delay forever*. Presentation to the International Solid State Circuits Conference. Retrieved from http://download.intel.com/research/silicon/Gordon_Moore_ISSCC_021003.pdf

Moreno, R., & Mayer, R. E. (2005). Role of guidance, reflection, and interactivity in an agent-based multimedia game. *Journal of Educational Psychology*, *97*, 117–128. doi:10.1037/0022-0663.97.1.117

National Research Council. (1996). *The National Science Education Standards*. Washington, DC: The National Research Council.

National Research Council. (2000). *The National Science Education Standards*. Washington, DC: The National Research Council.

NEA. (n.d.). *NCLB/ESEA: It's Time for a Change – Voices from America's Classrooms.* Retrieved from http://www.nea.org/esea/nclbstories/images/classroomvoices.pdf

Norman, D. A. (1993). *Things that make us smart*. Reading, MA: Addison-Wesley.

Office of Science Education. (2006). Curriculum supplement series. *National Institutes for Health web site*. Retrieved from http://science-education.nih.gov/customers.nsf/Supplements

Pasley, J. D. (1998). *APS Frontiers in Physiology Final Evaluation Report*. Chapel Hill, NC: Horizon Research Inc.

Roseman, J. E., Caldwell, A., Kurth, L., & Stern, L. (2000). *High School Biology Textbooks: A Benchmark-Based Evaluation.* AAAS Project 2061 Textbook Evaluations Reports. Retrieved from http://www.project2061.org/about/press/pr000627.htm

Singer, S. R., Hilton, M. L., & Schweingruber, H. A. (2005). *America's Lab Report: Investigations in High School Science.* Washington, DC: National Academy of Science. Retrieved from http://books.nap.edu/catalog.php?record_id=11311

Smith, P. S., Banilower, E. R., McMahon, K. C., & Weiss, I. R. (2002). *The National Survey of Science and Mathematics Education: Trends from 1977 to 2000.* Chapel Hill, NC: Horizon Research.

Thomas, L. G., & Livingston, M. (2004). Using video exhibits to support technology integration in teacher preparation and P-12 student learning. *Digitial Edge Project.* International Society for Technology in Education. Retrieved from http://cnets.iste.org/dedge/docs/FinalReport_DE_BellSouth.pdf

Universal Services Administrative Company. (2007). USAC provides demand estimate for funding year 2007 to FCC. *Schools and Libraries USAC web site.* Retrieved from http://www.universalservice.org/sl/tools/latest-news.aspx#030907

Weaver, G. C., Russell, C. B., & Wink, D. J. (2008). Inquiry-based and research-based laboratory pedagogies in undergraduate science. *Nature Chemical Biology, 4*(10), 577–580. doi:10.1038/nchembio1008-577

Wetzel, K. (1993). Models for achieving computer competencies in preservice education. *Journal of Computing in Teacher Education, 9*(4), 4–6.

Willis, J. W., & Mehlinger, H. D. (1996). Information technology and teacher education. In Sikula, J., Buttery, T., & Guyton, E. (Eds.), *Handbook of research on teacher education* (2nd ed., pp. 978–1029). New York: Macmillan.

ADDITIONAL READING

Baddeley, A. D., & Hitch, G. J. (1974). Working memory. In Bower, G. A. (Ed.), *The Psychology of learning and motivation: Advances in research* (*Vol. 8*, pp. 47–90). New York: Academic Press.

Beatty, A. (1997). *Learning from TIMSS: Results of the Third International Mathematics and Science Study, Summary of a Symposium.* Committee on Science Education K-12, National Research Council. The National Academies Press. Retrieved from http://www.nap.edu/catalog.php?record_id=5937

Blackwell, M. (2007). Letter RE: Estimate of demand for funding year 2007. *Universal Services Administrative Company Schools and Libraries.* Retrieved from http://www.universalservice.org/_res/documents/sl/pdf/2007-03-08-FY2007-Demand-Estimate.pdf

Clark, R., & Mayer, R. E. (2008). *E-learning and the science of instruction* (2nd ed.). San Francisco: Jossey-Bass.

Handelsman, J., Ebert-May, D., Beichner, R., Bruns, P., & Chang, A. (2004). Scientific teaching. *Science, 304*(5670), 521–522. doi:10.1126/science.1096022

Handelsman, J., Miller, S., & Pfund, C. (2007). *Scientific Teaching.* New York: W. H. Freeman and Company.

Harskamp, E., Mayer, R. E., Suhre, C., & Jansma, J. (2007). Does the modality principle for multimedia learning apply to science classrooms? *Learning and Instruction, 17*, 465–477. doi:10.1016/j.learninstruc.2007.09.010

International Society for Technology in Education. (1999). *Will new teachers be prepared to teach in a digital age? A national survey on information technology in teacher education.* Santa Monica, CA: Milken Exchange on Education Technology. Retrieved October 29, 2006 from http://www.milkenexchange.org/research/iste_results.html

Johnson, D. K., & Ratcliff, J. L. (2004). Creating coherence: the unfinished agenda. *New Directions for Higher Education, 125*, 85–96. doi:10.1002/he.141

Kaiser Family Foundation. (2005). Generation M: media in the lives of 8-18 year-olds. *Kaiser Family Foundation Web Site.* Retrieved from http://www.kff.org/entmedia/entmedia030905pkg.cfm

Mayer, R. E. (2004). Should there be a three strikes rule against pure discovery? The case for guided methods of instruction. *The American Psychologist, 59*(1), 14–19. doi:10.1037/0003-066X.59.1.14

Mayer, R. E. (Ed.). (2005). *Cambridge Handbook of Multimedia Learning.* New York: Cambridge University Press.

Mayer, R. E. (2008). *Learning and Instruction* (2nd ed.). Upper Saddle River, NJ: Merrill Prentice-Hall.

Mayer, R. E. (2008). Applying the science of learning: Evidence-based principles for the design of multimedia instruction. *The American Psychologist, 63*(8), 760–769. doi:10.1037/0003-066X.63.8.760

Mayer, R. E., & Massa, L. J. (2003). Three facets of visual and verbal learners: Cognitive ability, cognitive style, and learning preference. *Journal of Educational Psychology, 95*, 833–846. doi:10.1037/0022-0663.95.4.833

Mayer, R. E., & Moreno, R. (1998). A split-attention effect in multimedia learning: Evidence for dual-processing systems in working memory. *Journal of Educational Psychology: Applied, 90*, 312–320. doi:10.1037/0022-0663.90.2.312

Mayer, R. E., & Moreno, R. (1999). Cognitive principles of multimedia learning: The role of modality and contiguity. *Journal of Educational Psychology, 91*, 358–368. doi:10.1037/0022-0663.91.2.358

Mayer, R. E., Moreno, R., Boire, M., & Vagge, S. (1999). Maximizing constructivist learning from multimedia communications by minimizing cognitive load. *Journal of Educational Psychology, 91*, 638–643. doi:10.1037/0022-0663.91.4.638

Mayer, R. E., & Sims, V. K. (1994). For whom is a picture worth a thousand words? Extensions of a dual-coding theory of multimedia learning. *Journal of Educational Psychology, 84*, 389–460. doi:10.1037/0022-0663.86.3.389

McLaughlin, J. S. (2005). Classrooms Without Walls: a banana plantation, a turtle nest, and the random fallen tree. *International Educator, 14*(1), 52–54.

McLaughlin, J. S., & Johnson, D. K. (2006). Assessing the field course experiential learning model: Transforming collegiate short-term study abroad experiences into rich learning environments. *Frontiers: The Interdisciplinary Journal of Study Abroad, 13*, 65–85.

Paivio, A. (1971). *Imagery and verbal processes.* New York: Holt, Rinehart, and Winston.

Schmidt, W. H., McKnight, C. C., & Raizen, S. A. (1997). *A Splintered Vision: An Investigation of U.S. Science and Mathematics Education.* Boston, MA: Kluwer Academic Publishers.

Zervanos, S. M., & McLaughlin, J. S. (2003). Teaching biodiversity and evolution through travel course experiences. *The American Biology Teacher, 65*, 683–688. doi:10.1662/0002-7685(2003)065[0683:TBETTC]2.0.CO;2

Section 3
Inter-Institutional Collaboration

Chapter 7
Serving Rural Teachers Using Synchronous Online Professional Development

Shari L. Stockero
Michigan Technological University, USA

ABSTRACT

This chapter describes the design and implementation of a blended online synchronous teacher professional development course that was developed to meet the needs of rural educators. The author discusses how research on teacher learning influenced both the course design and instruction and then describes course activities and the ways in which the participants engaged in them. Specific features of the course that supported teacher learning are discussed, the instructor's and participants' perspectives on the course are shared, and evidence of teacher learning is presented. The chapter concludes with lessons learned and a discussion of potential areas of research related to supporting teacher learning in online environments.

INTRODUCTION

In an era when teacher qualifications and accountability for student achievement have increasingly come into the public view, providing high-quality teacher professional development has become more critical than ever. Fortunately, many teacher education programs have recognized this need and have taken on the challenge of developing high-quality, long-term learning experiences that build on what is known about teacher learning and effective professional development (e.g., Jacobs, Franke, Carpenter, Levi & Battey, 2007; Silver & Stein, 1996). Unfortunately, these programs often reach only a limited number of teachers, typically those who teach in larger urban schools where teachers participate as a school-based team or those who have easy access to a university where such programs are offered. Meeting the educational needs of rural teachers has been a greater challenge.

To address this need, a course was developed in which a group of rural secondary school mathematics teachers met in an online synchronous videoconference over one university semester. This

DOI: 10.4018/978-1-61520-899-9.ch007

chapter discusses the design, implementation and outcomes of this course. In particular, the chapter: (1) makes explicit the thinking behind the course—the course goals, design and content, including the research literature that influenced each; (2) describes the ways in which teachers participated in the course; (3) presents both the instructor's and the participants' perceptions of how the course supported learning; (4) describes the outcomes of the course in terms of teacher learning; and (5) discusses how the course could be redesigned to better support teacher learning.

BACKGROUND

To meet the needs of teachers who cannot easily travel to a university to complete coursework or attend professional development sessions to satisfy licensure requirements, teacher education programs have increasingly turned to distance education as a means of providing teacher learning opportunities. Many of the online courses described in the literature are asynchronous in nature; this model is beneficial in that it allows participants to complete coursework at their convenience, but may limit the kinds of professional development that can be offered and the sense of community that can be developed (Lock, 2006; Parr & Ward, 2006). Synchronous online courses tend to most often use text chats (e.g., Anagnostopoulos, Basmadjian & McCrory, 2005; Jin, 2005) or video conferencing (e.g., Rovai & Lucking, 2003) for real-time interactions among participants. Although these models might offer some advantages over asynchronous courses, there are still substantial limitations. Text chats, for instance, leave the participants essentially anonymous to one other, while traditional video conferencing often requires travel to a site where the necessary technology is available—which may be a substantial distance for some rural educators. Furthermore, all of these online models pose challenges to teacher educators who wish to engage teachers in substantive discussions about content and pedagogy in ways that are responsive to research on teacher learning (e.g., Ball & Cohen, 1999).

Although research on online learning has generally found no significant differences between student learning in online and on-campus courses (e.g., Caywood & Duckett, 2003; Phipps & Merisotis, 1999), it has also found that technology-based professional development is likely to be ineffective if it does not include substantial instructor-participant and participant-participant interaction (Lock, 2006; McLoughlin, 2002; O'Hanlon, 2007). This finding is not particularly surprising, as it parallels research findings on characteristics of quality teacher professional development in general that suggest there should be a focus on developing a strong learning community among the professional development participants (Darling-Hammond, Wei, Andree, Richardson & Orphanos, 2009). As Parr and Ward (2006) note, however, "(b)uilding a professional learning community is difficult to achieve within a school, let alone across schools, let alone virtually" (p. 790). To develop an effective learning community in an online environment, considerable groundwork must be laid and an intentional ongoing effort must be made to continuously promote this development. The establishment of trust and respect, in particular, are critical if teachers are to work collaboratively to advance their learning and improve their practice with others they know only virtually—especially in situations where teachers are asked to share artifacts of their own practice as part of the learning process.

In addition to the development of a professional learning community, a recent review of research on teacher professional development (Darling-Hammond et. al, 2009) found a number of other characteristics that are critical to teacher learning, which have also been echoed by others in the field (e.g., Ball & Cohen, 1997; Loucks-Horsley, Love, Stiles, Mundry & Hewson, 2003; Putnam & Borko, 1997). One major finding is that professional development should take place over time—in contrast to one-time workshops or seminars that were the norm for professional development of the past. Learning opportunities should also be closely connected to the work that teachers do. This could be accomplished by studying written or video cases of practices, studying artifacts of teachers' own practice, and providing opportunities for teachers to "try out" new ideas and techniques in their own classroom as part of the professional learning experience.

It has also been found that the most effective teacher professional development focuses on learning subject-specific content, rather than on general pedagogical issues, and has goals that are consistent with those of the individual teacher participants and the schools in which they work. Direct connections to the teachers' contexts make the learning immediately relevant to their classroom practice and supports the work teachers are required to do in their schools outside of the classroom.

The research on professional learning in general and aspects that are specific to distance education significantly influenced the design of the online course. In the following section, the issues that led to the development of the course are first discussed, followed by a description of the thinking behind the course design, including connections to the research literature.

The Course

Issues

The university that offered the online course is committed to supporting K-12 education, particularly through offering high-quality professional development opportunities to secondary school teachers in STEM-related (Science, Technology, Engineering And Mathematics) disciplines. In fact, over the years, the university has developed and delivered numerous graduate-level courses to hundreds of teachers from across the state and beyond, most of them grant-funded. Evaluators of these programs have consistently documented positive outcomes in terms of participants' increased content knowledge, knowledge of state and national standards, knowledge of diverse learners, and confidence in implementing new ideas into their instruction; more significantly, classroom observations have documented that teachers have integrated this learning into their classroom practice. In recent years, however, program personnel have experienced increased difficulty recruiting and retaining teachers in these professional development courses and programs, largely due to the university's remote location—over 500 miles from the urban centers of the state. Significant travel distances and the amount of time programs have required teachers to spend away from their families have caused many teachers to either not enroll or to drop out midway through grant programs.

To alleviate these problems, the teacher education department initially developed asynchronous online courses, delivering course content through web-based course management systems such as WebCT and Blackboard (Blackboard, Inc., 1997-2009). While this format continues to work well for some courses that are largely reading-based, it would not work as well in the type of course the instructor envisioned—one where teachers collectively studied artifacts of practice, analyzed students' understandings, and worked together as a community to develop content-specific pedagogies that would better support student learning. Thus, a blended online synchronous course was developed in order to enable the instructor to include activities in the course that more closely paralleled those that she would include in an on-campus course, using practice-based resources such as cases of practice and student written work as the foundation for the course instruction. While a course management system was still used in the course, it played a supplementary role to an interactive videoconferencing system that was used to host the course sessions.

Program and Participants

The course described in this chapter was the first course teachers were enrolled in as part of a two-year grant-funded professional development program focused on teaching algebra to a diverse student population. The program was developed in response to the state's new graduation requirements that expect all high school students to complete two years of algebra. Feedback from local teachers had indicated a widespread concern about how they would adapt their practices in order to help all students be successful—including many students who in the past may not have enrolled in higher-level mathematics courses. The overall goals of the professional development program were to introduce teachers to current research and thinking about the teaching of mathematics, to engage them in discussions about content-specific practices that would help them support student learning, to support them as they began to implement new ideas and study the outcomes in their own classrooms, and to help them take on leadership roles both in their local area and in the state.

Program participants were recruited from a rural area that geographically covers about one-third of the of a U.S. Midwestern state's land area, but contains only 3% of the state's population. This area was targeted because it includes a large number of small, rural school districts, most of which are not near a university and many that are small enough to have only a single full-time mathematics teacher serving their secondary school population. Thus, many of the teachers in the target area did not have site-based colleagues in their content area with whom to collaborate and could not easily access high-quality professional development.

The participants in the course were ten secondary school mathematics teachers, divided equally among males and females. They ranged from a first-year teacher to a veteran teacher with over 20 years of experience. Five of the participants held Master's degrees, one of whom was simultaneously working on completing an online doctorate degree at another institution. Half of the participants, including the first year teacher, were in mathematics departments with two or fewer teachers. Each of the teachers in these smaller schools had five or six different course preparations per day as part of their teaching assignment; one of these was teaching at an alternative education school. Some of the teachers had previously met one another at local meetings or workshops, but none of the teachers knew each other well or had collaborated in the past.

Course Goals and Design Principles

The goal of the online course was to engage teachers in discussions about content-specific pedagogical practices through the study of actual instances and artifacts of practices. Informed by research on teacher professional learning, there were four main principles that significantly influenced the course design: (1) the work was to be grounded in the teachers' practice so that it would be immediately relevant and connected to their work; (2) there would be a focus on developing a learning community that could become an ongoing professional support network for the participants after the conclusion of the grant program; (3) the course would focus on developing content-specific knowledge by concentrating on teachers' mathematical knowledge for teaching (Ball, Bass & Hill, 2004); and (4) the course content and instruction would need to respect the developmental learning trajectories (Simon & Tzur, 2004) of the teacher participants—from those with limited teaching experience, to those who were already beginning to reexamine their existing practices. The ways in which each of these principles was addressed in the course design are discussed in the following paragraphs.

The course was grounded in practice in a variety of ways. The early part of the course centered on analyzing cases of practice, in both written and video form—an approach that has been shown to support teacher learning in a number of important ways (e.g., Seago, 2004; Sherin, 2004; Sherin & van Es, 2005; Stockero, 2008). This work began with each teacher individually solving a mathematical task that was the focus of the case, after which they participated in a whole-group discussion. This discussion involved examining the ways individual teachers had thought about the task and predicting ways that students might approach it. To facilitate this discussion, each task that was chosen could be solved in multiple ways, using traditional mathematical procedures, as well as more visual methods. Classroom video clips and written cases of practice grounded the work of the course in actual instances of teaching. The cases that were used were not meant to be exemplars of practice, but rather, were chosen to raise issues and stimulate discussion about the teaching and learning of mathematics. The way the cases were used—the questions that were asked and the activities that teachers participated in around them—were based on research on practice-based professional development (e.g., Ball & Cohen, 1999) and were purposeful in using the specifics of practice to ground discussions about generalities. An important part of this work was using research-based frameworks such as *The Task Analysis Guide* (Stein, Smith, Henningsen & Silver, 2000) and *The Mathematical Task Framework* (Stein & Smith, 1998), which focus on the design and implementation of high-level mathematical tasks. These frameworks were introduced at the start of the course and were continually referenced as a way to keep course discussions focused on the new ideas that were being introduced in the course, rather than reverting to the story-sharing that often occurs when teachers engage in discussions of practice.

Based on the knowledge that "strong professional development communities are important contributors to instructional improvement and school reform" (Little, 2002, p. 936) and the instructor's perceived inability to achieve a strong learning community in previous asynchronous online professional development courses, this course was deliberately planned so that the continual development of a learning community would be central to the course design and activities. First, community development influenced the selection of the software that was to be used in the course—it had to provide a way for the participants to interact in an environment where they could both see and hear each other to avoid the anonymity and isolation that has been documented in online learning environments (e.g., Rice, 2006; Steinman, 2007). In addition, course activities were planned to allow the participants to directly interact with one other in real time, in both whole- and small-group discussions. The instructor deliberately structured and facilitated these interactions so that participants would get to know one other in a meaningful way during the course as they worked together to analyze teaching and learning and plan for instruction in their own classrooms.

The courses' emphasis on developing mathematical knowledge for teaching was influenced by Ball, Bass and Hill's (2004) set of content-specific pedagogical abilities essential to effective mathematics instruction. These abilities were developed in the course by providing opportunities for the participants to consider: the characteristics of good mathematical questions and tasks; what accurate and useful mathematical explanations might look like at the secondary-school level; how to represent ideas carefully and translate among mathematical representations; alternate interpretations of students' ideas; and how to respond productively to students' mathematical questions.

Simon and Tzur's (2004) set of design principles for planning mathematics instruction influenced the instructors' thinking about how to design and sequence the course activities in order to meet the wide range of needs of the teachers enrolled. Using this model, course design begins with identifying content-specific pedagogical understandings and abilities that are to be developed, which, in turn, form the basis for creating hypothetical learning trajectories that the participants are projected to follow as they work to meet the goals of the course. The instructor then designs a particular set of learning tasks that are anticipated to help achieve those goals. While the instructor planned a general sequence of learning activities that would be used during instruction prior to the start of the course, these tasks evolved on an ongoing basis in response to what the instructor learned about teachers' current understandings and learning needs. For example, during one case analysis in which the participants' attention turned to teacher questioning, it became apparent that most had not considered the ways in which their questions could constrain student thinking. This insight led the instructor to assign readings about teacher questioning that were discussed at the following course meeting; these provided a language that enabled the participants to subsequently talk about teacher questioning in a more productive way. This ongoing modification of the course in response to teacher learning is in contrast to the way that the design of many online courses is described in the literature, where learning modules are completely developed prior to the start of the course (Dykman & Davis, 2008).

Course Content

The blended online course began with a one-day face-to-face introductory meeting at a location geographically central to the participants. At this meeting, the participants completed grant paperwork, participated in introductory content-based activities, and were introduced to research-based frameworks that would be used to focus the online activities that took place in the remainder of the course. A significant focus of the course instructor during this meeting was on beginning to develop a professional learning community among the participants and to establish professional learning norms for the group that would be necessary to support productive online discussions. Thus, the day's activities were structured to allow for significant small- and whole-group interaction and sharing of ideas, during which the instructor worked to develop norms that included carefully listening to and considering others' ideas, using evidence and frameworks to support analyses, and developing a stance of inquiry about teaching and learning, rather than immediately drawing definitive conclusions about a teachers' instructional decisions or students' thinking. Although productive norms cannot be developed in a single day, this meeting provided a foundation for how the participants would interact in the subsequent online meetings.

Following the initial meeting, the course met online for four 3 ½-hour sessions that took place after the teachers' school work hours. Although more frequent, shorter sessions may have been ideal, the course instructor allowed the teachers in the course to have input into the course meeting times in order to accommodate family circumstances and school calendars, and to work around extra-curricular obligations that are common to teachers in small, rural districts. Complicating matters further was the fact that the teachers were living in two different time zones; thus, flexibility in scheduling was key to making the course work for everyone involved.

Prior to each course session, participants accessed course materials via the Blackboard course management system. Participants were often required to complete mathematics education readings about topics such as student discourse, mathematical justification, and mathematical tasks, and submit a brief online response or complete some other type of assignment before a class meeting. All assignments were submitted in Blackboard at least one day prior to the course meeting to allow the instructor time to read the responses and consider ways in which the teachers' current understandings should be incorporated into and addressed in the planned activities for the class session.

During the online course sessions, teachers participated in professional development activities that closely resembled those the instructor had previously used in on-campus courses. Examples of activities that were central to the course included sharing and discussing teachers' own mathematical thinking, examining student thinking, analyzing cases of practice, and discussing readings and research about pedagogical issues. Later in the course, participants worked together to help one another develop high-level mathematical tasks that were then used as the basis for a lesson in the teacher's classroom.

To ensure that the participants would try to implement ideas from the course into their classroom practice, the final course project required each teacher to design and teach a lesson in their own classroom that centered about the mathematical task they had developed. This took place following the final online course meeting. After the lesson was implemented, each teacher was required to write his or her own case of practice—similar to those that had been analyzed during the course. These cases were then shared and discussed with the other participants during a face-to-face meeting that concluded the course, using research-based frameworks to provide focus to the teachers' analyses of their own and their peers' practice. During this meeting, participants also completed final course paperwork, and collectively considered open issues that might be addressed in the second course in the professional development program. Although it is the instructor's opinion that this final face-to-face meeting was probably not necessary since all of the teacher were effectively navigating and participating in the online environment, the meeting was held since it had been scheduled at the start of the course.

Online Participation

Each individual teacher participated in the online course meetings at his or her home or school location by accessing the course on a computer with Internet access. This individual access was a critical component of the courses' success, since the participants were geographically spread out over a distance of more than 250 miles and no two teachers were from the same school. As part of the grant funding, each teacher was provided with a web-camera and a digital tablet that were used to access and participate in the course; they were shown how to do so at the initial course meeting. Participants were urged to set up the equipment and test their course access in advance of the first online meeting. The instructor made herself available for this testing at the participants' convenience, which seemed to be a critical support system for some teachers who had limited experience using computer technologies.

The course used the Marratech videoconferencing software (Marratech AB, 1998-2008), which was hosted by the university at the time that the course took place. This software displays an individual thumbnail video of each participant and the instructor. This thumbnail automatically becomes a larger video display for the participant who is currently speaking. Each teacher could see and hear both the instructor and the other participants in real time; in addition, teachers' names were displayed beneath their thumbnail video, which allowed participants to get to know one another more quickly and speak to one other by name. These features of the videoconferencing software are believed to have significantly contributed to the sense of community that was developed in the course.

From a teaching perspective, Marratech allows the instructor or participants to load presentations, word documents and images into the course to display on a whiteboard, as well as to share applications that are running on their computer desktop. The whiteboard also includes a number of communication tools. Early in the course, it was mainly the instructor who controlled the course content; later in the course, however, participants shared both their own and their students' work either by emailing it to the instructor in advance or by directly loading it to the whiteboard during a course meeting. Throughout the course, participants shared their mathematical thinking and other ideas by writing on their digital tablet, which displayed on the course whiteboard. The software also allows the whiteboards to be saved and the course meetings to be videotaped. Although these features of the software were not used on a regular basis during the course, they were used on occasions when individual teachers missed part of a course meeting.

One critical design feature that the software did not effectively support was small-group breakout sessions. To work around this issue, three additional course rooms were created that participants could move into for small-group meetings. The difficulty here was that in order to do so, the participants had to log out of the main course room and then into the small-group breakout room to which they were assigned; this also made it difficult for the course instructor to move between the groups to listen to and participate in small-group discussions. It should be noted that other videoconferencing software does include features that allow the instructor to create breakout groups and assign participants to them prior to a course meeting. During the meeting, the instructor can then quickly move participants from the main room into their small groups. The university has since adopted a new videoconferencing software program (Adobe Systems, Inc., 2001-2009) that includes this and other enhanced features.

Participants' and Instructor's Perspectives

The online learning environment was rated highly by both the teacher participants and by the course instructor. At the conclusion of the course, the participants were asked to assess the effectiveness of the online synchronous environment in meeting both their personal and professional needs. One participant noted that she liked the online course because of time and travel, and felt that "just as much learning occurred online as in face-to-face." Another said, "I have taken both real time online and asynchronous online classes and this was far better—equivalent to an onsite class." A third participant concurred, and went on to discuss issues that were quite significant in terms of course instruction:

The online learning was awesome! It was relaxing and thought provoking. The teacher did a wonderful job initiating conversation. She was well-organized, with documents and lessons and we could easily follow her. The group work online was also a great idea. I think this technology is effective and more teachers would be a part of this if they knew more about the online component!

This participant reflection raises an important issue for the online instructor: organization. Even though the course instructor had previously taught online courses—both asynchronous professional development courses for teachers and a synchronous calculus course for high school students—the level of organization necessary for a course such as this was significantly greater. The main reason for this was the length of time that the course met—3 ½ hours per session. This meant that the instructor had to be ready to load new electronic documents into the course in a seamless way as participants moved from one course activity to the next, and, in some cases, had to be ready with more than one activity in order to be responsive to the teacher learning that she observed during the session. In short, the instructor found it necessary to be thinking ahead to the next activity, while at the same time being engaged in the current activity in a way that allowed her to push participants' thinking and facilitate productive interactions among participants. In hindsight, it may have been more productive to have more frequent, shorter course meetings, as this would have made the preparation and organization more manageable and have given the instructor more opportunities to adapt instruction to the learners' needs. The course meeting times were chosen in order to be responsive to the learners' personal needs, however, which was also an important consideration in order to meet the program's goal of attracting and retaining teachers for the duration of the two-year grant program.

Although the participants' responses to the course were positive overall, this is not to say that there were not difficulties. A number of teachers had problems initially accessing the course, largely due to firewall issues at their schools or their own discomfort using online learning technologies. In all but one case, the firewall issues were resolved fairly quickly through communications between technology support personnel at the local schools and the university. One teacher never fully resolved the issues with his connection, however, and thus intermittently lost his connection and had to log back in to the course. Even the teachers who experienced such difficulties, however, had generally positive things to say about the course. One teacher, for instance, said, "I had lots of difficulty at first—old equipment and poor connection. But once everything worked, it was much better than driving." The participant with the most significant and ongoing problems noted that, "Although I had *many* problems with the physical connection, the intervals that I got to participate in were good. The added dimension of seeing/hearing the other participants was valuable (although I won't lie, it made for a long day)."

From the instructor's perspective, the course was particularly effective in developing a professional learning community that very closely paralleled those observed in effective on-campus courses. In their research focused on analyzing interactions in an online threaded discussion board, Waltonen-Moore and colleagues (2006) describe five levels of participation through which teachers advance: introduction, identification, interaction, involvement and inquiry. The teachers who participated in this course were able to quickly move past the introduction and identification stages—where participants meet and begin to relate to one another—and even in the first online meeting were observed to engage in interactions that indicated that a community of learners was evolving. For instance, the teachers talked directly to one other, rather than through the instructor, and addressed each other by name, responding to their colleagues' comments and offering alternative interpretations of the cases of practice that were being discussed. By the final online course meeting, participants were observed to be critical, yet respectful and supportive, in small-group discussions in which they discussed and modified the tasks their colleagues had developed and considered how to best implement these tasks in the classroom. Moreover, teachers regularly raised issues for the group to consider and were comfortable asking for advice when they were unsure about the best ways to use particular tasks with their students. When the participants met for the final course meeting and in the next course in the program, it was evident that they had developed positive collegial relationships. Some had even become friends and communicated with one another outside of the program. This is particularly important in this instance, as a number of the rural teachers in the course did not have collegial support in their own school buildings.

Teacher Learning

The program evaluation was not designed to measure teacher learning during this one course, but rather, to measure learning over the 2-year professional development program. Despite a lack of formal evaluation data, however, there is some evidence that the course was effective in meeting the goal of developing content-specific pedagogical knowledge. At the start of the grant program, immediately prior to the online course, seven of the participants were observed teaching a lesson in their classrooms. All seven of the lessons observed followed a similar pattern—the teacher introduced new ideas and provided examples on the board, and then students had time to try similar examples on their own or in small groups. There was some student participation and teacher questioning in some of the classrooms, but most of the interaction was focused on helping students recall procedures that they had previously learned, rather than on sharing novel mathematical thinking or developing new ideas. None of the classroom lessons were focused around rich mathematical tasks that required students to develop mathematical ideas or to extend ideas they had previously learned to new situations. In short, none of the teachers were observed to engage students in "doing mathematics" (Stein, Smith, Henningsen & Silver, 2000).

The cases that the teacher participants wrote for their final course project provide some insight into changes in their thinking and practice as a result of their work in the course. To complete the project, all of the teachers had to attempt to teach in a way that was substantially different from the teaching that was observed at the start of the program; the fact that they all did so was significant in itself. Although not all of the tasks that the participants initially planned to use in their classrooms were high-level tasks, all of them were modified during the small- and whole-class online interactions to include characteristics of high-level tasks. In fact, one participant noted that "some of the problems didn't seem higher order to me; however, with discussion, we made those problems reach that level. It just shows that collaboration and support can really help teachers."

In their analyses of the task implementation, nine of the ten participants were able to use a framework introduced in the course (Stein & Smith, 1998) to identify factors that either led to the maintenance or decline of the level of the task during the lesson. From the description of the lesson and excerpts of transcripts that were provided, the course instructor felt that eight of the nine were accurate analyses. Although four of the participants were unable to successfully implement the lesson they had planned, each was able to analyze why the level of the task declined during his or her implementation. One teacher for instance, wrote that she was too leading and reverted to choral responses from students, while another found that she essentially did the problem for her students once they began to struggle. Interestingly, three teachers noted that the normative behaviors in their classrooms actually inhibited the task implementation, since their students were not accustomed to working on mathematical tasks that did not have a defined procedure to follow and, as a result, tended to give up too easily. All three of these teachers reflected that it would be important to rethink their expectations for students and the norms for their classroom prior to the start of the next academic year. Thus, although not all of the teachers were successful at teaching in a new way, they were able to view their practice differently, which provided a solid foundation for the work in subsequent courses in the program.

FUTURE RESEARCH DIRECTION

The course described here was developed as part of a professional development grant for rural mathematics teachers, and thus, conducting research around the course delivery and learning outcomes was not a central focus. During implementation of the course, however, it became apparent that there are numerous avenues for fruitful research focused on the design and implementation of online teacher professional development courses.

In the course described, no teachers dropped out during the semester, which is in contrast to the significant drop-out rates described in the distance education literature (Phipps & Merisotis, 1999; Rice, 2006). This raises questions related to teachers' motives for enrolling in online courses, attributes of successful online teacher-learners, and features of online teacher education courses that teachers perceive to be more or less effective in meeting their personal and professional learning needs. It may be the case, for instance, that this course was perceived differently than other online courses because the face-to-face synchronous interactions more closely resembled those the participants were accustomed to in previous teacher education courses.

The instructor's prior research has focused on the use of practice-based materials, and in particular on the use of video cases in teacher education; this significantly influenced the design of this course. Teaching this course has raised the issue, however, of whether the types of learning outcomes that have been observed in on-campus courses are achieved to the same degree in an online environment. In more general terms, there is a need for research focused on issues related to transferring elements of effective teacher professional development that have been studied in site-based environments to an online environment where the interactions among participants are mediated by the technologies used in the course.

Finally, if online teacher professional development is to be used to bring high-quality learning opportunities to an audience of underserved teachers who are great distances from the site where the professional development is offered, researchers must consider ways to study the impact of professional development not only on teacher knowledge, but also on their classroom practice. Classroom observations will be used as one measure of the impact of this professional development program on teachers' practice, but this is only practical because the participants are all within 200 miles of the university—a distance that still poses some challenges in terms of time and resources. To measure course impact and study more general issues related to online teacher learning, researchers will need to be creative in using technology to not only deliver instruction, but to collect data that can be used for course and program evaluation, as well as for more formal research on teacher learning in online environments. As technologies continue to advance, the possibilities for their creative use are endless; it is our task to think about how to use them with teachers in ways that meet our needs as researchers, while at the same time are easy for teachers to engage with as they work to improve their practice.

CONCLUSION

The blended online synchronous course described in this chapter was developed specifically to meet the needs of a group of rural mathematics teachers. Although it was designed in a mathematics context, many of the design principles and lessons learned apply equally to teacher professional development courses in other content areas. Most importantly, if online teacher professional development is to be effective and result in improved teaching and learning, teacher educators must consider not only how to deliver content via electronic means, but must also consider how to engage teachers in learning opportunities that are responsive to research on effective teacher professional development. This involves integrating what is known about best practices in distance education with best practices in teacher professional development in order to design teacher education courses that include both general and content-specific elements that support teacher learning. One such element the instructor of this course, as well as others, have found to be particularly critical to online teacher professional development is a focus on developing a professional learning community in which teachers are able to discuss and debate the difficult issues they face in their daily work with colleagues who they trust and are supportive of them, yet are still able to push their thinking in productive ways. This does not happen spontaneously; in this course, it had to be nurtured by the instructor in ongoing, deliberate ways, since the participants did not know each other and were not physically together. If this community is not developed in an online course, not only will learning be compromised, but feelings of isolation and disconnectedness could cause teachers to withdraw from the online course.

The course described in this chapter is just one example of a blended online synchronous course that resulted in positive learning outcomes, and was perceived by both the instructor and participants as meeting their learning needs. As technologies continue to evolve and we learn more about supporting teacher learning in general, and in an online environment in particular, teacher educators must be creative in thinking about how to meet the professional learning needs of teachers who traditionally may not have had access to high-quality professional development. In this example, the instructor designed the course to parallel in an online environment the types of activities she had previously used in on-campus courses. Future technologies, however, could offer the potential to not only parallel on-site courses, but to actually enhance teacher learning. If online learning is to reach its full potential, we need continue to think beyond what is, to what could be, and then collaboratively share and study emerging best practices in online teacher learning.

REFERENCES

Adobe Systems, Inc. (2001-2009). *Adobe Acrobat Connect Pro*. San Jose, CA: Adobe Systems, Inc.

Anagnostopoulos, D., Basmadjian, K. G., & McCrory, R. S. (2005). The decentered teacher and the construction of social space in the virtual classroom. *Teachers College Record, 107*(8), 1699–1729. doi:10.1111/j.1467-9620.2005.00539.x

Ball, D. L., Bass, H., & Hill, H. C. (2004). Knowing and using mathematical knowledge in teaching: Learning what matters. In A. Buffler & R. C. Laugksch (Eds.), *Proceedings of the 12th Annual Conference of the Southern African Association for Research in Mathematics, Science and Technology Education*. Durban: SAARMSTE.

Ball, D. L., & Cohen, D. K. (1999). Developing practices, developing practitioners. In Darling-Hammond, L., & Sykes, G. (Eds.), *Teaching as the learning profession: Handbook of policy and practice* (pp. 3–32). San Francisco: Jossey-Bass.

Blackboard, Inc. (1997-2009). *Blackboard Learning System*. Washington, DC: Blackboard, Inc.

Caywood, K., & Duckett, J. (2003). Online vs. on-campus learning in teacher education. *Teacher Education and Special Education, 26*(2), 98–105. doi:10.1177/088840640302600203

Darling-Hammond, L., Wei, R. C., Andree, A., Richardson, N., & Orphanos, S. (2009). *Professional learning in the learning profession: A status report on teacher development in the United States and abroad*. Dallas, TX: National Staff Development Council.

Dykman, C. A., & Davis, C. K. (2008). Online education forum—part three: A quality online educational experience. *Journal of Information Systems Education, 19*(3), 281–289.

Jacobs, V. R., Franke, M. L., Carpenter, T. P., Levi, L., & Battey, D. (2007). Professional development focused on children's algebraic reasoning in elementary school. *Journal for Research in Mathematics Education, 38*(3), 258–288.

Jin, S. H. (2005). Analyzing student-student and student-instructor interaction through multiple communication tools in web-based learning. *International Journal of Instructional Media, 32*(1), 59–67.

Little, J. W. (2002). Locating learning in teachers' communities of practice: Opening up problems of analysis in records of everyday practice. *Teaching and Teacher Education, 18*, 917–946. doi:10.1016/S0742-051X(02)00052-5

Lock, J. V. (2006). A new image: Online communities to facilitate teacher professional development. *Journal of Technology and Teacher Education, 14*(4), 663–678.

Loucks-Horsley, S., Love, N., Stiles, K. E., Mundry, S., & Hewson, P. W. (2003). *Designing professional development for teachers of science and mathematics* (2nd ed.). Thousand Oaks, CA: Corwin Press, Inc.

Marratech AB. (1998-2008). *Marratech (version 6.1.2)*. Stockholm, Sweden: Marratech AB.

McLoughlin, C. (2002). Learner support in distanceand networked learning environments: Ten dimensions for successful design. *Distance Education, 23*(2), 149–162. doi:10.1080/0158791022000009178

O'Hanlon, C. (2007). The teacher becomes the student. *T.H.E. Journal, 34*(11), 21–22.

Parr, J., & Ward, L. (2006). Building on foundations: Creating an online community. *Journal of Technology and Teacher Education, 14*(4), 775–793.

Phipps, R., & Merisotis, J. (1999). *What's the difference? A review of contemporary research on the effectiveness of distance learning in higher education*. Washington, DC: Institute for Higher Education Policy. Retrieved April 3, 2009 from http://www2.nea.org/he/abouthe/distance.html

Putnam, R. T., & Borko, H. (1997). Teacher learning: Implications of new views of cognition. In Biddle, B. J., Good, T. L., & Goodson, I. F. (Eds.), *International Handbook of Teachers and Teaching* (*Vol. 2*, pp. 1223–1296). Dordrecht, The Netherlands: Kluwer Academic Publishers.

Rice, K. L. (2006). A comprehensive look at distance education in the K-12 context. *Journal of Research on Technology in Education, 38*(4), 425–448.

Rovai, A. P., & Lucking, R. (2003). Sense of community in a higher education television-based distance education program. *Educational Technology Research and Development, 51*(2), 5–16. doi:10.1007/BF02504523

Seago, N. (2004). Using video as an object of inquiry for mathematics teaching and learning. In Brophy, J. (Ed.), *Using video in teacher education* (pp. 259–286). Oxford, UK: Elsevier.

Sherin, M. G. (2004). New perspectives on the role of video in teacher education. In Brophy, J. (Ed.), *Using video in teacher education* (pp. 1–28). Oxford, UK: Elsevier Ltd.

Sherin, M. G., & van Es, E. A. (2005). Using video to support teachers' ability to notice classroom interactions. *Journal of Technology and Teacher Education, 13*(3), 475–491.

Silver, E. A., & Stein, M. K. (1996). The QUASAR Project: The Revolution of the Possible in mathematics instructional reform in urban middle schools. *Urban Education, 30*(4), 476–521. doi:10.1177/0042085996030004006

Simon, M. A., & Tzur, R. (2004). Explicating the role of mathematical tasks in conceptual learning: An elaboration of the hypothetical learning trajectory. *Mathematical Thinking and Learning, 6*(2), 91–104. doi:10.1207/s15327833mtl0602_2

Stein, M. K., & Smith, M. S. (1998). Mathematical tasks as a framework for reflection: From research to practice. *Mathematics Teaching in the Middle School, 3*(4), 268–275.

Stein, M. K., Smith, M. S., Henningsen, M. A., & Silver, E. A. (2000). *Implementing standards based mathematics instruction: A casebook for professional development*. New York: Teachers College Press.

Steinman, D. (2007). Educational experiences and the online student. *TechTrends, 51*(5), 46–52. doi:10.1007/s11528-007-0069-x

Stockero, S. L. (2008). Differences in preservice mathematics teachers' reflective abilities attributable to use of a video case curriculum. *Journal of Technology and Teacher Education*, *16*(4), 433–458.

Waltonen-Moore, S., Stuart, D., Newton, E., Oswald, R., & Varonis, E. (2006). From virtual strangers to a cohesive online learning community: The evolution of online group development in a professional development community. *Journal of Technology and Teacher Education*, *14*(2), 287–311.

Chapter 8
Synergy: Service Learning in Undergraduate Instructional Technology Courses

Jacqueline M. Mumford
Walsh University, USA

Elizabeth Juelich-Velotta
Walsh University, USA

ABSTRACT

Synergy describes a situation where the combined efforts are greater than individual parts. Service learning ties together academic content, in this case instructional technology, while providing service. This chapter offers an orientation to an exceptionally rewarding service learning activity in an instructional technology course. Based upon a case study and extensive literature review, this chapter provides best practices for fostering the synergy between service learning and instructional technology courses. This approach increased teacher candidates' exposure to diversity, served community needs, and facilitated candidate practice of skills from instructional technology class.

INTRODUCTION

In instructional technology courses, teacher candidates are taught to use a variety of tools for instruction. Some instructional technology courses require field experience where pre-service teacher candidates observe and interact with in-service teachers and students in schools. A service learning model provides candidates with an opportunity to put the theory they are learning in the classroom into practice while serving the community. Service learning sites provide unique field opportunities for teacher candidates to work with diverse student populations. The resulting experience can be both rich and rewarding.

Service learning is an activity that meets identified community needs and connects course content with real life experiences. By exposing instructional technology undergraduate teacher candidates to service learning, significant benefits are possible. Howard (1998) also indicated that academic service learning is a synergistic model where the students' experiences in community settings are just as valuable to the students' learning experience as any other element within the course. Citing a reciprocal relationship between service and learning, he posited

DOI: 10.4018/978-1-61520-899-9.ch008

that the service experiences of his students both "inform and transform the academic learning and the academic learning informs and transforms the service experience" (p.22). This chapter will explore the benefits of this approach to instructional technology courses through literature review and a case study.

This chapter will:

- Explain the synergistic relationship between instructional technology and service learning in undergraduate teacher preparation.
- Define service learning through both a historical and teacher preparation lens.
- Investigate stakeholder responsibilities and benefits of service learning.
- Detail a case study from a small, private, Midwestern university.
- Discuss best practices, documentation, and integration of experiences.
- Provide recommended readings.
- Establish an agenda for future research.

THE NECESSITY AND COMPLEXITY OF FIELD EXPERIENCES

The National Council for Accreditation of Teacher Education (NCATE) defines field experience as "A variety of early ongoing field-based opportunities in which candidates may observe, assist, tutor, instruct, and/or conduct research. Field experiences may occur in off-campus settings such as schools, community centers, or homeless shelters" (2008, p. 86). Field experiences are considered critical to teacher preparation programs (McIntyre, Byrd, & Foxx, 1997). This experiential work provides an opportunity for teacher candidates to interact in an authentic instructional setting. Candidates teach, facilitate learning, and connect theory from classes to actual practice in their field placements. Such field experiences promote increased emotional involvement and intrinsic motivation for candidate success (Casey & Howson, 1993). By integrating field experience partnerships between K-12 schools and universities, positive results have been reported (Clark, Foster & Mantle-Bromley, 2005).

Although field experience has been a longstanding hallmark of teacher education, integrating field experience into educational technology was a relatively new concept just a decade ago. Many reports surfaced in the late 1990s indicating that a restructuring of technology preparation toward integrative models (theory and practice) was necessary in order to prepare teachers for the digital age (Larson & Clift, 1996). According to one report from Willis and Mehlinger, 1996:

Most pre-service teachers know very little about effective use of technology in education and leaders believe there is a pressing need to increase substantially the amount and quality of instruction teachers receive about technology... [T]he virtual universal conclusion is that teacher education, particularly pre-service, is not preparing educators to work in a technology-enriched classroom. (p. 978).

Field experiences integrating technology were recognized as solutions to the deficits in teacher technology skills (Brush, Igoe, Glazewski, Ku, & Smith, 2001). In a 1999 paper, Strudler and Wetzel detailed programs that provided pre-service teachers with technology experiences in the field prior to student teaching. In reaction to the reports and recommended solutions, models were developed that provided teacher candidates with authentic experiences focusing on effective use of instructional media (Dexter & Reidel, 2003; National Council for the Accreditation of Teacher Education [NCATE], 2008).

More recently, teacher preparation programs began confronting another issue: preparing teacher candidates to teach in diverse settings. Public schools are becoming more diverse, while the teachers remain predominantly White, female, and middle-class (Swartz, 2003). There is a certain "cultural discontinuity" (Irvine, 2003) that may produce negative interactions and reinforce teacher candidate stereotypes. This cultural discontinuity creates a divide between the teachers and the students they are teaching. The literature indicates that teachers need to have more field experiences with diverse student populations in order to understand students and offer better instructional experiences (Graybill, 1997; Pransky & Bailey, 2002/2003). Research indicates that field experiences in culturally diverse urban settings encourage teacher candidates to teach in culturally responsive ways (Barnes, 2006; Gay, 2000).

MAKING THE CASE: A CASE STUDY ON INTEGRATING SERVICE LEARNING

In an effort to address the technology deficit, as well as the need for diverse experiences, a program was developed and implemented in the undergraduate teacher preparation program at a small, private, Midwestern university. Service learning is a general education requirement for all undergraduate students at this institution. Instructional Technology is a required core course for all teacher candidates.

Since fall 2006, every teacher candidate in Instructional Technology has been required to complete a minimum of ten hours of structured service learning field experience. This service learning field experience for instructional technology was piloted in three phases. In every phase, teacher candidates completed structured pre-service reflections, kept reflective logs, and participated in service share sessions in class. Service shares will be discussed further in the case study narrative. These experiences tied the theory of instructional technology and pedagogy to the practice of working in a diverse setting with students via service learning.

There was a distinct lack of substantive research and literature on integrating service learning with instructional technology courses. In the literature review process, no research on this specific connection with undergraduate students was located. However, significant information on service learning was available. With a goal of investigating the synergy of service learning and instructional technology, the guiding question for this process was: "How can service learning be integrated effectively into undergraduate teacher preparation through instructional technology coursework?"

SERVICE LEARNING FUNDAMENTALS: A REVIEW OF THE LITERATURE

Prior to implementing the case study, a thorough investigation into service learning was completed. This included reviewing the history, definitions, concepts, models, and best practices of service learning. It was essential to have a clear understanding of this method in order to design an integrated service learning experience in educational technology. The following section highlights critical aspects of service learning pedagogy.

Establishing a Working Definition of Service Learning

The term service learning has infiltrated the vocabulary of most college campuses today. As a result of the desire to improve the scholarship of teaching and learning and to produce educated citizens who can think critically and solve problems, service learning programs and courses have developed and expanded over the last few decades. But just what does the term service learning mean and how is it different from other forms of experiential education and service?

Many definitions and methods of service learning exist in the literature base from the field, but commonalities exist amongst them. For the purpose of this chapter, the NCATE definition will be used. Service learning is defined as:

A teaching/learning method that integrates community service into academic courses, using structured reflective thinking to enhance learning of course content. Through meaningful service, candidates are engaged in problem solving to create improved schools and communities while developing their academic skills, their sense of civic responsibility, and their understanding of social problems affecting children and families. When used as a pedagogical strategy, service learning can help candidates understand the culture, community, and families of students, as well as the connections between the school and the community (2008, p.91).

Service Learning Foundations

The term service learning first surfaced in the 1960s. During that time period, Robert Sigmon emerged as a leader within service learning and coined three principles that would serve as the foundation for future service learning work (Mintz & Hesser, 1996). Sigmon's (1979) principles were:

1. Those being served control the service(s) provided.
2. Those being served become better able to serve and be served by their own actions.
3. Those who serve also are learners and have significant control over what is expected to be learned (p. 10).

Sigmon's principles highlight the centrality of reciprocity, capacity building, and community-defined need. Reciprocity exists due to the symbiotic relationship between the server and the served. As the expert on the community needs, the community should be the ones to define the 'what' and 'how' of the service. Additionally, the service is not meant to perpetuate the dependency on the servers, rather the service should help build capacity for the served to better help themselves (Council for the Advancement of Standards in Higher Education, 2006).

The 1980s were marked with increased growth in the national service movement as the Campus Outreach Opportunity League (1984) and Campus Compact (1985) were formed (National Service Learning Clearinghouse, n.d., History). With a desire to create high quality service programs and to aid in institutionalization of service learning, the National Society for Experiential Education (NSEE) collaborated with seventy organizations and the Johnson Foundation to convene a group at Wingspread (Mintz & Hesser, 1996). The result of this group was the *Principles of Good Practice for Combining Service and Learning*, or otherwise called the Wingspread Principles (Porter Honnet & Poulsen, 1989).

The group outlined the following principles for combining service and learning:

1. Engages people in responsible and challenging action for the common good.
2. Provides structured opportunities for people to reflect critically on their service experience.
3. Articulates clear service and learning goals for everyone involved.
4. Allows for those with needs to define those needs.
5. Clarifies the responsibilities of each person and organization involved.
6. Matches service providers and service needs through a process that recognizes changing circumstances.
7. Expects genuine, active, and sustained organizational commitment.
8. Includes training, supervision, monitoring, support, recognition, and evaluation to meet service and learning goals.
9. Insures that the time commitment for service and learning is flexible, appropriate, and in the best interest of all involved.

10. Is committed to program participation by and with diverse populations. (8)

More than a decade after the Wingspread Principles were drafted, the rapid progression of service learning led to new pedagogical principles that built on the Wingspread Principles. Jeff Howard (2001), Editor of the Michigan Journal of Community Service Learning, outlined ten principles for service learning pedagogy. They are:

1. Academic credit is for learning, not for service.
2. Do not compromise academic rigor.
3. Establish learning objectives.
4. Establish criteria for the selection of service placements.
5. Provide educationally-sound learning strategies to harvest community learning and realize course learning objectives.
6. Prepare students for learning from the community.
7. Minimize the distinction between the students' community learning role and classroom learning role.
8. Rethink the faculty instructional role.
9. Be prepared for variation in, and some loss of control with, student learning outcomes.
10. Maximize the community responsibility orientation of the course (pp. 16-19).

Service Learning Stakeholders

When deciding to integrate service learning, faculty must consider whether service learning will enhance the course learning outcomes. Service learning, as a pedagogical tool, engages students in active learning and allows them to put theory into practice while serving others. The benefits, however, are not exclusive to the students or the community partner. Although there is additional work associated with creating service learning courses, faculty members can also benefit tremendously from the experience. Synthesizing the work of the Morgridge Center for Public Service at the University of Wisconsin – Madison (2008), Table 1 outlines the benefit of service learning for stakeholders: faculty, students, and community partner.

One of the most important components of making good service learning partnerships is effective communication amongst stakeholders. Each entity needs to understand the other stakeholders' needs, expectations, responsibilities, and roles. Faculty members have the pressure of teaching, scholarship, and service within the time context of a semester or quarter. Community partners have the focus of serving clients, staffing, funding needs, etc. within the unique timeline specific to the services they provide. Having a conversation prior to entering into a partnership will make the service learning more effective, smooth, and successful. Building off the work of the Council for the

Table 1. Service learning stakeholder benefits

Faculty Benefits	Student Benefits	Community Benefits
Enhances teaching through organization's service learning experience	Provides an opportunity to apply course content	Supplements the human resources to meet the community needs
Strengthens relationships with students	Improves critical thinking	Raises awareness about the organization's mission needs, and population served
Broadens topics for research and publication	Gain valuable work experience	Provides the organization a connection to the the community
Demonstrates commitment to university	Explore career interests	Identifies prospective employees and volunteers

Table 2. Service learning stakeholder responsibilities

Faculty Responsibility	Student Responsibility	Community Responsibility
Listen to community partner needs	Understand their role and function within the organization	Create an environment conducive to learning
Develop clear, strong, and course-specific learning objectives	Manage time effectively as to accomplish the goals and/or work	Orientate and train the students
Create meaningful reflection opportunities	Learn by engaging, discussing and reflecting	Serve as partner and co teacher
Know the skill level of the students and inform the community partner	"Do no harm"	Provide honest communication to the faculty member
Ensure academic rigor	Represent the college/university well	Understand the university timeline

Advancement of Standards in Higher Education (2006), Cress, Collier, Reitenauer, and Associates (2005), and Howard (2001), Table 2 outlines each stakeholder's responsibilities.

While considering stakeholder responsibilities, addressing student rights is crucial for higher education institutions. Service learning takes place via the sphere of academics, but the classroom extends beyond the college campus, thus acquiring unique features. As a result, it is important to note that students have "rights" when it comes to service learning courses. Cress, Collier, Reitenauer, & Associates (2005) and Heffernan (2001) note that students have a right to:

- Know what is expected for the service learning and how it will be graded.
- Work with a community partner in a safe environment.
- Have the opportunity to apply knowledge for the benefit of others.

In order to have the most beneficial and educational service learning, it is important not to overlook safety; if the students don't feel safe, they won't be able to learn. Everything from travel associated with the service to the actual physical environment of the service site needs to be discussed with students to aid in preparation. Some students arrive to college having experienced little exposure to diverse settings or economically depressed communities. While not all service learning takes place in these types of communities, environments in which students work with homeless, tutoring programs, and other social services do frequently have similar characteristics. Discussing what to expect; helping students reflect on their fears, expectations, and prejudices; as well as outlining safety procedures, will help prepare students to gain more from the experience.

PRINCIPLES OF GOOD PRACTICE

There are many aspects to consider when designing a service learning course. Fortunately, abundant resources and research are available to inform practice. To implement service learning into instructional technology courses, components like reflection, learning outcomes, and syllabi require attention.

Reflection

When incorporating service learning within a course, reflection is a critical component. Students will have new, eye-opening, and challenging experiences via service learning; thus, it is important to help them process the experience as it relates to academics, career pursuits, and life. Through their service, students may be confronted with circumstances, behaviors, and human experiences that force them to re-examine previously held ideas or theories. Old frameworks for analyzing experiences may not suffice.

Eyler and Giles found that "the centrality of reflection to the academic enterprise had a significant impact on problem solving and critical thinking and on the complexity of students' problem analysis and issue understanding" (1999, p.174). In a survey of 22,236 undergraduate students, Astin, Vogelgesang, Ikeda, and Yee (2000) found that class discussion, encouraged by the professor, was "the second most significant factor in a positive service learning experience" (p.iii). Similarly, Mabry found that while there was no difference between groups in her study with different frequency of out of class reflection, there was greater academic benefit for students who reflected at least weekly in class (1998). Some modes of reflection are: writing (journals, reflective papers, directed writings, case studies); activities (role playing, skits, interviewing peers); multimedia (photo or video essay, on-line discussions, wikis or blogs, poster boards); and telling (presentations, class discussions, meetings with faculty). Each of these modes offers a different way for the students to process and learn from their service learning experience.

Syllabus and Learning Outcomes

It is important not to overlook the power of the syllabus and learning outcomes when creating a service learning course. The syllabus is seen as the contract between the students and faculty member and serves to prepare students for the experience that will unfold over the semester. Additionally, students need to see the connection between the service learning and the academic course content or learning outcomes. Faculty can demonstrate that connection via the course learning objectives and description of the service learning project.

The Council for the Advancement of Standards, in describing the role of the service learning syllabus, recommends that the following components be included in the syllabus:

- Needs that the service will address.
- Desired outcomes of the service and learning for all participants.
- Assignments that link service and academic content.
- Opportunities to reflect on one's personal reactions to the service and learning experiences.
- Logistics (e.g., time required, transportation, materials required).
- Nature of the service work.
- Roles and responsibilities of students and community members.
- Risk management procedures.
- Evaluation of the service and learning experiences and assessment of the degree to which desired outcomes were achieved (2006, p. 305).

A CASE STUDY ON SPARKING SYNERGY: THE ROAD TO BEST PRACTICES

Based on the benefits of the service learning practices outlined above, three class sections of an initial teacher preparation course were selected to incorporate service learning. The average class size was 17; with two-thirds of the candidates being female and one-third male. Instructional Technology is generally the second course in education for the majority of students; the first course being a survey of school and society that requires several observation hours. None of the students had formal service learning experience at the university prior to taking this course.

The guiding research question was how to incorporate service learning effectively into undergraduate instructional technology courses. Spanning four semesters, this case study illustrates three separate phases of implementation for all instructional technology students, detailing successes and challenges. The study takes place at a small, private Midwestern university. It is important to note that teacher candidates in this NCATE accredited program may pursue licensure in five different bands including Early Childhood (Pre-K through Grade 3), Middle Childhood (Grades 4-9), Adolescent to Young Adult (Grades 7-12), Multi-Age Physical Education, and Intervention Specialist (special education).

Phase One: Hi-Tech Environment

In fall 2007, undergraduate candidates in the teacher preparation program began their course with an innovative component—ten required hours of service learning. Prior to the semester, arrangements had been made with a local school district to place these candidates in classrooms and labs where they could tie the theory of instructional technology to practice. Placements were also aligned with their intended licensure bands.

According to the Ohio Department of Education (ODE) District Report Card for 2007-2008, the local school district selected for this phase consisted of 4,100 students (ODE, 2008). This school district's enrollment was 1,347 students at the high school, 1,025 students at the middle school, and 1,547 students at the seven elementary schools. The ratio of students to teachers was 17:1. Demographically, the district was 94% Caucasian, 2% Multiracial, 2% Asian, and 2% Black. The district reported 13% of the students had disabilities, and the overall attendance rate was 96%. Only 14% of the students in the district were economically disadvantaged. The district had recently received the second-highest recognition from the state, a designation of "Excellent." The expenditure per pupil was $7,424. The school district was rich in technology, and all classrooms had at least one networked computer. Most classrooms had a data projector, and each school had at least one Smart Board™ interactive whiteboard. There were multiple brand-new computing labs in each location.

Prior to the start of classes, the instructor met with the cooperating schools. The instructor and cooperating teachers discussed expectations, curriculum, learning goals/outcomes, and needs. Upon completion of that discussion, the course syllabus was created. Because service learning was integral to the course and a general education requirement at the university, teacher candidates would not be able to pass the course if the service component was not successfully completed. A service learning contract between the teacher candidates, site, and faculty member was implemented. Please note that in subsequent semesters, an additional liability waiver for travel was added, based on administrative policy.

Scheduling teacher candidates for service learning times was challenging. With several different schools comprising this district and each school having its own unique schedule, teacher candidates were challenged to balance service learning hours and their academic schedules. The university schedule for course times as well as academic calendar did not match any schedules at the partner schools. A system of creating sign-up sheets displaying time options was created to address schedule issues, although many candidates expressed stress and frustration because some schools were on block scheduling that conflicted with candidate coursework on campus.

Qualitative data was gathered to analyze candidate expectations and growth. Since service learning literature discussed the emphasis on reflections prior to their first site visit, candidates were asked to do a pre-service reflection. These reflections were brief open-ended essays covering candidate feelings, perceptions, and attitudes regarding service and technology. This first pre-service reflection format was unstructured. Due to the broad scope of responses, in subsequent semesters a more structured format of the pre-service reflection activity was implemented. The goal was to improve focus and ensure that all teacher candidates addressed specific questions.

Pre-service reflection essays offered insight to inform class discussions, reading materials, and instructor intervention. The themes that emerged were that the candidates:

1. Did not see themselves as technology experts.
2. Had high comfort levels with certain technology applications (Facebook®, MySpace®, Microsoft Word®, PowerPoint®, Internet searches, music, etc.).
3. Felt their high school experiences did not include teachers modeling effective technology.
4. Expressed apprehension regarding interaction with students at the partner site.
5. Believed effective teachers made school fun, and technology was the answer.

As the semester unfolded, the emphasis on reflection continued. Teacher candidates completed a log of activities, accomplishments, epiphanies, or other notable occurrences throughout the service learning experience. The cooperating teacher verified participation and completed an evaluation of each candidate's work. Two of the teacher candidates did not complete their service hours which resulted in a failing grade.

At the conclusion of this service learning experience, teacher candidates wrote extensive reflections based on a departmental service rubric. For assessment of learning outcomes, a rubric was created by a task-force within the Division of Education to evaluate candidate reflections. The five criteria for the teacher candidate final reflection essays included:

1. What happened? (Objective statements without interpretation describing population, setting, demographics, and activities)
2. What was learned about the candidate's licensure area?
3. What are the candidate's reactions, feelings, impressions, and ideas? (An analysis of the experience)
4. What about the future? (Theoretical issues, content knowledge, dispositions that could apply to future teaching)
5. What two Specialized Professional Association (SPA) or State Teacher Standards could be applied to strengthen the service learning experience?

All candidates in the undergraduate instructional technology course were required to create a Microsoft PowerPoint® electronic portfolio that showcased their semester of coursework. A significant portion of this presentation required candidates to detail their experiences, growth, and learning as a result of this service component. This course generated interest from the broader campus community. Administrators and other faculty members attended student presentations to learn more about the synergy.

When the semester concluded, the instructor analyzed student reflections and comments. Each electronic portfolio presentation was reviewed, as well as any notes taken on verbal comments from the candidates' presentations. Five themes emerged. Participants in this service learning course:

1. Developed a sense of efficacy regarding the use of technology.
2. Observed effective use of technology.
3. Benefitted from working with students and technology in an authentic environment.
4. Appreciated exposure to new high-tech equipment (SMART Board™ interactive whiteboards, audience response systems, and specialized software).
5. Established bonds with the students they were tutoring.

In spring 2008, given the same placement, results were parallel. The instructor this time handed out periodic service share worksheets to candidates for completion in class. Service share sessions were discussion/activity times set aside in specific class sessions where teacher candidates shared information on their experiences in service learning. Candidates completed forms consisting of open-ended questions about what was happening in their service work, how they were connecting class content to their service experience, and any challenges or successes. These worksheets were reviewed by the instructor. Closer attention was paid to each candidate's experience and follow-up calls or instructor visits were made to service sites to facilitate better cooperation and improve experiences. However, at the close of spring 2008, it was apparent that the challenges from fall 2007 remained.

Teacher candidate comments confirmed that appropriate placements were critical to success. Candidates who were matched with cooperating teachers excited and skilled with instructional technology had very positive experiences. The candidates assigned to cooperating teachers who were not confident in their ability to use technology were either given menial tasks (photocopying, lunchroom supervision/tutoring) or given too much responsibility (primary instructor for technology lessons). Additionally, many students jokingly remarked that the service site (school) had better technology than their own university campus. The instructor reviewed data. It was clear that the experience had benefits, but the design of the service component was not the right fit. Two questions arose:

1. How can negative experiences be avoided?
2. Are candidates providing true service in an environment already rich in resources?

After thorough discussion at the university, it was decided that a greater focus on service and diversity would be beneficial to the teacher candidates. Investigation for alternative placements began.

Phase Two: Shifting Focus - Service and Diversity

In fall 2008, the instructional technology course sections partnered with an after-school urban outreach enrichment program sponsored by the university and an urban church for K-4 youth. Candidates with licensure bands addressing early childhood, middle childhood, and intervention specialist participated in that program. Candidates with adolescent to young adult licensure bands assisted with an alternative high school program in the same building. This combination of service learning field placements made it possible for all licensure areas to be accommodated.

According to the Urban Outreach Report (Smith, 2009), the urban outreach site consisted of 32 students in regular attendance. The student to teacher ratio was approximately 5:1. Demographically, data indicated that 47% of the students were White, 34% Hispanic, 16% Black, and 3% did not disclose. Approximately 75% of the students served were economically disadvantaged. Although some students had disabilities, no data was gathered that semester on that topic. Over 90% of the students were at the early childhood licensure band level at this site (grades one through three). Regarding technology, this site offered seven older non-networked computers and 2 non-networked printers.

The adolescent to young adult licensure band service option was at a "last chance" high school in the same building. The mission of this school was to serve at-risk youth including drop-outs, near drop-outs, adjudicated youth or others with low achievement. This charter school did not meet any of the state requirements and was listed at the lowest designation, "academic emergency," on the state report card (ODE, 2008). The high school had approximately 88 students (J. Cole, personal communication, August 27, 2008). The ratio of students to teachers was 10:1. Demographically, the district was 46% Black, 42% Caucasian, and 12% Unspecified. The school reported 46% of the students had disabilities. The attendance rate was 65%. At least 56% of the students in the district were economically disadvantaged (ODE, 2008). Regarding technology, most classrooms had at least one networked computer, and 2 classrooms had data projection.

In addition to the instructional technology course, several other university courses participated in the after school urban outreach initiative. The location of these facilities was in an economically disadvantaged area, candidate safety was a concern. To prepare the candidates for working with a more diverse population, a mandatory evening orientation session was scheduled and delivered prior to beginning the service hours; an asynchronous version was also available to candidates.

A few schedule concerns arose from the design of this service learning partnership. The enrichment program was an after-school program offered only on Tuesdays, Wednesdays, and Thursdays between the hours of 4:00 and 6:00 PM. Several candidates had evening or afternoon classes at those times. Others candidates were athletes or had employment/activity conflicts. With the program running over a 12 week period, many candidates reported stress based on scheduling issues.

Candidates signed service learning contracts and wrote pre-service reflection essays; however, the reflections were modified to include questions on diversity and poverty. Most answers about technology were parallel to previous semesters. However, the incorporation of diversity and poverty questions into this exercise yielded interesting data. Candidates:

1. Enjoyed community service and helping others.
2. Expressed concerned about interactions with poor people.
3. Worried about how low socio-economic status impacted teaching and learning.
4. Lacked prior experience with racially and economically diverse populations.

Throughout the semester, candidates completed a log of their experiences, as well as answered periodic service share worksheets to inform the instructor of their activities and progress. These worksheets helped the instructor adjust lessons to more closely tie the service experience to the theory and objectives of the course. Additionally, based on comments from candidates' reflections, several readings on the culture of poverty were introduced and discussed in class.

Upon analysis of student reflections and comments at the end of the semester, the instructor saw some substantive growth with regard to diversity, empathy, and volunteerism. Seven core candidate observations emerged. The participants:

1. Reported that they felt they had made a difference in students' lives at the service sites.
2. Expressed interest in volunteering more.
3. Witnessed the effects of poverty.
4. Realized trust and respect had to be earned from the students.
5. Adapted activities to meet the needs of their diverse students.
6. Experienced a great deal about different cultures, economic status, and values.
7. Developed bonds with the students they served.

Some shortcomings did appear regarding the limited technology available. Although the initial project at the enrichment site was to set up and install a non-networked computer lab, some candidates raised concerns that there was not much connection to instructional technology thereafter. Additionally, some reported that they felt there were too many university service students for the number of youth participants. Candidates felt that they could not tie classroom theory to practice since there was a lack of opportunity for personal interaction with the partner students.

Upon analysis, the course instructor found the experience extremely rich and positive with respect to diversity, but the candidates' experiences lacked a focus on instructional technology. Experiences under the previous structure (Phase 1) afforded candidates observation of cooperating teachers modeling effective technology use but lacked a true sense of service. Phase 2 offered candidates the opportunity to truly serve others in need, but lacked sufficient technology exposure. It was decided that an alternative site (Phase 3) would be sought to address both concerns.

Phase Three: Merging Service Learning, Diversity, and Instructional Technology

In spring 2009, the instructor and Director of Service Learning contacted a local non-profit organization that worked closely with an urban school district to implement after-school programs. At this location, 95% of the students attending the partner schools were below the poverty level. Further, 100% of the students participating in the non-profit organization's programs were below the poverty level (T. Bigler, personal communication, January 8, 2009). The non-profit also offered several support services (food, clothing, counseling, etc.).

The urban school district directly served by this non-profit consists of almost 11,000 students. Regarding enrollment, there were seventeen elementary schools with a total of 5,090 students, six middle schools totaling 2,528 students, and four high schools totaling 3,361 students. Nine of the schools in the district are listed as charter, alternative, or collaborative locations. The non-profit partner was specifically affiliated with a neighborhood area serving approximately 400 students. The student to teacher ratio was 19:1. Demographically, 54% of the students were Black, 24% White, 20% Multiracial, and 2% did not specify. The combined district reported 19% of the students had disabilities. The attendance rate was 95%. The district expenditure per pupil was $9,916. The school received a mid-level designation of "Continuous Improvement" from the state (ODE, 2008). Regarding technology in the non-profit center, there were multiple computers and printers in a networked lab, a digital music lab, library, large art/media classroom, and access to additional resources in the adjacent school building.

Collaboration between the non-profit Education Director and course instructor outlined expectations, needs, schedule options, and responsibilities for participants. Candidates were offered a sign-up sheet of various service times throughout the week between 10am and 5pm. This schedule addressed earlier concerns regarding candidate schedule conflicts mentioned in Phases 1 and 2. The Education Director delivered an orientation that prepared candidates for their work in an impoverished ethnically diverse neighborhood. The orientation included safety, rules, regulations, best practices, and other administrative issues.

Once again, candidates signed a service learning contract and liability waiver. They completed pre-service reflections, kept time logs, and participated in structured in-class service share sessions. Additionally, the final presentation and e-portfolio requirements were continued. Communication between the service partner and instructor was open and regular.

In spring 2009, candidates completed their service learning instructional technology experiences at the third site. Although some candidates felt that they had signed up for dates and times where there was not as much interaction with students, the overall response was very positive. Candidates reported that the activities they completed addressed both traditional and electronic media including:

1. Organizing and evaluating media (books, software, etc.).
2. Developing a cataloging system for media.
3. Tutoring on computers.
4. Working one-on-one with students to create mixed media projects.

5. Creating instructional and tutoring materials (bulletin boards, flashcards, PowerPoint® presentations).
6. Developing thematic units incorporating technology.
7. Supporting instruction with technology.

In previous semesters, service share activities were primarily written and insular. In this phase, four structured service share sessions were conducted verbally in class. Candidates began to build off of each other's experiences and openly discuss theory and practice connections collaboratively. The instructor used a variety of active learning methods to facilitate the reflections.. Active learning is defined by Bonwell and Eison as: "instructional activities involving students in doing things and thinking about what they are doing." (2001, p.2).

One example of active learning was an asynchronous discussion on SAKAI, an Internet-based open-source learning management system. An online discussion was conducted, focusing on "repurposing" equipment/materials as well as critically evaluating such materials. The instructor posted a question asking students to consider their service site and how they could "repurpose" or "re-use" existing equipment in innovative ways to bring media rich experiences to impoverished schools. Several candidates were able to locate and share that they could create a low-cost interactive whiteboard—much like the SMART Board™ interactive whiteboard used in the course, by using an infrared pen ($8) and a Nintendo Wii™ remote (aka "WiiMote") ($40). Candidates downloaded free software and tested their idea. Although instructional technology candidates commented that it was not as good as the classroom SMART Board™, they used research from the *WiiMote Project* (http://www.wiimoteproject.org) to successfully build and evaluate their own low-cost interactive whiteboard (Chung Lee, 2009).

The service opportunity in Phase 3 demonstrated the synergy between providing true service and applying instructional technology content. Candidates openly discussed how to work with limited budgets but still bring rich technology options to their students. The candidates connected with the idea of technology being a tool, but recognized that not all schools would have the 'latest and greatest' equipment. Instead, they had learned to find innovative solutions to increase student learning with somewhat non-traditional technology tools.

In final presentations and reflections, candidates expressed high levels of satisfaction and growth as a result of this experience. Several commented that they had found projects that they planned to implement in their own classrooms. They also indicated that they had new appreciation for serving diverse learners. The majority of candidates felt they would continue to volunteer for the facility in the future.

At the conclusion of the semester, candidates' reflections and final presentations offered an interesting combination of the positive outcomes from previous semesters, as well as shed light on some new affordances. Overall, eight specific themes emerged. Candidates reported that they:

1. Saw great benefit from working with students and technology.
2. Developed bonds with the students they were tutoring.
3. Made a difference in students' lives at the service partner sites.
4. Expressed interest in volunteering more.
5. Witnessed the effects of poverty and expressed an increased understanding of the importance of education all children and creative ways of introducing technology.
6. Adapted activities with technology (traditional and electronic) to meet the needs of their diverse students.
7. Learned a great deal about different cultures, economic status, and values.
8. Developed bonds with students.

Beyond Phase Three

The instructor found the format of Phase Three to be the most effective. Plans are to continue to nurture the partnership with the local non-profit organization in order to improve services to all stakeholders. Course activities are being added in order to further strengthen the connections between service learning and instructional technology. Experience from the three phases has led to the continuation of best practices for this course--including pre-service reflections, verbal service shares, clearly stating expectations/outcomes, schedule flexibility, student diversity, and adequate technology. In the spirit of continuous improvement, evaluation will be ongoing.

Recent research offers a great deal of information on the implication of social justice as it ties into this service learning and instructional technology study. Currently social justice is not an explicit part of service learning at the university, though it is part of the underlying foundation. Unfortunately, it was not one of the specific main goals of the experience during the case study period. In the next phase, the instructor will focus more on social justice and its implications by incorporating additional readings and discussion points.

SOLUTIONS AND RECOMMENDATIONS

Based on the literature review and established best practices noted earlier, it is critical for the instructor to focus on the 'how' and 'why' of integrating service learning into instructional technology. At the same time, it is critical to ensure that the design of the service learning course will meet all stakeholder needs. Recommendations for those who wish to pursue service learning in instructional technology are:

- Incorporate meaningful pre-service reflections.
- Prepare students through orientations on the service site as well as safety.
- Select an appropriate site based on course learning objectives.
- Provide an opportunity and environment for meaningful direct service.
- Incorporate frequent and varied reflections with peers and faculty member.
- Maintain flexibility as service learning is not controlled by the instructor but discovered through the journey.
- State requirements and outcomes/objectives for service on the syllabus.
- Require all stakeholders to sign service contracts.
- Communicate effectively with all stakeholders and maintain a dialog.
- Evaluate and revise throughout the process.

FUTURE RESEARCH DIRECTIONS

This initial case study has yielded several agendas for future research topics addressing different stakeholder impacts. A series of potential research questions surfaced, spanning three domains: University Students, Community Partner Site, and Faculty. Although the entire list is not exhaustive, the researcher will work with the Director of Service Learning, community partner(s), and faculty to formulate additional research projects. The following list offers some emergent questions relating to each of the domains.

University Students

- What is the impact of service learning on university students regarding skills, knowledge, and implementation of instructional technology (quantitative and qualitative approaches)?

- How can candidates better understand poverty and its effects?
- Does the synthesis of service learning and instructional technology impact teacher candidates in their first year of practice?
- Does the service learning experience make candidates more comfortable in selecting diverse schools for their first year of practice?
- How does in-class discussion of service learning affect the experience for the service learning students?
- How many hours are optimal to achieve enhancement of course learning objectives via service learning?
- How do educators better prepare students to work in diverse educational environments?

Community Partner Site

- What are the academic, emotional, and social impacts of service learning on the constituents (students) from the community site through which the university students served?
- Are service projects able to meet a need identified by the community partner?
- How can the partnership be improved?
- What time commitment is sufficient to meet service partner needs?

Faculty

- What are the benefits for the faculty member teaching the service learning course?
- Is teaching and learning improved based on the service learning experience?
- Does the faculty member have a stronger relationship with the students?
- What are the incentives for teaching a service learning course?
- How can institutions of higher education better support service learning faculty?
- How can social justice be effectively integrated into an instructional technology course in a service learning format?

CONCLUSION

In conclusion, combining service learning with an undergraduate technology course requires a great deal of preparation and planning but yielded rich results. This chapter provided an overview of critical service learning information, review of current literature, and discussion of best practices. Combining service learning with instructional technology offers teacher candidates valuable experiences while tying the theory from the classroom to practical experience serving others. Effectively implementing service learning can meet the deficit previously found in field experience for instructional technology courses while preparing teacher candidates for diverse educational settings.

REFERENCES

Astin, A. W., Vogelsang, L. J., Ikeda, E. K., & Yee, J. A. (2000). *How service learning affects students*. Los Angeles: University of California, Higher Education Research Institute.

Barnes, C. J. (2006). Preparing preservice teachers to teach in a culturally responsive way. *Negro Educational Review*, *57*(1/2), 85–100.

Batchelder, T., & Root, S. (1994). Effects of an undergraduate program to integrate academic learning and service: cognitive, prosocial cognitive and identity outcomes. *Journal of Adolescence*, *17*, 341–356. doi:10.1006/jado.1994.1031

Bonwell, C., & Eison, J. (1991, September 1). Active learning: Creating excitement in the classroom. *ERIC Digest*. (ERIC Document Reproduction Service No. ED340272) Retrieved August 18, 2009, from ERIC database.

Brush, T., Igoe, A., Brinkerhoff, J., Glazewski, K., Ku, H., & Smith, T. C. (2001). Lessons from the field: Integrating technology into preservice teacher education. *Journal of Computing in Teacher Education*, *17*(4), 16–20.

Casey, B., & Howson, P. (1993). Educating preservice students based on a problem-centered approach to teaching. *Journal of Teacher Education*, *44*(5), 361–369. doi:10.1177/002248719304400506

Chung Lee, J. (n.d.). Low-cost multi-point interactive whiteboards using the WiiMote. *WiiMote Project*. Retrieved on February 2, 2009, from http://www.cs.cmu.edu/~johnny/projects/wii/

Clark, R. W., Foster, A., & Mantle-Bromley, C. (2005). *Hybrid educators and the simultaneous renewal of schools and the education of educators*. Seattle, WA: Institution for Educational Inquiry.

Council for the Advancement of Standards in Higher Education. (2006). *CAS professional standards for higher education* (6th ed.). Washington, DC: Author.

Cress, C. M., Collier, P. J., & Reitenauer, V. L. (2005). *Learning through serving: A student guidebook for service-learning across the disciplines*. Sterling, VA: Stylus Publishing.

Dexter, S., & Riedel, E. (2003). Why improving preservice teacher educational technology preparation must go beyond the college's walls. *Journal of Teacher Education*, *54*(4), 334–346. doi:10.1177/0022487103255319

Eyler, J., & Giles, D. E. (1999). *Where's the learning in service learning?*San Francisco: Jossey-Bass.

Gay, G. (2000). *Culturally responsive teaching: Theory, research, and practice*. New York: Teachers College Press.

Graybill, S. W. (1997). Questions of race and culture: How they relate to the classroom for African American students. *Clearing House (Menasha, Wis.)*, *70*, 311–319.

Heffernan, K. (2001). *Fundamentals of service learning course construction*. Providence, RI: Campus Compact.

Howard, J. (Ed.). (2001, Summer). Service-learning course design workbook. Ann Arbor, MI: OCSL Press.

Howard, J. P. F. (1998). Academic service learning: A counternormative pedagogy. In Rhoads, R. A., & Howard, J. P. F. (Eds.), *Academic Service Learning: A Pedagogy of Action and Reflection* (pp. 24–29). San Francisco: Jossey-Bass.

Irvine, J. (2003). *Educating teachers for diversity: Seeing with a cultural eye*. New York: Teachers College Press.

Larson, A., & Clift, R. (1996). Technology education in teacher preparation: Perspectives from a year-long elementary education program. *Educational Foundations*, *10*(4), 33–50.

Mabry, J. B. (1998). Pedagogical variations in service-learning and student outcomes: How time, Contact, and reflection matter. *Michigan journal of community service learning, 5*, 32-47.

McIntyre, J., Byrd, D., & Foxx, S. (1997). Field and laboratory experiences. In Sikula, J. (Ed.), *Handbook of research on teacher education* (pp. 171–193). New York: Simon and Schuster Macmillan.

Mintz, S. D., & Hesser, G. W. (1996). Principles of good practice in service-learning. In Jacoby, B. (Eds.), *Service-Learning in Higher Education: Concepts and Practices*. San Francisco: Jossey-Bass.

Morgridge Center for Public Service. (2008, June). *Faculty introduction to service-learning/community-based research.* University of Wisconsin Madison. Retrieved February 18, 2009, from http://www.morgridge.wisc.edu/faculty/facultyservicelearning.html

National Council for Accreditation of Teacher Education. (2008). *NCATE handbook*. Washington, DC: NCATE. Retrieved from http://www.ncate.org/documents/handbook/handbook.pdf

National Service-Learning Clearinghouse. (n.d.). *History.* Retrieved February 17, 2009, from http://www.servicelearning.org/what_is_service-learning/history/index.php

Ohio Department of Education. (n.d.). *District report cards* [Data file]. Retrieved from http://ilrc.ode.state.oh.us/Districts/Default.asp

Porter Honnet, E., & Poulsen, S. J. (1989). *Principles of good practice for combining service and learning*. Retrieved February 10, 2009, from http://www.johnsonfdn.org/principles.html

Pransky, K., & Bailey, F. (2002/2003). To meet your students where they are, first you have to find them: Working with culturally and linguistically diverse at-risk students. *The Reading Teacher, 56*, 370–383. doi:10.1598/RT.56.4.3

Sigmon, R. L. (1979, Spring). Service-learning: Three principles. *Synergist, 8*(1), 9–11.

Smith, C. (2009). *Urban outreach report.* Unpublished raw data.

Swartz, E. (2003). Teaching white preservice teachers. *Urban Education, 38*(3), 255–278. doi:10.1177/0042085903038003001

Willis, J., & Mehlinger, H. (1996). Information technology and teacher education. In Sikula, J., Buttery, T., & Guyton, E. (Eds.), *Handbook of research on teacher education* (2nd ed., pp. 978–1029). New York: MacMillan.

ADDITIONAL READING

Anderson, J. (1999). *Service-learning and teacher education*. (ERIC Document Reproduction Service No. ED421481). Retrieved January 3, 2009, from http://www.ericdigests.org/1999-1/service.html

Brownell, K. (1997). Technology in teacher education: Where are we and where do we go from here? *Journal of Technology and Teacher Education, 5*(2/3), 117–138.

Brush, T. (1998). Teaching preservice teachers to use technology in the classroom. *Journal of Technology and Teacher Education, 6*(4), 243–258.

Brush, T., Glazewski, K., Rutowski, K., Berg, K., Stromfors, C., & Van-Nest, M. (2003). Integrating technology in a field-based teacher training program: the PT3@ASU project. *Educational Technology Research and Development, 51*, 57–73. doi:10.1007/BF02504518

Bullock, D. (2004). Moving from theory to practice: an examination of the factors that preservice teachers encounter as the attempt to gain experience teaching with technology during field placement experiences. *Journal of Technology and Teacher Education, 12*, 211–237.

Clift, R. T., Mullen, L., Levin, J., & Larson, A. (2001). Technologies in Contexts: Implications for Teacher Education. *Teaching and Teacher Education, 17*(1), 33–50. doi:10.1016/S0742-051X(00)00037-8

Conderman, G. (2003). Using portfolios in undergraduate special education teacher education programs. *Preventing School Failure, 47*(3), 106–111. doi:10.1080/10459880309604438

Danielson, C. (1996). *Enhancing professional practice: a framework for teaching*. Alexandria, VA: Association of Supervision and Curriculum Development.

Davis, N., Kirkman, C., Tearle, P., Taylor, C., & Wright, B. (1996). Developing teachers and their institutions for IT in education: An integrated approach. *Journal of Technology and Teacher Education*, *4*(1), 3–18.

Enterline, S., Cochran-Smith, M., Ludlow, L., & Mitescu, E. (2008). Learning to teach for social justice: Measuring change in the beliefs of teacher candidates. *New Educator*, *4*(4), 267–290. doi:10.1080/15476880802430361

Erickson, J. A., & Anderson, J. B. (1997). *Learning with the community: Concepts and models for service-learning in teacher education. AAHE's series on service-learning in the disciplines*. Washington, DC: American Association for Higher Education.

Evans, N. J., Forney, D. S., & Guido-DiBrito, F. (1998). *Student development in college: Theory, research, and practice*. San Francisco: Jossey-Bass.

Gollnick, D. M., & Chin, P. C. (1990). *Multicultural education in a pluralistic society* (3rd ed.). Columbus, OH: Merrill.

Goodlad, J. (1994). *Educational renewal*. San Francisco: Jossey-Bass Publishers.

Gray, M. J., Ondaatje, E. H., Fricker, R. D., & Geschwind, S. A. (2000). Assessing service-learning results from a survey of Learn and Serve America, Higher Education. *Change -New Rochelle then Washington, D.C.*, *32*, 30-39.

Jacoby, B. (1996). *Service-learning in higher education: Concepts and practices*. San Francisco: Jossey Bass.

Kolb, D. A. (1984). *Experiential learning: Experience as the source of learning and development*. Englewood Cliffs, NJ: Prentice-Hall, Inc.

Kurth, D., & Thompson, A. D. (1998). *Case-base approach to facilitate integrating technology into teacher education*. Paper presented at annual meeting of the Society for Information Technology and Teacher Education, San Antonio, TX.

Laffey, J., & Musser, D. (1998). Attitudes of preservice teachers about using technology in teaching. *Journal of Technology and Teacher Education*, *6*(4), 223–242.

Moursund, D., & Bielefeldt, T. (1999). Will new teachers be prepared to teach in a digital age? A national survey on information technology in teacher education. *Milken Family Foundation*. Retrieved from http://www.Milkenexchange.org/

National Service-Learning Clearinghouse. (n.d.). *History*. Retrieved February 17, 2009, from http://www.servicelearning.org/what_is_service-learning/history/index.php

Nitschke-Shaw, D. (1998). *Teacher education service-learning guidebook*. Bedford, NH: Campus Compact for New Hampshire.

Payne, R. K. (2009). Poverty does not restrict a student's ability to learn. *Phi Delta Kappan*, *90*(5), 371.

Pelligrino, J., & Altman, J. (1997). Information technology and teacher preparation: Some critical issues and illustrative solutions. *Peabody Journal of Education*, *72*(1), 89–121. doi:10.1207/s15327930pje7201_5

Powell, R. R., Zehm, S. J., & Garcia, J. (1996). *Field experience: Strategies for exploring diversity in schools*. Englewood Cliffs, NJ: Merrill.

Smaldino, S. E., Lowther, D. L., & Russell, J. D. (2008). *Instructional technology and media for learning*. Upper Saddle River, NJ: Pearson Merrill Prentice Hall.

Strudler, N., & Wetzel, K. (1999). Lessons from exemplary colleges of education: Factors affecting technology integration in preservice programs. *Educational Technology Research and Development*, *47*(4), 63–81. doi:10.1007/BF02299598

Umbach, P. D., & Kuh, G. D. (2006). Student experiences with diversity at liberal arts colleges: Another claim for distinctiveness. *The Journal of Higher Education*, *77*(1), 169–192. doi:10.1353/jhe.2006.0008

Vaughan, R., Seifer, S., & Vye Mihalynuk, T. (2004). *Teacher education and service learning*. Retrieved January 3, 2008, from National Service-Learning Clearinghouse Web site: http://www.servicelearning.org/instant_info/fact_sheets/k12_facts/teacher_ed/index.php?search_term=vaughn,%20R

Waterman, A. (1997). An overview of service-learning and the role of research and evaluation in service learning programs. In Waterman, A. (Ed.), *Service Learning: Applications from Research*. Mahwah, NJ: Lawrence Erlbaum Associates, Publishers.

Chapter 9
Finding Our Way While Leading the Way

Gloria Latham
RMIT University Melbourne, Australia

Julie Faulkner
RMIT University Melbourne, Australia

ABSTRACT

This chapter will follow two teacher educators at RMIT University in Melbourne in their quest to lead and enable others to lead as they capture and critically reflect upon the constructs that frame the creation and implementation of a virtual primary school for pre-service teachers. The school is now six years old and has moved through numerous iterations, but remains guided by theories of Christensen (1997) and Boler (1999). That is, pre-service teachers, through their interactions with the virtual school, are challenged to question and rethink assumptions through sustained innovations and the disruption of habituated practices in learning and teaching. As the school has evolved, the authors have also had to rethink assumptions and build strong theoretical frameworks to support change.

BACKGROUND

At RMIT University's School of Education we struggled with ways to support and challenge pre-service teachers to think in fresh ways about learning and about teaching. The proliferation of digital technologies offers considerable potential to reconceptualise schooling and yet so often emerges as 'old frameworks on new realities' (Senge, Scharmer, Jaworski and Flowers 2004, p. 84). On professional practice, pre-service teachers often experience little of the 'New Learning' argued for by research and leading educators (Papert 1993; Bigum 1995; ACDE 2001; Oblinger, 2003) We wondered whether beginning teachers were merely perpetuating an old model of schooling based on the model they had experienced, even when presented with new ideas about learning. Adopting new thinking can be problematic when novice teachers enter the teaching profession with at least 12 years of being a school learner. They come with intimate knowledge and firmly ingrained images of the practices of schooling from direct experience and from the

DOI: 10.4018/978-1-61520-899-9.ch009

media. Common practices in schools and repeated popular culture narratives tend to reinforce traditional beliefs and assumptions about learning, and of how schools are organized with beliefs being deeply connected to identity formations around teaching. We searched for a way to negotiate these tensions within an environment that most of our pre-service teachers were familiar with – a digital setting.

FRAMING QUESTIONS WITHIN A MULTIMODAL ENVIRONMENT

As our pre-service teachers encounter new kinds of learners in traditional classrooms on their teaching placements, they are presented with difficult teaching challenges. Disengaged learners struggling with content which has little connection with their worlds require approaches beyond 'one size fits all' pedagogies. The pressures of standardised testing add to a perceived gap between learning theory and learning realities. Within the context of needed change and pre-service teacher anxieties over establishing the teacher role, we created a new context for addressing some of these issues – a virtual school called Lathner Primary (http://www.dlsweb.rmit.edu.au/education/lathnervirtualschool/index.htm Password: Explore). Unlike many existing digital versions of schools, this was not a space intended to replace or simply complement university teaching. Simulations as learning environments are often being used in teacher education (Risco, 1995; Gibson, 2002; Ferry, Kervin, Cambourne, Pulisi, Jonassen & Hedberg, 2004). Existing simulations seek to replicate school settings in order to have pre-service teachers study them in some detail through discussion and role play. In 2001 America had 14 virtual schools that appear to replicate existing schools. However, as these simulations are pre-programmed, they often become static representations of schools. Our virtual primary school was to differ in that we wanted this school to be dynamic and reflect ideas around what schools might become in response to New Learning challenges.

To realise our aims, we underpinned the design of the virtual classroom with the theories of Christensen's 'disruptive innovations' (1997) and Boler's 'pedagogy of discomfort' (1999). Schools have changed over the past two decades to respond to some of the current and emerging demands on learners, yet it the very nature of these changes that require greater attention. Clay Christensen argues that the changes that have been undertaken are sustaining innovations; changes that better support the present system and make it more effective. Christensen advocates far more radical change that he terms 'disruptive innovations'. Innovations of this kind are systemic and dramatically alter the existing culture.

In concert with Christensen, Boler (1999) argues that a pedagogy of discomfort enables us to see differently. Her definition includes both 'an invitation to inquiry as well as a call to action' (p. 176). In the process of examining 'cherished' beliefs and assumptions, we are likely to experience 'defensive anger, fear of change, and fears of losing our personal and cultural identities' (p. 176). As pre-service teachers typically embark on an education degree with the expectation that educators will unproblematically build their teaching identities, the process of breaking down some of the premises supporting those identities can be confronting. Boler argues that such a practice is ethically justified in the interests of willingly inhabiting 'a more ambiguous and flexible sense of self' (p. 176). This is an aim we embraced but needed to sustain through careful planning and resource design.

The virtual school was intended to become both a sustained innovation (that of educational reform) and a disruptive innovation (an upheaval from the known to the new). Schlechty (2005) argues that a disruptive change, such as giving students autonomy, may require the role of teachers and the authority of that role to be redefined. It appeared to us that initially both innovative and sustained thinking were needed to take our pre-service teachers from where they are to never before imagined possibilities. 'While invention is the first occurrence of an idea for a new product or process, innovation is the first attempt to carry it out into practice' (Fagerberg 2004, p.2). It was our intent to use the potential of ICT to play out what New Learning looks like, sounds like, and feels like in a school context so that our pre-service teachers could see the benefits in the theoretical knowledge and the relationship of new approaches to practices for 21st century learners.

In formulating the design of Lathner Primary, we wanted our pre-service teachers to experience the same school environment so that they would have authentic purposes to dialogue with one another. We wanted the exterior of the school to look fairly similar to the school they may have attended, with surprises emerging with every click. Brenda Laurel (1991) believes in the importance of surprise and reversal elements, stating that 'the discovery process becomes more interesting when the information found is not what the user might have expected' (p. 90). In the case of reversal or a surprise that reveals the opposite of what might have been expected, a learner's interest might be heightened, or a path might be changed. Laurel suggests that to focus solely on information delivery, we risk missing the opportunity to view web design as an engagement and performance. Duffy (2003) asks us to turn surprises into questions. She believes that unexpected occurrences can stimulate unlearning and raise questions that may in time alter existing mindsets (Latham 2007).

FACING RESISTANCE

Once we had undertaken further research and formulated clearer thinking around the design of the virtual school, we took our ideas to a web graphic designer and a programmer from the Educational Media Group at RMIT. We were not at all certain what was possible. Could we design and program a virtual school that was dynamic? Would the designers and programmers be prepared to explore new ways of conceiving the technology? Would we be able to understand their technical language? Would they be able to understand ours? Initially many of the design concepts we proposed were challenged. We realized we were asking them to break rules. For instance, they had been taught to provide a site map to guide visitors. We were adamant that we did not want a site map because we wanted visitors to get lost and encounter surprises along the way, rather than be directed in their journey. Maxine Greene's (1973) concept of 'teacher as stranger' was enacted to allow pre-service teachers' entry to an experience as anthropologists might experience unfamiliar surrounds. Therefore, while the designer and programmer wanted to make the visitors comfortable navigating the site, we wanted to provide some discomfort in order for participants to become critically conscious of the culture of this virtual school and provide opportunities to start to question 'fixed, customary modes of seeing'(p.8). It was our hope that even the familiar might be viewed differently. During these initial meetings with the Educational Media Group they shared the learning objects they had created for other areas in the university and we realised that most would not suit the primary school we envisaged, as they were far too static and promoted certainty. We wanted our pre-service teachers to recognize and accept the uncertainties in teaching and learning.

Fortunately after many long meetings, the designer and programmer started to acquire shared understandings with us. We engaged in needed compromise while still embracing the ideals of the school. At our end, we began to realise some of the technological constraints with the user interface. In time, the project was scoped and a designer and programmer were contacted to work on the virtual school project. They hired people who were knowledgeable, flexible, imaginative, playful and forward thinking. These people asked to read about some of the theorists who had inspired our thinking and as a team, we continued to meet regularly and discuss ideas. Although time consuming, these meetings were fruitful and necessary to continue to clarify our thinking and generate new directions.

Permission was sought and granted to photograph the exterior and interior of an old and somewhat neglected local primary school in Melbourne. It was important to show our pre-service teachers that 21st century ideas could occur in old structures as these buildings may well be their reality. The designers began gutting the existing classrooms, staircases, offices and playground areas to create a virtual wonderland of shifting perceptions, sounds and movements. For instance there are trap doors, leaves blowing, flying cupcakes, vegetables growing, a claw foot bathtub and dinosaurs emerging from the walls. These extinct creatures remind us that old ideas are still lurking.

The use of Flash-related technologies - Zoomify and Flashpaper - appear over time as the users enter each room. Images and signs on the walls change several times. This encourages participants to revisit the places again and again. This act of revisiting lived experience is not possible in the actual classroom, yet returning to the experience virtually and viewing parts over time through a range of lenses is essential in promoting reflective practices that might one day transform teaching.

LATHNER PRIMARY SCHOOL

We recognized the influence and importance of the wider context for understanding and accepting change. It is often when there is instability or threat, that change is sought. The digital innovation allowed us to create carefully orchestrated scenarios to invite pre-service teachers into the life of a school educating towards change. One scenario, for instance, plants the seeds for needed change and begins building alternative stories for how learning can be conceived in this school. The pre-service teachers learn that several converging circumstances prompt the need for some radical rethinking about the direction of Lathner Primary. For the past several years the teachers at the school had been informally annotating changes in students' behaviours and general attitudes towards learning. They often spoke about children's shorter attention spans, incessant comments about being bored, tired and unmotivated. The teachers also felt that the students were far less compliant, often refusing to do what they were told. The staff members at the school were finding more students disruptive while others just tuned out. The rewards and punishments given out were not working. In fact they were creating even greater divisions between students. The staff generally agreed that the abilities and knowledge base of the students in recent years were greater than ever before but the students were not performing to their potential and were increasingly difficult to manage. The job of teaching was becoming highly stressful.

We created new stories about Lathner Primary, a school that was under threat of closure. The virtual Principal, Brian Treadwell, was about to retire; he felt tired, worn down by the difficulties the school faced and he was no longer willing to fight to save this school. He describes the passage of change:

A once middle class predominantly Anglo Saxon population became a far more multicultural community with greater mobility, and quite varied economic levels. There were more rental properties than ever before and more families in financial need. There were also fewer children in the area and the population of Lather Primary was rapidly declining. So, this once stable and somewhat predictable school community was in the midst of a sizable change.

Along with these two major shifts, five virtual teachers retired or transferred schools. Two of these teachers admitted they had become unable to cope with the daily student demands. One long standing, highly traditional virtual teacher, Eileen Trigony, remained at Lathner Primary. She would represent teachers who hold onto patterned ways of teaching. Mrs Trigony refuses to adopt the new pedagogies and holds tightly to her formal and highly disciplined teacher-centered approach. Yet we also did not want to polarise this teacher and paint her as a stereotype of the 'old guard'. Eileen Trigony reveals some of the reasons behind her resistance and her fear of letting go of known practices. Pre-service teachers learn to recognize more of the complexities of changing beliefs.

In a series of folders in the virtual school we reveal that a new group of beginning teachers was hired along with one more experienced teacher, each bringing their unique orientations and personalities to teaching and learning and new challenges to existing staff. These teachers breathed new life and energy into a somewhat tired and troubled school. One of these new virtual teachers was Anna Jones, one of the mentors for our pre-service teachers. At staff meetings Anna, in particular, kept asking questions, important questions about some of the existing and enduring beliefs and practices at the school. From this group of new teachers with current pedagogies and critical questioning came renewed energy for change in the Principal and several members of staff. Slowly the school started a process of bettering existing conditions. A series of sustained and disruptive innovations were planned, agreed upon and actualised, drawing staff and the wider community into ongoing communities of practice.

Through this renewal process it became apparent that staff did not always know why they were perpetuating particular philosophies and practices. One teacher writes:

Clearly many of our practices were no longer effective and yet we were clinging to them because, I suppose, these practices were what we knew and they were also who we were. A few teachers started to read some current research on new pedagogie. (Latham et al 2006, p.54).

THE TEACHERS' NARRATIVES

Lathner Primary evolved in response to our developing pedagogical aims and pre-service teacher feedback. As mentioned earlier, some of the less comfortable aspects of our teaching lay in the negotiation of critical pre-service teacher feedback. Students initially found the content of the virtual school overwhelming. They often experienced technical difficulties accessing the site. They found 25 Grade 4/5 students too many and too virtual to grasp.

We reduced the class size to 20. Over time, we focused less on the school as a whole or the children in one grade and more on the class teachers, and the ways in which they were moving their teaching to new times. For instance, Anna Jones's profile was built in lectures, tutorials, online through her professional journal and in her interactions with the pre-service teachers, other colleagues, parents and students. From her professional journal Anna Jones explains some of the tensions she experiences daily:

I realise that most of the questions are coming from me lately – I'm slipping back a little as I try and take the students on to where I want them to go, not where they are interested in going. I don't feel I can always relinquish that control. Tomorrow I'm going to consciously try a different starting point from their questions, and see where that goes ...

We deliberately created a virtual teacher who keeps facing her traditional past, slipping back to habitual modes of operating but still seeking needed change. Anna Jones is a highly reflective practitioner and a teacher/researcher. She became the kind of questioning reflective teacher we encourage our pre-service teachers to become.

Along with this we built and strengthened the school and community around the school to give credence to the pedagogical and physical shifts in this school and in this classroom. For instance, the staff was far more responsive to what learners bring to the learning and the wealth of expertise brought by the community around the school. The virtual Principal, Brian Treadwell, successfully applied for funds to renovate the playground in the school. The students in each grade are working on designs for the new playground and the family committee has put in a vegetable garden with the children's support. As the viewer navigates through the virtual school, the children's models and designs for the playground can be accessed in progress. Brian Treadwell recognizes the vital importance of utilising the resources of the community and of building a supportive community.

The authors purposefully made Lathner Primary a school on the edge. Thrown into this foreign territory, our pre-service teachers continue to discuss teaching and learning in this environment and how they might best meet the needs of their students. Our novice teachers form a teaching and learning community by talking face to face in and outside of university tutorial sessions, and writing online about the same school, the same classroom and the same students. 'Experts' are invited into the virtual environment to add a rich layer of learning and further support pre-service understanding of the school community. Pre-service teachers' interactions with authors, for example, provide appreciation of authors' work and the research undertaken while writing a text. They also deepen comprehension about some of the complexities inherent in the text. These discoveries are discussed and interrogated in some detail, both online and in face to face tutorials. We introduced two blogs to the online site. One of the blogs acts as a newsletter to parents and other family members and is designed, written and edited by the 4/5 F students. The second blog gives the visitor background information on the school and its creation. The following is taken from the Creating Lathner Primary blog:

We decided to name this direction 'Opening windows, Opening doors'.

In this spirit, students are often taught by teams rather than a single teacher, teams that include their peers and friends of the school. We are opposed to teaching behind closed doors. Teachers are being given increased opportunity to visit one another's classrooms, in order to learn from one another. The principal, Brian Treadwell, takes many teachers' classes while they visit other rooms. This gives him a much stronger understanding of what children at the school need.

Teachers are encouraged to move learning out to the wider community and to invite members of the community into the school to share their stories, their knowledge and their skills. We recognize that some of these changes can be threatening to teachers as they may feel they are under constant scrutiny. We are working hard to help our teachers understand that they are being watched because they have a great deal to offer others. We want our teachers to know that we not only trust them, we also value what they bring and we want to learn from them.

These innovations in our school are opening up and stimulating new kinds of conversations in the staffroom (through the big coffee mug in the office) about teaching and learning.

RESEARCHING THE ZONE OF DISCOMFORT: STUDENT RESISTANCE

I was confused...I still haven't explored the school to its full potential but I realize I need to get lost and be open to new ideas and experiences. (Karl)

Boler (1999) argues that the first sign of the success of a pedagogy of discomfort is 'quite simply, the ability to recognize what it is that one doesn't want to know, and how one has developed emotional investments to protect oneself from knowing' (p. 200). This discomfort asks students to leave the familiar waters of learned beliefs and explore the riskier critical depths of ethical and moral differences. Pre-service teachers responding to the virtual school for the first time, wrote comments which reflected both the apprehension and exhilaration of venturing in to new territory:

To be honest, my initial reaction isn't a positive one. I feel reluctant and hesitant to give it a go because it's unlike anything I've done before. I'm used to the 'normal' way of doing things and tend to have trouble accepting change. (Rebecca)

Wow! This online form of learning of a virtual school is one I have never experienced before. The fact that it's set in what looks like a whole school setting is great ... It seems to cover very practical topics which will be relevant to us when we are out there teaching. I wonder how much of it is real, from real teachers. (Jennifer)

Learners are often reluctant to embrace new teaching practices and therefore we recognized the need to scaffold risk-taking, using as many available modes as possible. We also needed to interrogate and share our own risk taking.

For instance, Julie shares her risk taking in the online forum:

My challenge as a lecturer is to allow for silences - moments of awkwardness even - when I could try and gauge what students were thinking, or not understanding. When I go to observe pre-service teachers in action now, I find that sitting at the back of the class watching students helps me pick up little things that pass among students I never saw at the front of the classroom: comments and questions the teacher doesn't hear, expressions of revelation or confusion, blank workbook pages. To stop explicitly teaching when I have covered the material and shift from my teaching to the students' learning (which some fear as giving up control) is the area of my teaching I need always to keep in focus, looking for the little signs of understanding/not understanding.

Support is offered through sequencing lecture material as a continuous narrative and complementary tutorial activities, accessing the research literature in timely ways, and sharing peer knowledge in structured online forums and tutorial group discussion. These all serve to extend existing levels of understanding.

Guided ventures to connect what learners already know to less familiar territory we term 'sustained' innovation, while having pre-service teachers enter an unpredictable learning environment without a map is intended to be more *disruptive* in effect. Lathner Primary explores the potential of digital technology for both sustained and disruptive innovation, thus expanding spaces for rethinking routine pedagogical approaches. Moreover, we recognized that we, as teacher educators, also needed to take risks along with our students. We want to challenge traditional thinking through designing something completely new, yet we were cognisant of student feedback. We had to learn how to manage feedback that could be critical and negative; when to review and rework aspects of the virtual school and when to understand that frustration and criticism were an integral part of learning to deal with something unfamiliar and disruptive. The need for a responsive approach to our learners reminded us of Boler's (1999) assertion that, ideally, a pedagogy of discomfort represents 'an engaged and mutual exchange' (p. 200).

Lathner Primary School as an environment in progress has been 'growing in', as past and current pre-service teachers with digital skills add content and animate the school. They have augmented the website with children in conversation audio-taped from actual primary classrooms. In this sense, the virtual school is far from a static concept. Over the past six years since its initiation, the narratives have evolved, and will continue to evolve according to our analysis of need through our future ideas in relation to the resources available.

As we continue to build Lathner Primary School online and face to face, we depended largely on anecdotal responses from participants to evaluate the extent to which our aims are being achieved. We increasingly realise the need for more systematic, comprehensive feedback as part of an action research methodology. This involves planning, acting, reflecting, evaluating, and initiating additions and improvements which have assisted in expanding and strengthening our virtual school over time (Kemmis & McTaggart, 1988; Burns, 1999). As a process-oriented collective approach, action research helps us to contextualize our research knowledge by monitoring our teaching and students' learning over time, making informed and systematic decisions about change.

Our research focus continually shifts as we modify the virtual school and the subjects that surround it. For instance, in the last iteration we gave far greater emphasis to disrupting habitual and unexamined practices as we encouraged risk-taking. In this process of change we undertook three actions to support pre-service teachers:

- We presented a virtual school community that takes risks to enable their school to remain viable and flourish;
- We presented pre-service teachers with a mentor, albeit virtual, who values, supports and practises risk taking;
- As lecturers we identified and shared (with one another and with our students) ways in which we engage in risk-taking;

Even with a range of support structures in place, the analysis of pre-service teachers' abilities to cope with disruption and risk-taking is revealing. Many students describe risk taking apprehensively: 'It scares me,' one felt, as others articulated *'letting go of the reins', 'giving up control,' 'needing structure,' 'needing to know what works.'*

Allison expresses her fear of taking and not taking risks this way:

I know I need to push myself and explore new knowledge and ways of doing things. However there is so much at risk; the children and their education, my professional reputation and employment. Too many times I have asked myself, 'What if?' Maybe I should be asking 'What if I don't?

Ben, a peer, responds to Allison with the following:

I think it's important to not fall in the trap of always wondering 'what if' because that time could be better spent ... There are always going to be times when the risk we take doesn't work... I am sure that the successful risks will heavily outweigh the failed ideas...Personally, I want to try and eliminate the 'if only' as much as possible. A great way to do that is to take risks, preferably educated ones at that.

Bronwyn's comments below are reflective of the schooling system she inhabited:

Having just been spat out at the end of the kindergarten, primary school and high school/VCE assembly line, I asked myself as a learner, was I ever encouraged to take risks?

Sarah (6/08) sums up her learning as a pre-service teacher at Lathner Primary to her mentor, Anna Jones, she said:

When I first met Eileen Trigony [the most conservative teacher in the school] last term, I realized ... that this is what I'm like. Not to say Eileen isn't a wonderful teacher, but her teaching style has nothing to do with the philosophy of the school and the culture you created in your classroom that I now love so much. This got me thinking that I need to change and try a different approach to teaching to be better able to engage students to learn...

RESOLUTIONS AND RENEWED COMPLICATIONS: HOW WE ARE NEGOTIATING THE TECHNOLOGY

As pre-service teachers have a placement in the same classroom of the virtual school, they have reason to form a community of practice to build knowledge and learn from one another. Some staff in the School of Education are adopting classes in the virtual school and embedding content into the school that align with their courses, so they too have formed communities of practice. As well, some of the graduates who embrace the ideas inherent in the School have remained in touch to receive support, to return and talk to pre-service teachers, to dialogue with one another and to share successes and challenges. Yet resistance remains and we increasingly need greater understanding of pedagogical change. We also need to move slowly, to have ongoing dialogue and encourage students, staff and practising teachers to take greater ownership over the technology, the content and the pedagogy.

The school's growth in scope and complexity over the past few years has encouraged us to continue developing the concept, believing that it has the potential to offer rich learning and teaching understandings to other disciplines. While our concept is a populated classroom set in a primary school, the details of the space and texture of responses could transfer to a myriad other environments where more reflective practices are sought by critical educators from all sectors. However, the challenge remains in terms of immersing not only pre-service teachers, but also our colleagues into a New Learning context. The technical culture of teaching is not highly receptive to sharing knowledge. While the interchange of resources and ideas should be a teaching goal, the reality is that teachers are often isolated in classrooms and time poor. Ironically, but perhaps not unexpectedly, we have experienced more enthusiasm and willingness to use the virtual classroom from peers in other states than those who work closely with us. In this sense, we continue to build an expanding community of practice through communication technologies.

Carefully orchestrated and selected technology and how and when it is utilized has, by necessity, allowed the virtual school to remain dynamic, enriched by formative feedback and active staff, student and teacher involvement. We remain committed to the development of a digital resource which offers choice to those who engage with it: to reinforce learner comfort or, more productively, to disrupt and challenge habituated practice. The discovery of proliferating ways of achieving this has driven the growth of the School, and reinforced Boler's (1999) claim that in a generative mode of enquiry, there is no one 'right' resolution or ideology. Continued research into pre-service teachers' areas of discomfort will provide us with increasingly clearer understandings of how deep change in education might occur, and our role in encouraging and leading this process.

REFERENCES

ACDE. (2001). New Learning: A Charter of Australian education. ACDE: RMIT University.
Bigum, C. (1995). Schools and the internet: reinventing the 1980s? Paper delivered at IARTV seminar, Melbourne 24 May 1995.

Boler, M. (1999). *Feeling power: Emotions and education*. New York: Routledge.

Burns, A. (1999). *Collaborative Action Research*. Cambridge, UK: Cambridge University Press.

Christensen, C. M. (1997). *The innovator's dilemma: When new technologies can cause great firms to fail*. Boston: Harvard Business School Press.

Duffy, F. M. (2003). I think, therefore I am resistant to change: What we know - or think we know - is our biggest roadblock to learning. *Journal of Staff Development*, *24*(1).

Fagerberg, J. (2004). Innovation: A Guide to the Literature. In Fagerberg, J., Mowery, D., & Nelson, R. (Eds.), *The Oxford Handbook of Innovations* (pp. 1–26). Oxford, UK: Oxford University Press.

Ferry, B., Kervin, L., Cambourne, B., Turbill, J., Puglisi, S., Jonassen, D., & Hedberg, J. (2004). Online classroom simulation: The 'next wave' for pre-service teacher education? In R. Atkinson, C. McBeath, D. Jonas-Dwyer & R. Phillips (Eds.), *Beyond the comfort zone: Proceedings of the 21st ASCILITE Conference* (pp. 294-302). Retrieved from http://www.ascilite.org.au/conferences/perth04/procs/ferry.html

Gibson, S. E. (2002). Using a problem based multimedia enhanced approach in learning in the social studies classroom. *Australian Journal of Educational Technology*, *18*(3), 394–409.

Greene, M. (1973). *Teacher as stranger: Educational philosophy for the modern age*. Belmont, CA: Wadsworth.

Kemmis, S., & McTaggart, R. (1990). *The Action-research planner*. Geelong, Victoria: Deakin University.

Latham, G. Blaise, M., Dole, S., Faulkner, J., Lang, J., Malone, K. (2006). Learning to teach: New times, new practices. Melbourne, Australia: Oxford University Press.

Latham, G. (2007). *New Learning: Building surprise through the virtual*. Melbourne RMIT University.

Laurel, B. (1991). *Computers as theatre*. Reading, MA: Addison-Wesley Publishing Company. Oblinger, D. (2003). Boomers, gen-Xers and millennial: Understanding the new students. *EDUCAUSE Review*, *38*(4), 37–47.

Linch & E. G. Stutevant (Ed.). *Growing Literacy* (pp. 173-187). Pittsburgh: PA. College Reading Association.Schlechty, P. C. (2005). *Creating the capacity to support innovations*. Occasional Paper No. 2. Louisville, KY: Schlechty Centre.

Papert, S. (1993). *The Children's Machine: Rethinking School in the Age of the Computer*. New York: Basic Books.

Risco, V. (1995). *Using videodisc based cases to promote pre-service teachers problem solving and mental model building*. In W. M.

Senge, P., Scharmer, C. O., Jaworski, J., & Flowers, B. S. (2004). Presence: Human purpose and the field of the future. Cambridge, MA: SoL (The Society for Organizational learning, Inc.).

Zeichner, K. M. (1996). *Reflective teaching: An introduction*. Mahwah, NJ: L. Erlbaum Associates.

Section 4
Assessment and Accreditation

Chapter 10
Creating Electronic Evidence Rooms for NCATE Accreditation:
Using College LiveText Solutions

Natalie Johnson-Leslie
Arkansas State University, USA

ABSTRACT

For nearly a century the clarion call for more accountability at all levels of education across the USA has been made. As a result, we find accreditation bodies (national, regional and specialized), in the USA being independent of the Department of Education. In this chapter, the focus will be on creating electronic evidence rooms for The National Council for the Accreditation of Teacher Education (NCATE). NCATE was developed over 50 years ago requiring concrete evidence that teacher candidates are prepared rigorously to acquire the relevant body of knowledge and field experiences needed for them to be successful teachers. With technological advances, NCATE accredited institutions are given the charge to produce electronic evidence rooms as a means of show-casing tangible evidence of students, departments and colleges of education progress. This chapter will provide a comprehensive overview of how electronic evidence rooms are created using College LiveText Solutions for NCATE accreditation.

INTRODUCTION

In this chapter, student learning, as demonstrated by teacher candidates' is documented in the electronic evidence rooms for The National Council for Accreditation of Teacher Education (NCATE) accreditation. With the ubiquity of technologies electronic evidence rooms are created using a variety of media. The medium of focus for creating such electronic evidence room, for this chapter, is College LiveText Education Solutions™ (CLT™) (www.livetext.com). CLT™ features a repository of state standards and benchmarks to help educational institutions assess, measure, and report standards usages linked with student competencies outlined by NCATE. Part of the vision of any College of Education is the recognition that high-quality student learning is correlated with high-quality preparation that are attuned to simultaneous renewal strategies (Goodlad, 1994).

DOI: 10.4018/978-1-61520-899-9.ch010

This renewal is akin to changes in knowledge and skills being made at all levels impacting the education of children, pre-service and in-service teachers. One critical aspect of the knowledge and skills teacher candidates are expected to leave college with include but is not limited to the; use, integration, and application of computer technology. Both faculty and students are expected to use technology inclusive of CLT™ to archive evidence for NCATE. Instructors use CLT™ to develop and assess student learning outcomes. Simultaneously, students use CLT™ to create artifacts including; projects, lesson plans, and their electronic portfolio sample. The administrators then collate reports that account for the overall evidence of teacher candidates' performance outlined in the teaching and learning standards guiding the curricular (see Figure 1).

Figure 1 shows the web of activities that are carried out by the various stakeholders involved with the accreditation process. Specifically, the four primary objectives of this chapter are: evaluating how electronic evidence rooms are created and utilized; establishing a historical contextualization of accreditation in the USA; outlining the general principles and policies of accreditation; and addressing the issues, problems, and current trends in creating electronic evidence room for NCATE accreditation by using CLT™ to support technology leadership in teacher education.

Figure 1. The electronic evidence room web of activities for NCATE accreditation

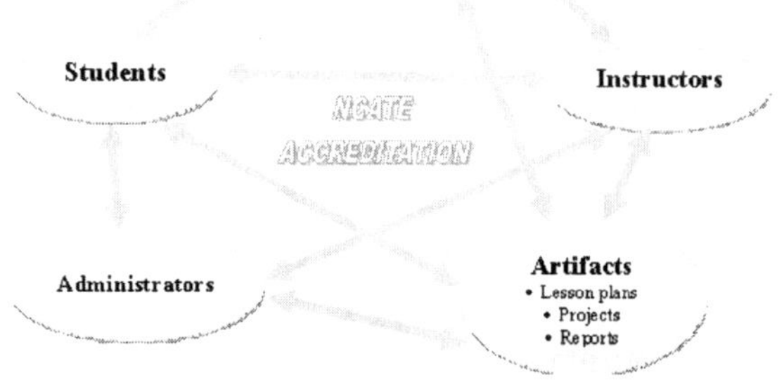

BACKGROUND

What is an Electronic Evidence/ Resource Room?

An electronic evidence room is defined as a purposeful environment in cyberspace guided by a common set of rules, techniques and tools for collecting, examining, preserving, retrieving and presenting data that has been processed electronically and has been stored on computer media. An electronic evidence/ resource room makes it easy for the review of evidence anytime, anywhere instead of waiting to wade through and reviewing hard-copy evidence (Wong, 2007). In this chapter, electronic evidence rooms are the electronic sites created by teacher candidates, faculty and administrators that contain documents based on specific standards of achievement as directed by the university and NCATE standards.

The Creation of Electronic Evidence Rooms

The advent of widespread electronic document handling, including word processing as well as electronic and voice mail and facsimile transmission, has revolutionized the areas of business, criminology, finance, and education globally (Wong, 2007; Hamilton, 2009). Interestingly, there is a plethora of literature regarding the creation of electronic evidence rooms in business, finance, and criminology. However, the review of literature revealed a sacristy of documentation regarding electronic evidence rooms. This chapter is important in technology leadership in order to fill the gap in the literature. In electronic evidence rooms, documents at all stages of development are accessible in unprecedented quantities, iterations and timeliness. In education specifically, many paper forms of transactions and evidences of accomplishment have been replaced with electronic means. These electronic documents are easily stored and retrievable. Electronic evidence rooms provide a wealth of potential evidence that educators and accreditation agencies welcome as an indication that teacher candidates meet the expected standards of performance.

Electronic files hold a wealth of information. Today, 93% of business documents exist only in electronic databases (Wong, 2007). In education, this trend continues to increase and more and more educational institutions are moving rapidly towards electronic evidence. There is a new paradigm in education regarding data storage and retrieval. In fact, data is everywhere and paper printing is only a partial glimpse of the underlying data. Paper evidence also becomes clunky and time consuming to sift through especially when there is a large amount of data.

In this chapter, the creation of electronic evidence rooms was for the expressed purpose of documenting the progress of teacher candidates against NCATE standards. Hence, the electronic evidence room is two tiered and must meet the following criteria: relevance, authenticity, originality, and free from unfair prejudices (Hamilton, 2009). Tier one encompasses students providing artifacts from which the institutional data is collated, analyzed, and reported. *First*, teacher candidates purchase access to the College LiveText portal to create their electronic evidences that must be relevant based on the class requirement. By relevance, teacher candidate's electronic evidence must meet the requirements outlined. There are checks and balances to ensure data relevance. Instructors ask students to produce artifacts that are relevant to the standards of performance expected of a teacher candidate. *Second*, each artifact is then assessed by class instructors based on a predetermined set of grading criteria. If there is a need for modification, teacher candidates are given the opportunity to do so. Hence, only relevant artifacts created by teacher candidates whose authenticity can be verified would be included in student's electronic evidence room.

Third, authenticity addresses maintaining data integrity. Hence, it has to be proven without a doubt that the artifacts teacher candidates display in the electronic evidence room is a true and accurate representation of each teacher candidate's performance. Authenticity is verified by teacher candidates signing and uploading an authorship form displayed in Appendix A, as part of their electronic evidence.

Fourth, in teacher education programs teacher candidates are encouraged and expected to produce original work. Therefore, candidates apply their knowledge in producing work that clearly shows their understanding of the various concepts taught. Originality also encompasses that teacher candidates acknowledge the sources they obtain the information from. Again, verification of student's original work is obtained through the signing and uploading of the (Family Educational Rights and Practices Act of 1974 (FERPA) and access document shown in Appendix B. *Finally*, work must be free from unjust biases as best as possible. Each individual has some degree of prejudices; however, in the artifacts students selected for the electronic evidence must not be laced with prejudices. After the compilation of teacher candidate's electronic evidence these evidences are further assessed in tier two.

Tier two of the electronic evidence room addresses the collation, analysis and reporting of the data to the accreditation agency. In College LiveText, the advanced reporting features allow faculty to assess the data and send an official report to program administrators. This official report is then mined by the administrators who analyze the data and produce the final report for NCATE. The final report is accessed by NCATE board of examiners from the electronic evidence room prepared by school administrators who historically, are accountable for teacher candidates meeting and exceeding the criteria outlined by NCATE.

History of the Development of Electronic Evidence Room

Over the last five years, changes in how evidence of student performance is evaluated, collated and reported has benefitted from the ubiquity of technology. In the state of Arkansas, one of the largest preparers of teacher candidates adopted the software College LiveText as the means of creating electronic evidence rooms. In any given year, up to 900 students are prepared for licensure in the college. Licenses are in the areas pre-school to four years old (PK-4); fourth to eighth grade (4-8) and secondary education (7-12) students for teachers to serve in both public and private schools. With the large number of teacher candidates being prepared each year, it is imperative that a reliable and reputable system for collating and reporting data was selected. To ensure quality preparation that is in keeping with NCATE accreditation standards, authentic assessments of candidate's learning was of paramount importance in selecting the software (Astin, 1985). Traditional paper-based evidence of teacher candidate's performance gave way to electronic forms of evidence. These electronic forms of evidence also were in keeping with the NCATE requirements in providing authentic, original, prejudice free, and relevant evidences that program standards were being met adequately by students being prepared to become teachers (Johnson-Leslie, in press)

Historically, since the 2003-2004 academic year, all teacher candidates were required to develop and maintain electronic documents compiled as an electronic portfolio to showcase their academic performance over the course of their study. Teacher candidates began the process of creating their electronic evidence rooms as part of their introduction to teaching courses—their initial gateway into the teacher education program (see Figure 2 for general guidelines for creating and maintaining electronic evidence rooms).

Figure 2 shows the steps in the process of students creating electronic evidence rooms. At level 1, admission to the teacher education program, the initial review of electronic evidence is conducted as part of the admission process to the Teacher Education Program. In level II, pre-teacher intern review the second review is completed prior to submission of the Pre-Teacher Intern Review application to the Office of Professional Education Programs or placement office. In Level III, admission to the student internship, review is completed prior to submission of the application for admission to the student internship and a copy of the electronic evidence assessment submitted with the validation of internship review to the office of professional programs. Level IV, the final level program exit, has the review completed near the conclusion of the internship experience of teacher candidates. The official performance report is collated by the instructors and submitted for the institutional report to the administrators. Administrators then compile all the electronic evidence and formulate the report that will be populated for NCATE's Board of Examiners to review as electronic evidence that pre-service teachers do meet the requirements as outlined by the accreditation standards used to measure students' success to become effective teachers (Institutional Report Continuing Accreditation, 2008; Johnson-Leslie, in press).

The creation of the electronic evidence rooms by teacher candidates was one means of facilitating the seamless integration of technology in students' preparation to become teachers as well as having students become actively engaged with technology. Based on the capacity that computer

Figure 2. General guidelines for creating and maintaining electronic evidence rooms

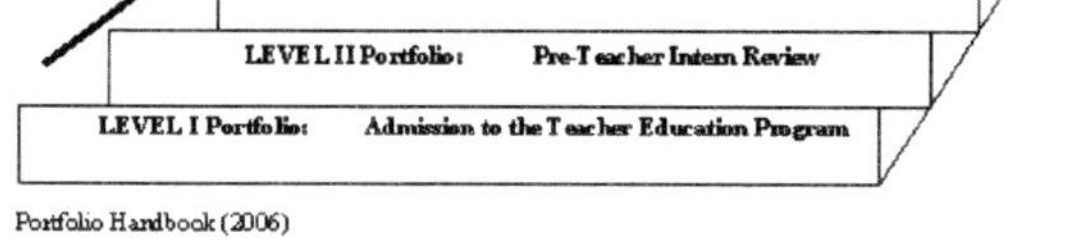

Portfolio Handbook (2006)

technology allows, students also were required to use multimedia technology including recording, editing, and incorporating text, images, audio, and video in the production of their electronic evidence room.

Selecting the Electronic Evidence Room System

After a rigorous process of evaluating software for the creation of electronic evidence room, in fall 2002, CLT™ was introduced and adopted in the college of education as the portal that would best facilitate the development and maintenance of electronic evidence for students, instructors and administrators. According to Don Maness, Associate Dean in the College of Education, as cited in LiveText Solutions, inc., (2004)

After looking at a number of online portfolio applications that met our requirements, we were convinced that LiveText not only provides the most advanced functionality, but it was also very customer focused with regards to service, user feedback, and that continual effort to improve and expand its services.

As mentioned in the above quote, several e-portfolio applications were surveyed before selecting CLT™ as the most comprehensive and cost effective electronic evidence creation system suitable for the needs and context of teacher candidates. In subsequent pages of this chapter, a detailed description of CLT™ with its standards database among other relevant features will be described. The focus will now be on contextualization of accreditation—a main element of this chapter.

HISTORICAL CONTEXTUALIZATION OF ACCREDITATION

What is the primary difference between higher education in the United States of America (USA) and higher education in many other countries? Research reveals that there is no centralized government control over higher education in the USA (Education Encyclopedia, 2009), when compared with other nations. How has United States emerged as having one of most highly recognized system of higher education with no centralized government control? The rigorous process of accreditation, that is responsible for assessing an institution's quality and integrity help to provide the checks and balances for ensuring that graduates from institutions of higher education possess the necessary skills, knowledge, and competencies required to practice in any given field. Accreditation can be loosely defined as quality control while providing protection from governmental interference and simultaneously ensuring academic freedom.

The need for a quality control system emerged in the late 1800's when colleges and universities began mushrooming in the USA with no regulatory system in place. Commonly acceptable standards for admission and graduating became important to parents, educators and the public. Institutions deemed as having higher quality clamored for governmental regulation to reduce competition. Around 1870, the Bureau of Education commissioned the Carnegie Foundation to evaluate these institutions. The Carnegie Foundation recommended that if institutions of higher education wanted to be regulated they would have to do that task themselves (Black & Smith, 2001).

Harvard one of the earliest institutions of higher education partnered with the Massachusetts Classical and High School Association to form the first regional accreditation association "The New England Association of Schools and Colleges." Between 1885 and 1923 there were six regional accrediting associations across the USA. Each association differed in size, scope, and traditions but they provided a general or basic framework for quality control. As time and the need developed, this basic framework was further developed and common standards that led to the formulation of the accreditation process were negotiated. Hence, today there is a degree of coherence and continuity that has the ability to respond to the sometimes changing accreditation process that serves as a tool of communication and discussion forum for national and regional accrediting bodies (Education Encyclopedia, 2009).

Since 1954, the U. S. Department of Education officially recognized NCATE as a regional accrediting body for institutions that prepare teacher candidates and other professional personnel for work in all levels of education, pre-kindergarten through college (Pre K-16). The main thrust of NCATE, a non-profit, non-governmental organization is the issue of accountability. Based on the issue of accountability NCATE develops standards, policies, and procedures that must be followed and achieved in order that institutions receive the stamp of approval from NCATE. This stamp of approval indicates that the accredited institution produces competent, caring, and qualified teachers and other professional school personnel who can help all students learn. Student learning is the ultimate educational accomplishment in U.S. education system (Professional Standards Accreditation of Teacher Preparation Institutions, 2008). In essence, NCATE provides guidelines for the general policies and practices that govern accreditation (Cibulka, 2008; Education Encyclopedia, 2009).

GENERAL PRINCIPLES AND PHILOSOPHY OF ACCREDITATION

Across the USA, educational institutions can voluntarily select any accreditation body for evaluating their programs and degrees offered. Thus, self-regulation through the rigorous process of accreditation embodies a traditional U.S. philosophy of self-governance, representative, flexible, and responsive system. Accreditation serves to enhance educational quality throughout the USA and the world at large help to maintain and improve the effectiveness of institutions, ensuring that these institutions meet the overarching standards established by the higher education community, and simultaneously serves as a common denominator of shared values and practices among the diverse institutions.

The stamp of approval, that is, accreditation by the NCATE signifies that an institution has the resources, programs, and services sufficient to accomplish and sustain the goal of preparing teacher candidates for service in public and private schools (www.ncate.org). In other words, accreditation signifies that such an institution maintains clearly measurable educational objectives that are consistent with the mission of the institution as well as degrees/programs offered (Commission on Colleges of the Southern Association of Colleges and Schools, 2004).

Accreditation can be seen as both a process and a product as it relies on integrity, thoughtful and principled judgment, rigorous application of requirements, and a context of trust from all parties. More often than not, accreditation can be seen as a having four main principles (1) An evaluation of an institution's effectiveness in the fulfillment of its own mission; (2) compliance with the requirements of the accrediting body, (3) continuing efforts to enhance the quality of student learning and its programs and services, and (4) providing a means of continuing accountability to constituents and the public (www.ncate.org). These four principles are shown in Figure 3

As shown in Figure 3, based upon reasoned judgment, the principles of accreditation are based on institutional effectiveness, student learning, compliance, and accountability. Each principle is not independent of the other. With reference to Gergen's (1999) analogy, the focus is on the game of chess rather than on the component pieces for the game to be relevant. Therefore, it is the sum, or the product of all four principles that results in institutions earning the status of being accredited, than simply focusing on each component part.

What is the end-product of accreditation? The product of accreditation is generally a public statement of an educational institution's ability to continually provide effective programs and services based on agreed-upon standards (Professional Standards Accreditation of Teacher Preparation Institutions, 2008). Embedded in this public statement is an affirmation that the institution is committed to pursue its educational mission. The bedrock of this overall educational mission is comprehensive as it protects the right of faculty members to teach, investigate, and publish freely; and the right of students to access opportunities for learning and for the open exchange of ideas without fear of discrimination (Holmberg, 1997). Furthermore, exercising these rights should not interfere with the broader obligation of the educational institution to offer enhance student learning, which is one of the sound principles of evidence based accreditation.

Evidence based accreditation has been one of the hallmarks of NCATE accreditation since its inception (Cibulka, 2008). As a result, teacher education programs have over the years provided these evidences of student learning in multiple formats. Paper-based portfolio evidence was the classic medium used for decades to provide evidence of student learning for teacher candidates. With the ubiquity of technology, the requirements have not changed. However, technology media is now used as the primary medium to provide electronic evidence of the performance of teacher candidates. In essence, technology has been used to successfully replace the paper-based portfolios that generally provided rooms full of evidence for the NCATE accreditation teams to evaluate during visits. Technology has not solved all the issues that may arise. However, it has revolutionized the ways in which electronic evidence is provided. Not-with-standing, the positive effects of technology in providing electronic evidence, there are issues, problems and trends that teacher education programs need to wrestle with as they create electronic evidence rooms for NCATE.

Figure 3. Four Main Principles of Accreditation

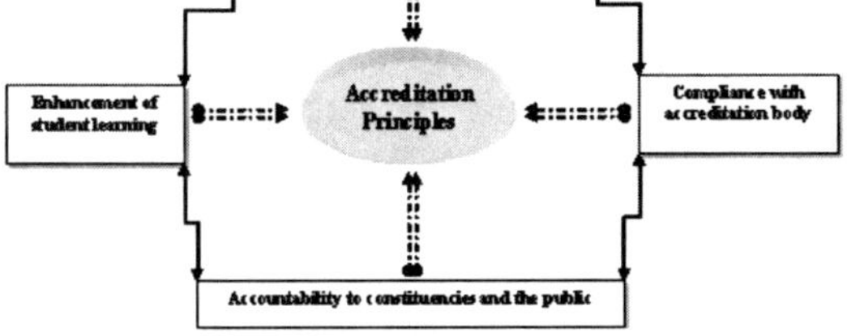

MAIN FOCUS OF THE CHAPTER

The Issues in Creating Electronic Evidence Room for NCATE Accreditation: Using College LiveText Solutions to Support Technology Leadership in Teacher Education

The issue of evidence-based accountability continues to be a key concern in education. Thus, sweeping changes in America's educational system including the No Child Left Behind (U.S. Department of Education, 2003) initiative has led colleges and universities to be more accountable in accurately measuring and reporting student learning competencies. To support and measure these reforms, state and federal legislators as well as accreditation agencies have issued many standards and guidelines. For education reform to be effective there must be simultaneous renewal (Goodlad, 1994), that include the reform of teacher preparation as well as schools in order that the ultimate goal of improved student learning will result from high standards of teaching and learning. It is through the rigorous processes of accreditation, licensing, and advanced board certification that improvement in student learning will be realized (Professional Standards Accreditation of Teacher Preparation Institutions, 2008).

NCATE has over the years designed standards and guidelines that are essential. These standards help to advance the reform of and ensure that accreditation, licensing, and advanced certification requirements are compatible with the needs for advancing quality assurance in education on the whole. In this section of the chapter, three issues will be elucidated (1) standards guiding performance, (2) epistemological foundations, and (3) advantages of technology use.

Standards Guiding Performance

NCATE has six standards that guide the preparation of teacher candidates in teacher education programs as shown on Table 1.

As shown in Table 1, the six standards for guiding student performances are not prescriptive. Teacher preparation programs select the specific curriculum and course work for teacher candidates to meet the standards outlined. Each standard clearly delineate the general performances expected by all teacher candidate to accomplish during their preparation.

Standard 1: Candidate Knowledge, Skills and Dispositions

This is the bedrock for preparing teacher candidates. Teachers must have a solid knowledge base of the content they will teach. This knowledge must not be inert but practical and applicable in demonstrating the content, pedagogical, and professional knowledge, skills, and dispositions necessary to help all students learn. Content knowledge and pedagogical content knowledge (the art of teaching) are important for teacher candidates to develop expertise. Both encapsulate effective instruction, meaningful learning experiences, utilizing valid and reliable forms of assessment strategies, and creating positive environments that support student learning.

Standard 2: Assessment System and Unit Evaluation

Part of the knowledge base teacher candidates are expected to master includes the creation and selection of valid and reliable assessments. In order to use these assessments effectively in the classroom it is important that the broader education unit has an assessment system in place. The purpose of this assessment system is to collect and analyze data on applicant qualifications as well as on the performance of each teacher candidate. Teacher candidates must show competence before gaining acceptance in the teacher education program (evidence by Praxis 1 and any other competency standardized exams scores); during preparation (monitored by the rigorous course and field work pre-service teacher candidates are expected to complete); and recommendation for licensure prior to graduation before they go out to be in-service teaching. For rigor and depth of preparation the assessment system should be inclusive of multiple assessments including performance-based assessments.

Table 1. NCATE's 6 standards guiding performances

Standard 1	Candidate knowledge, skills and dispositions
Standard 2	Assessment system and unit evaluation
Standard 3	Field experiences and clinical practice
Standard 4	Diversity
Standard 5	Faculty qualifications, performance and development
Standard 6	Unit governance and resources

Standard 3: Field Experiences and Clinical Practice

All teacher preparation programs are expected to design and implement multiple field and clinical experiences so that teacher candidates can further develop and demonstrate the knowledge, skills and dispositions they were taught. The clinical experiences serve as a capstone for teacher candidate's learning at different stages in their preparation. The clinical practice is both extensive and intensive for teacher candidates. They are required to demonstrate competence in their professional role as teachers during these experiences. Teacher candidates must plan, organize, implement, and evaluate meaningful activities that facilitate student learning. In addition, they have to demonstrate the ability to manage their classroom that comprises of students—some having special needs and others from diverse ethnic, racial, gender, and socioeconomic groups.

Standard 4: Diversity

The issue of diversity can sometimes be difficult to manage. Teacher preparation programs are expected to design, implement and evaluate both curriculum and experiences for candidates to acquire and apply knowledge, skills and dispositions that are fundamental to the diverse learning styles of learners. Furthermore, the issue of diversity includes the expectation that teacher candidates have the opportunity to interact with other teacher candidates, faculty, in-service teachers, administrators and P–12 students from diverse groups.

Standard 5: Faculty Qualifications, Performance and Development

In order to prepare teacher candidates to be successful in the classroom, the faculty members teaching them are expected to be highly qualified demonstrating best professional practices in scholarship, service and teaching. It is conventional wisdom that teachers generally teach how they were taught, hence, it is important that teacher candidates are exposed to effective role models who have exceptional expertise in their content area. Of great importance is the need for supervising faculty members to have professional experiences in school settings in the areas they supervise. In other words, these supervisors must be licensed teachers in the field they teach or supervise.

As professionals, all education faculty members are expected to be engaged in conducting scholarly work and service to the institution and the wider community. Standard five also outlines that teacher education faculty must collaborate with faculty from other institutions as well as P–12 school practitioners. This collaboration will serve as a catalyst to improve teaching, learning and the preparation of teacher candidates. Prior to going out into classrooms of their own, teacher candidates need multiple experiences in the classroom, observing, learning, assisting and being mentored by veteran teachers. Mentorship is extremely important during this process. Part of the requirement for maintaining their positions in teacher education programs, it is expected that each faculty performance is evaluated to document and further encourage professional development and growth for faculty.

Standard 6: Unit Governance and Resources

The final governing standard outlined by NCATE addresses the area of governance and resources on the whole. Both are important for adequately preparing teacher candidates. Thus, the teacher education unit is expected to have the budget, personnel and facilities, including information technology resources to prepare teacher candidates to meet professional, state and institutional standards. The budget allocations are expected to be proportional to comparable units on campus in terms of number of faculty, support personnel, support programs, and faculty workloads to name a few. It is also expected that facilities support the use of information technology by both teacher candidates and faculty. Most importantly, faculty and teacher candidates need to have access to current and sufficient curricular and library resources and electronic information for them to be prepared holistically for the teaching profession (www.ncate.org).

In sum, NCATE has provided teacher preparation programs with general guidelines to govern how teacher candidates are prepared for teaching. There must be a solid base for candidate knowledge, skills, and dispositions; effective assessment system and unit evaluation must be in place to provide checks and balances in the unit. Each teacher candidate must experience multiple opportunities for meaningful field experiences and clinical practice as part of their training. Diversity is a key issue that teacher candidates need to be grounded in so they are better prepared to handle the diversity in today's classroom. Qualified faculty members are expected to provide solid teaching and learning strategies for teacher candidates to emulate and adapt to fit the needs of their students. All these activities must be carried out in units where there is good governance as well as needed resources. Together these resources, both tangible and non-tangible help to shape students epistemological views as they are prepared to become teachers.

The Epistemology of Teacher Candidates Creating Electronic Evidence

Is there a relationship between epistemology and teacher candidates' ability to provide electronic evidence in their work? Is this epistemological connection made known to teacher candidates? Does NCATE require teacher candidates to demonstrate their epistemological grounding in the electronic artifacts they present? In this section of the chapter, a clear description regarding teacher candidate epistemological foundation in creating electronic evidence will be elucidated as a key issue.

First, an outline of the constructivist view that influences how teacher candidates develop, select, and reflect on electronic evidence in shaping their epistemological roots will be explained. The basic premise of constructivism is grounded in the tenets of Gergen (1999) who posits that reality is a social construction by the individuals who have experienced such. Earlier proponents of constructivism such as Dewey, Piaget and Vygotsky also positioned constructivism in each individual's unique set of experiences. The early work of Dewey grounds education in experiential or activity based learning. Such learning seeds both knowledge and ideas as emerging from specific situations that occur in a social context. Classrooms provide the social context whereby teacher candidates are engaged in a community of learners questioning, discussion and problem solving as they build their knowledge together (Dewey, 1966).

Like Dewey, Piaget's posits that constructivism is anchored in how learners formulate their knowledge based on the experiences they encounter in social settings. In other words the development of the mind is fundamental to the knowledge the learner will acquire. According to Piaget (1973) "To understand is to discover, or reconstruct by rediscovery, and such conditions must be complied with if in the future individuals are to be formed who are capable of production and creativity and not simply repetition" (p. 92). As Piaget worked with children he learned that they went through multiple phases of mental development as they accept and reject ideas. It is in the social context that the students discover relationships and ideas that are meaningful to them. Similarly, teacher candidates make meaning of ideas and situations in the social context they are immersed in as they prepare to become teachers.

Vygotsky (1978) is another important proponent to the concept of constructivism. He purported that individuals learned concepts based on the everyday activities they encounter. Hence, learners draw on prior and new experiences in order to formulate or construct their reality. Each experience impact and is impacted by the other, creating an interwoven fabric of experiences from which the teacher candidate can build their knowledge base. As teacher candidates create electronic evidence rooms, they construct their knowledge based on their prior and current experiences in the teacher education program. For example, based on the 4 gateways, teacher candidates have to select the relevant artifacts to include in their evidence rooms that may have been constructed in former years. The choices they make are influenced by their current set of reality. This reality is fashioned by outside impacted by cultural, historical, political, and social norms influences within a specific context and time frame as shown in Figure 4.

Figure 4 indicates that one's epistemological point of view does not operate in a vacuum. Rather, it is shaped by external forces that the individual has no control over. Even though the relationship between teacher candidates' epistemological standing and the requirement to provide electronic evidence may not be overtly articulated through coursework and even discussions across the curriculum, the choices teacher candidates make are greatly influenced by the wider learning environment that are involved in within the confines of context and time (Darlston-Jones, 2007). Therefore, the information available, the teaching strategies utilized, types of assessments required, issues in the society as they relate to history, politics, culture and social norms all shape teacher candidates views and decisions. Each teacher candidate interprets and makes sense of his/her world. In providing electronic evidence, the training, requirements related to standards and experiences of teacher candidates also will determine what they represent in the electronic evidence room. Thus, we see the unique *differences* of teacher candidates evident in their creative work in presenting artifacts relevant to the learning goals. Furthermore, there will be some essential *sameness* evident because of the use of CLT™ and the advantages it brings as the technology media housing teacher candidates' electronic evidences (Ashworth, 2003).

ADVANTAGES OF USING TECHNOLOGY TO CREATE ELECTRONIC EVIDENCE ROOMS

Advances in Technology around the Globe have Revolutionized all Aspects of Education

Computer-based instruction has been widely used over the past three decades and these technologies have dramatically changed the way information is gathered, research is conducted, and how communication is conducted with others all over the globe (Wang, 2005). Considering all the changes technology has ushered into the realms of education what are the advantages for teacher candidates to use this medium for creating electronic evidence rooms? Do we really need the use of technology for accreditation purposes?

Teacher candidates are expected to utilize technology in their preparation and implementation of lessons in the classroom. Even though technology usage is not explicitly mentioned in the NCATE

Figure 4. How teacher candidate develop their epistemology

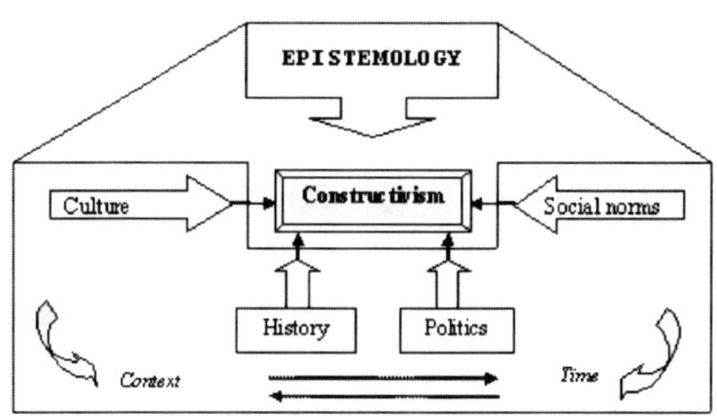

standards, there is a furrowing expectation in today's technological age to use technology. In fact, since 1998, the International Society for Technology in Teacher Education (ISTE) has provided standards for improving teaching and learning skills for all stakeholders including (students, teachers, and administrators) to help measure proficiency and set achievable goals for the knowledge, skills, and attitudes needed for success in today's digital age (www.iste.org). What are the hallmarks of a new education leader? According to Kenezek (2008) the hallmarks of a new education leader entails being comfortable as a co-learner with others using technology efficiently, moving ahead with the global community with advances in technology, and demonstrate a vision of integrating technology in the curricular for the development of technology skills of others.

Teacher candidates are being prepared to be new leaders in the field of education and technology is being utilized as a means of helping to prepare these teachers for the awesome tasks teachers have ahead of them. There are advantages for using technology to provide electronic evidence of their learning during their preparation as teacher candidates. Technology helps them to:

- Allows students to concentrate on problem formulation and solution analysis
- Solve problems by enhancing critical and divergent thinking skills
- Facilitates demonstration and the use of multi-media
- Develop their visual and geometrical understanding
- Provides opportunities to advance ideas concretely
- Shows students creative abilities
- Explore concepts thoroughly
- Utilizes space efficiently

As today's teacher candidates continue to 'grow up digitally' there is a vast array of technology available for their usage—electronic gadgets from i-pods to i-phones (Alley, Blocher & Markel, 2008). The digital technologies available help fuel teacher candidate's wealth of knowledge and information. In fact, requiring teacher candidates to demonstrate their use of technology by producing electronic evidence using CLT™ is an excellent means of demonstrating students critical thinking, reasoning, and problem-solving capabilities. In this chapter, the electronic evidence provided outlines a logical way to help students manage the process of planning, learning, making sound judgment, collaborating and communicating, demonstrating the achievement of competencies; and illustrating the balanced view of how teacher candidates construct their knowledge and epistemology (Barrett, 2000; Bergman, 2004; Fiedler & Baumbach, 2008; Johnson-Leslie, in-press).

The electronic evidence rooms demonstrating students work in CLT™ are more than file cabinets of students work. An ideal electronic evidence room allows for flexible input, organization (objects/artifacts can be hierarchically organized in folders), retrieval (objects can be easily searched using key terms), and display (items can be grouped and permission granted to intended audience) (Barrett, 2000). When these criteria are followed, an electronic evidence room becomes a very versatile tool to meet the needs of all potential participants in the process (students, faculty, administrators as well as accreditation evaluators. When students create their electronic evidence rooms, they link the artifacts and contents to specific learning objectives that demonstrate student learning and linked to accreditation standards used to measure students' performance (Brown, 2002). Accompanying the many advantages available when planning electronic evidence rooms are problems that must be solved in order that electronic evidence rooms can provide the true evidences necessary.

TheProblems in Creating Electronic Evidence Room for NCATE Accreditation: Using College LiveText Solutions to Support Technology Leadership in Teacher Education

Considering the general needed startup expenses, copyright issues, objectionable materials and other potential disadvantages of technology, much research has been conducted regarding the effectiveness and workable strategies for creating electronic evidence rooms, in general (Wang, 2005). Specifically, problems that could possibly occur when creating electronic evidence room for NCATE accreditation include but is not limited to; reporting accomplishment of standards, authenticity of work, legal issues surrounding the viewing of students work in an electronic room, timely completion of activities and artifacts for review, and reporting clearly how teaching strategies are linked to student learning and accomplishment. These problems lead to the following questions: What strategies are used to measure outlined standards and guidelines? How are standards usage and accomplishments reported? How is authenticity of student's work verified? How do departments of teacher education link standard usage and accomplishments with student competencies? Are there legal issues that surround the display of students' work in the electronic room? What measures are in place for the timely completion and reporting of data? These questions are answered in this chapter as a means of providing concrete evidence for accreditation purposes.

REPORTING ACCOMPLISHMENT OF STANDARDS

CLT™ has a built-in selection of Specialty Professional Association (SPA) as well as state and school standards. SPAs are national associations representing the education profession, such as NAEYC, the Association for Childhood Education International (ACEI), Teachers of English to Speakers of Other Languages (TESOL), and National Council of Teachers of Mathematics (NCTM). NCATE is a coalition of more than 30 such associations. Approximately 20 of these SPAs have NCATE-approved standards that are embedded in CLT™. For example, Figure 5 shows how to access and add the ISTE standards in CLT™.

Figure 5 shows an example of how to obtain a specific standard set available in CLT™. Teacher candidates can select subject area, grade level as well as keywords for a specific lesson or requirement. Following this categorization, the number of standards that are applicable can be added as shown in Figure 6.

As shown in Figure 6, there were 91 ISTE standards that addressed computer usage (indicated by the arrow). The teacher candidate would select 1-5 standards by placing a check mark in the appropriate box then clicking the button to ADD only the relevant standards for the assignment or task. Teacher candidates would then address the selected standards explicitly as part of the work they display in the electronic evidence room.

AUTHENTICITY OF STUDENT WORK AND LEGAL ISSUES

Teacher candidates need to do their own work and present such as part of their training to be professionals. Hence, evidence has to be provided that indicate authenticity of work. One of the strategies in place to ensure authenticity is having students complete and sign an authorship form that indicates the work presented is that of the teacher candidate (see Appendix A for a copy of the authorship form). A second form serves as giving permission to faculty members to gain access to grading teacher candidate's work. In addition, this form satisfies the FERPA and ensures compliance. See

Figure 5. Accessing ISTE standards in CLT™

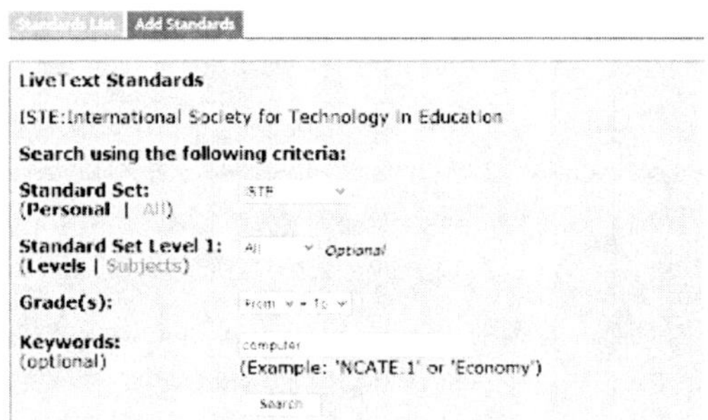

Appendix B for a copy of the access form. Both the authorship as well as the access and security forms are important to authenticate the work of teacher candidates.

TIMELY COMPLETION OF ACTIVITIES AND ARTIFACTS FOR REVIEW

Teacher candidates are expected to demonstrate their learning by selecting relevant artifacts that clearly show how they meet the outlined standards. Teacher candidates are expected to show their growth in learning over the course of their study. Hence, there is a time-line in place to help teacher candidates remain on task. As a result, at each level of their training, they upload electronic evidence of their accomplishment. Without this deliberate strategy of having a time-line in place, all the electronic evidence would not be in place to meet the deadline for accreditation.

After teacher candidates reflect on, select and upload their artifacts, they submit their work for review by selected faculty members. The faculty members who are able to review students work are given permission to review the work. In keeping with FERPA requirements, these faculty members cannot share teacher candidate's work with anyone else. Additionally, there were specific rubrics built in CLT™ that faculty members use to grade the performance of teacher candidates. These rubrics are used to ensure reliability among the graders and ensuring that the standards as outlined by NCATE will be adequately met (see Appendix C for a sample rubric). With consistency among graders, the reports generated will be both valid and reliable.

REPORTING ACHIEVEMENT

Expectations for preparing teachers have risen over the years. Teachers are held responsible for evaluating student achievement, ensuring that all students master a broad array of 21st Century learning skills to function in the global community (Cibulka, 2008). NCATE is expecting valid and reliable data that clearly shows student learning and accomplishment of the learning goals.

Each teacher education unit compiles the aggregated data to give the big picture of the performance of teacher candidates arranged under each standard. There are general standards writing teams preparing the reports that help to

Figure 6. Adding specific standards

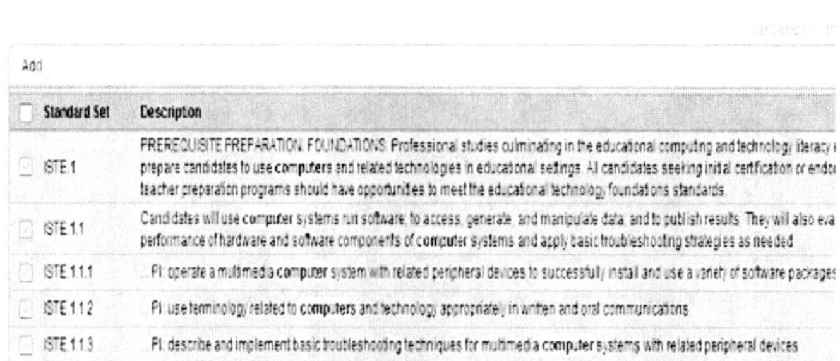

provide evidence of accomplishment by teacher candidates. Standard writing teams organize their reports in a cohesive and understandable way so that Board of Examiners (BOE) from NCATE can find the evidence readily.

First, a plan for the design of the electronic evidence room for each standard is developed. The plan is very detailed indicating a map of the site, labels and the format of the document proving the evidence. *Second*, there has to be a website designed with hyperlinks for ease of movement from artifact to artifact that conveys the evidence. *Third*, electronic evidence has to be clearly organized around the standards and each specific element of the standard. Clear connections have to be made between the evidence and the standards units are graded on. *Fourth*, there must be ease of movement between and among electronic evidence for ease of navigation during review.

Teacher education departments report their data that is collated in CLT™. For example, based on NCATE standard 1that addresses Candidate Knowledge, Skills, and Professional Dispositions, teacher candidate's performance on the Praxis II content test is one of the artifact displayed to show teacher candidate's performance to satisfy this standard. Figure 7 shows a sampling of students' performance on the Praxis II exam. The data was collected and generated in CLT™.

Figure 7 shows a snap shot of the performance of students at the three levels early childhood, mid-level and secondary programs from 2005-2008. This data shows the trend of student performance over the time period. Conclusions that can be drawn from the data displayed on Figure 7 include: an overall pass mark of 91%-92% over this 3 year period; Percent wise, early childhood majors have a consistently high rate of passes ranging from 95%-100%; the secondary program students are not all passing Praxis II content test, having scores ranging from 88%-92%. This trend indicates that the secondary program need to better prepare students in the standard 1 addressing content knowledge, so more secondary teacher candidates will succeed at passing Praxis II content exam.

THE TRENDS IN CREATING ELECTRONIC EVIDENCE ROOM FOR NCATE ACCREDITATION: USING COLLEGE LIVETEXT SOLUTIONS TO SUPPORT TECHNOLOGY LEADERSHIP IN TEACHER EDUCATION

The key trend in Colleges of Education for creating electronic evidence room for NCATE accreditation include the use of electronic portals such as

Figure 7. Pass rates on Praxis II content

Pass Rates on Praxis II Content Tests for Initial Teacher Preparation
For Period 2005 -2008

Praxis II Content Exams	2005-2006			2006-2007			2007-2008			Totals		
	Pass	Total	% Passed	Pass	Total	% Passed	Pass	Total	% Passed	Pass	Total	% Passed
Overall Pass Rate for Unit	268	293	91%	397	438	91%	294	315	93%	959	1046	92%
Early Childhood	91	96	95%	111	114	97%	77	77	100%	279	287	97%
Middle School	43	45	96%	63	69	91%	42	47	89%	148	161	92%
Secondary Programs	134	152	88%	223	255	87%	175	191	92%	532	598	89%

CLT™ Educational Solutions; excel spreadsheets; regular websites among other portals. As part of the trends, the electronic evidence rooms must be clearly labeled; artifacts must be clearly identified and have hot links; be attractive; easy to navigate; current; relevant and above all show concrete evidence of student learning. Furthermore, the trend of starting to work intently on accreditation issues close to the time of visits from the BOE is very common across multiple institutions. In addition, after the successful accreditation, many institutions tend to 'relax' for a number of years until the next accreditation draws near. The two latter trends could lead to rushing to collect quality data over a shorter period of time than is desirable.

The use of CLT™ can help to reduce the time lag between collecting data for accreditation processes. For example, data can be collected in an ongoing process before, during and after accreditation using CLT™. This way, no data will be lost and there will be robust data available at all times ready for the generation of reports to be displayed in the electronic evidence room.

Many institutions do follow the trend of hiring specific faculty and workers to compile the data for NCATE accreditation. In fact, many colleges of education have an office designated to focus on preparing for NCATE. This trend helps to ensure that the reports are generated in a timely and efficient manner and presented in an orderly and understandable manner in the designated electronic evidence room.

SOLUTIONS AND RECOMMENDATIONS

Unquestioningly, accountability of teacher candidate's learning will continue to be a focal point in the future in spite of the current issues, problem and trends. There clearly is a need in education for a detailed and textured discourse at all levels regarding the creation of electronic evidence rooms, how they work and how information is stored and retrieved. There is no doubt that technology is here to stay. Hence, the field of education is required to maintain the trend in requiring teacher candidate to utilize technology optimally as a tool in the teaching and learning processes. The bottom line is that technology works and allows teacher candidates to create electronic evidence rooms that display their work and indicates the degree to which they meet the benchmark standards as outlined by the respective accreditation agencies.

The research shows that based on the trends in education given the right conditions effectively using technology portals inclusive of CLT™ has the potential to:

- Help teacher candidates relate academics to practices in the classroom
- Motivate and engage learners based on the tenets of constructivism
- Accelerate, enrich, and deepen basic skills
- Increase the viability of teacher candidates
- Foster needed connections
- Contribute to change
- Strengthen teaching

With these potentials in mind, three recommendations are suggested:

1. Maintain the rigor in meeting accreditation standards through in-depth preparation of teacher candidates. This is key in producing effective teacher candidates who are creative both naturally and intellectually; divergent and productive thinkers who are fluent in their ability to generate many ideas, flexible in producing a wide variety of relevant ideas, original in thoughts and practices, effective in problem solving. Problem solving is important as the teacher candidates must invent new ways to solve problems in creating and utilizing electronic evidence rooms as well as in the use of technologies. Accreditation

agencies are evaluating teacher candidates not simply on knowledge acquisition, but also on utilization of the knowledge acquired.

2. Encourage students to develop their epistemology as it relates to the development of their electronic evidence. Earlier in this chapter teacher candidates' epistemological grounding was addressed briefly. It is recommended that a deliberate act of helping teacher candidate's recognize and develop their epistemological foundation should be firmly established. In addition, as part of the rigor mentioned in the first recommendation, teacher candidates also need understand their epistemological views to the extent where they can clearly see its impact on their thinking processes and how such underpins the approaches they utilize in creating electronic evidences to meet NCATE requirement.
3. Maintain a continuous data base between accreditation visits The research showed that many times the data collection process slows between accreditation visits. In some institutions effective measures are in place to reverse this trend by maintaining electronic evidence rooms at different levels over the period of time. Furthermore, some institutions follow the trend of having an office designated to prepare evidences for NCATE accreditation Board of Examiners. In so doing, faculty members are not stretched thin with the added responsibility when the time draws near for NCATE's visit, because there is a constant stream of accountability in-between visits. This is a preferred option rather than ending up in a stressful situation close to the time of an accreditation visit.

FUTURE RESEARCH DIRECTIONS

In the last five decades, accountability in higher education has reached a crescendo. Institutions of higher education have taken this call seriously and voluntarily have accreditation bodies evaluate their programs and progress. With the many advances in technology, this task has been enhanced with sophisticated means of collecting, analyzing and reporting progress. Some research has been conducted in the accreditation process. However, there is a place for more research action, both qualitative and quantitative. Based on the contents of this chapter, the future research proposed include but is not limited to: further exploration of the how learners develop their epistemological views as it relates to technology; compare and contrast CLT™ portal for collecting and reporting data with other systems available; explore the advantages and disadvantages of creating electronic evidence rooms versus the paper and pencil portfolios; surveying teacher candidates who prepare electronic evidence rooms during their preparation to find out their thought processes; and conducting comprehensive literature reviews on key accreditation topic areas and using the consensus on the priority areas for research.

These areas for future research will be highly beneficial to educators, researchers and doctoral candidates who are constantly in search of research topics. Addressing these topics will foster action in the research community addressing accountability and accreditation leading to expanded knowledge and literature in the field. The push for accountability has opened the door to set institutions firmly on a path where self-regulation of academic quality through accreditation is significantly important. NCATE provides such a system of accountability to teacher education programs preparing teacher candidates.

CONCLUSION

This chapter offered practical ideas regarding how electronic evidence rooms for NCATE accreditation using CLT™ solutions that focuses on student learning, assessment, and accreditation are created. Thus, institutions are provided with the most advanced, complete, and user-friendly web-based tools for developing, assessing, and measuring student learning. Furthermore, institutions can provide its students, faculty, administration, and stakeholders the best assurance of its commitment to accountability, continuous improvement, and excellence in education.

The clear delineation of the development and utilization of electronic evidence room provides a stable background for readers. The historical contextualization clearly outlines the growth and development of the accreditation process in the USA. The four general principles and philosophy of accreditation anchors the chapter on the tenet of accountability. The issues, trends, and problems highlighted are not novel approaches. However, each undergirds the importance of having a plan in place to meet accreditation standards. Using the CLT™ integrated solutions media for accreditation purposes helps to provide needed technology leadership in teacher education the main thrust of this book. The audience reading this book will find the contribution of this chapter to be useful, practical, insightful, and above all supportive of technology leadership in teacher education.

REFERENCES

Alley, P., Blocher, M., & Markel, S. (2008 March). *The road to electronic assessment: An examination of one college's systematic process for evaluating and recommending electronic portfolio software*. Paper presented at Society for Information Technology & Teacher Education, Las Vegas, Nevada.

Ashworth, P. (2003). The origins of qualitative psychology. In Smith, J. (Ed.), *Qualitative psychology: A practical guide to research methods*. Thousand Oaks, CA: Sage.

Astin, A. (1985). *Achieving educational excellence: A critical assessment of priorities and practices in higher education*. San Francisco: Jossey-Bass.

Barrett, H. (2000). Create your own electronic portfolio using off-the-shelf software to showcase your own or student work. *Learning & Leading with Technology*. Retrieved June 5, 2005, from http://electronicportfolios.com/portfolios/iste2k.html

Bergman, T. (2004). *Feasible electronic portfolios: Global networking for the self-directed learner in the digital age*. Retrieved June 5, 2008, from, http://www.mehs.educ.state.ak.us/portfolios/why _digital _portfolios.html.

Black, S., & Smith, E. (2001). The integrity of the council accreditation process. *Journal of Family and Consumer Sciences*, *93*(3), 52–62.

Brown, J. (2002). *Growing Up Digital: How the Web Changes Work, Education, and the Ways People Learn*. United States Distance Learning Association. Retrieved on March 10, 2009, from http://www.usdla.org/html/journal/FEB02_Issue/article01.html

Chuang, H. (2007). Making connections: n international student's perspective. In Thompson, A., Chuang, H., & Sahin, I. (Eds.), *Faculty mentoring: The power of students in developing technology expertise* (pp. 59–69). Charlotte, NC: Information Age Publishing.

Cibulka, J. (2008). Quality teaching: Moving forward to strengthen NCATE accreditation. *The Newsletter of the National Council for Accreditation of Teacher Education*, *18*(1), 1–6.

College LiveText Educational Solutions. (2009). Retrieved from http://www.livetext.com

Commission on Colleges of the Southern Association of Colleges and Schools. (2004). *Principles of Accreditation: Foundations for Quality Enhancement*. Retrieved April 1, 2009, from http://www.sacscoc.org/pdf/PrinciplesOfAccreditation.PDF

Darlaston-Jones, D. (2007). Making connections: The relationship between epistemology and research methods. *The Australian Community Psychologist*, *19*(1), 19–27.

Dewey, J. (1966). *Democracy and Education.* New York: Free Press. Educational Encyclopedia. (2009). *Accreditation in the United States: Higher Education*. Retrieved June 17, 2009, from http://education.stateuniversity.com

Fiedler, R., & Baumbach, D. (2008 March). *Portfolio as a Comprehensive Exam: Instigating Change*. Paper presented at Society for Information Technology & Teacher Education, Las Vegas, Nevada.

Gergen, K. (1999). *An invitation to social construction*. London: Sage.

Goodlad, J. (1994). *Educational renewal: Better teachers, better schools*. San Francisco: Jossey-Bass.

Hamilton, W. (2009). *Electronic evidence PowerPoint V6*. Retrieved June 17, 2009, from http://www.slideshare.net/williamfhamilton/electronic-evidence-powerpointv6final.

Holmberg, S. (1997). Is accreditation worth the trouble? *Education Weekly, 16*, 32. Institutional Report Continuing Accreditation. (2008). *College of education professional education unit*. Jonesboro, AR: Arkansas State University.

Johnson-Leslie, N. (in press). Comparing the efficacy of an engineered-based system (College LiveText) with an off-the-shelf general tool (Hyperstudio) for developing electronic portfolios in teacher education. *Journal of Educational Technology Systems, 37*(4), 385-404.

Knezek, D. (2008). *Providing leadership and service to improve teaching and learning by advancing the effective use of technology in education.* Retrieved November 12, 2008, from http://www.iste.org/AM/Template.cfm?Section=About_ ISTE*LiveText Solutions, Inc.* (2004). Retrieved from http://www.livetext.com U. S. Department of Education. (2003). *No Child Left Behind.* Retrieved October 9, 2008, from http://www.ed.gov/news/pressreleases/2003/12/12092003.html

Piaget, J. (1973). *To Understand is to Invent.* New York: Grossman. *Professional Standards Accreditation of Teacher Preparation Institutions.* (2008). Retrieved from http://www.ncate.org/institutions/publicationsbooks.asp?ch=49&book=standards

Vygotsky, L. (1978). *Mind in Society: The Development of Higher Psychological Processes.* Cambridge, MA: Harvard University Press.

Wang, L. (2005). The advantages of using technology in second language education: Technology integration in foreign language teaching demonstrates the shift from a behavioral to a constructivist learning approach. *T.H.E. Journal*, *32*(10), 38.

Wong, A. (2007). *Adapting to the E-world.* Retrieved June 15, 2009, from http://www.lawcrossing.com/article/1429/Adapting-to-the-E-world/

ADDITIONAL READING

Barnes, R. (2005). Moving towards technology education: factors that facilitated teacher's implementation of a technology curriculum. *Journal of Technology Education, 17*(1), 6–18.

Byrd, G., & Shedlock, J. (2003). The association of academic health sciences libraries annual statistics: An exploratory twenty-five-year trend analysis. *Journal of the Medical Library Association, 91*(2), 186–202.

Cary, C. (1909). Proposed changes in the accrediting of high schools. *The School Review*, *17*(4), 223–235. doi:10.1086/435326

Childress, V. (2006). Teaching about technology: An introduction to the philosophy of technology for non-philosophers. *Journal of Technology Education*, *17*(2), 76–78.

Chrzastowski, T. (2003). Making the transition from print to electronic serial collections: A new model for academic chemistry libraries? *Journal of the American Society for Information Science and Technology*, *54*(12), 1141–1148. doi:10.1002/asi.10318

Eldredge, J. (2000). Evidence-based librarianship: An overview. *Bulletin of the Medical Library Association*, *88*(4), 289–302.

Feldhusen, J. (1993). A conception of creative thinking and training. In *S. G. Anderson*. M.C. Murdock.

Firestone, R. L., & Trefinger, D. J. (Eds.), *Nurturing and developing creativity: The emergence of a discipline* (pp. 31–50). Norwood, NJ: Ablex Publishing Company.

Flowers, J. (2001). The value of humor in technology education. *Technology Teacher*, *50*(8), 10–13.

Foster, P., & Wright, M. (2001). How children think about design and technology: Two case studies. *Journal of Industrial Teacher Education*, *38*(2), 40–64.

Frank, M. (2005). A systems approach for developing technological literacy. *Journal of Technology Education*, *17*(1), 19–34.

Gattie, D., & Wicklein, R. (2007). Curricular value and instructional needs for infusing engineering-design into K-12 technology education. *Journal of Technology Education*, *19*(1), 6–18.

Grizzell, E. (1927). The accrediting of secondary schools in the middle states and Maryland. *The School Review*, *35*(7), 496. doi:10.1086/438547

Harris, D., & Herrington, C. (2006). Accountability, standards, and the growing achievement gap: Lessons from the past half-century. *American Journal of Education*, *112*(1), 209–238. doi:10.1086/498995

Lewis, T. (2005). Creativity—A Framework for the Design/Problem Solving Discourse in Technology Education. *Journal of Technology Education*, *17*(1), 35–52.

Linnell, C. (2006). An adventure living with simple technology: A review of better off flipping the switch on technology. *Journal of Technology Education*, *17*(1), 88–89.

Luther, J. (2002). White paper on electronic journal usage statistics. *The Serials Librarian*, *41*(20), 118–119.

Montgomery, C., & King, D. (2002). *Comparing library and user related costs of print and electronic. journal collections*. Retrieved October 21, 2002, from http://www.dlib.org.dlob/october02/montgomery/ 10montgomery.html

Morse, D., & Clintworth, W. (2000). *Comparing patterns of print and electronic journal use in an academic health science library*. Issues in Science and Technology Librarianship.

Opfer, V., Henry, G., & Mashburn, A. (2008). The district effect: Systemic responses to high stakes accountability policies in six southern states. *American Journal of Education*, *114*(2), 299–332. doi:10.1086/521242

Phillips, K. (1985). *A progression of technology in industrial arts education in technology education: A perspective on implementation* (pp. 15–18). Reston, VA: International Technology Education Association.

Savage, E., & Sterry, L. (1990). *A conceptual framework for technology education*. Reston, VA: International Technology Education Association.

Schillerand, K., & Muller, C. (2000). External examinations and accountability, educational expectations, and High School Graduation. *American Journal of Education*, *108*(2), 73–88. doi:10.1086/444235

Steinke, L., & Putnam, A. (2007). Why should I stay? Factors influencing technology education teachers to stay in teaching positions. *Journal of Technology Education*, *19*(1), 81–98.

Superfine, B. (2005). The politics of accountability: The rise and fall of goals 2000. *American Journal of Education*, *112*(1), 10–43. doi:10.1086/444513

Valli, L., Croninger, R., & Walters, K. (2007). Who (else) is the teacher? Cautionary notes on teacher accountability systems. *American Journal of Education*, *113*(4), 635–662. doi:10.1086/518492

Van Dunk, E., & Dickman, A. M. *American Journal of Education*, *111*(4), 617–621.

Vergari, S. (2005). School choice and the question of accountability: The Milwaukee experience by

KEY TERMS AND DEFINITIONS

Accountability: In this chapter accountability is defined as the being responsible or answerable to others.

Accreditation: accreditation can be loosely defined as quality control while providing protection from governmental interference and simultaneously ensuring academic freedom.

College Livetext Solutions: Electronic portfolio portal that makes it easy to create an on-line portfolio. Designed to be flexible; allows customization; has the capacity to store, retrieve, collage, analyze and report data.

Electronic Evidence Room: An electronic evidence room is defined as a purposeful environment in cyberspace guided by a common set of rules, techniques and tools for collecting, examining, preserving, retrieving and presenting data that has been processed electronically and has been stored on computer media.

Epistemology: Contextualized as a theory of knowledge is the branch of that is concerned with the nature and scope of knowledge acquisition and utilization

NCATE: The National Council for the Accreditation of Teacher Education (NCATE)

Teacher Candidates: Students who elect to become teachers

Chapter 11
The Online Exhibit Room: Complement to NCATE Accreditation

Lesia Lennex
Morehead State University, USA

Brianna Swetnam
Morehead State University, USA

Heather Flynn
Morehead State University, USA

ABSTRACT

National Council for the Accreditation of Teacher Education (NCATE) reviews offers a serious challenge for many educational institutions. The educational program must provide, through the Internet, documentation for the six NCATE standards. What should be included, when should the process begin, and how is it accomplished? This chapter will provide detailed development of Americans with Disability Act compliant Web (Section 508) sites, detail technical construction of Web sites for an online exhibit room, and examine features such as Adobe Flash animation and appropriate online databases. This chapter gives special attention to the construction of sites that welcome prospective students, highlight the cultural diversity of its campus/institution, and provide relevant information quickly to any site visitors. This chapter represents the best ideals and practices of NCATE-accredited Web sites, and will effectively instruct teacher education candidates and instructors in appropriate electronic methods.

INTRODUCTION

This chapter will provide detailed development of Americans with Disability Act compliant Web (Section 508) sites, detail technical construction of Web sites for an online exhibit room, and also discuss additional Web features such as Adobe Flash animation and appropriate, accessible online databases. A National Council for the Accreditation of Teacher Education (NCATE) site should have multiple purposes including marketing and current educational unit news. The authors pay special attention to the development of Web sites that welcome the visitor with culturally diverse, relevant content. This chapter represents the best ideals and practices of NCATE accreditation Web sites, and will effectively instruct teacher education candidates and instructors in appropriate electronic methods.

This chapter will also explore how, with the appropriate application of technology and artifacts,

DOI: 10.4018/978-1-61520-899-9.ch011

a Web page can become an engaging tool that enables visitors to delve into the unique heritage of a region that is directly responsible for shaping university practices and student life. However, these pages need not be limited to the accreditation committee. A Web site is a unique marketing tool to both recruit potential candidates and retain graduate candidates. In circumstances where a campus visit is inadvisable geographically, potential candidates would need only to browse the Web to find the latest news, program, and faculty information.

NCATE BACKGROUND AND REQUIREMENTS

Educational reform in the United States includes transformation of teacher preparation programs as a basic tenet. NCATE is the accrediting body for American teacher education institutions. Founded in 1954, NCATE standards hold that all children can and should learn, and all recent graduates from teacher education programs should be able to professionally assist P-12 children in learning. Teacher education candidates should receive a "foundation of professional and pedagogical knowledge upon which to base instructional decisions" (Professional Standards, 2008, p. 4) regarding teaching issues and curriculum including the areas of diversity, assessment, and up-to-date content knowledge.

Five groups worked together to create the agency: the American Association of Colleges for Teacher Education (AACTE), the National Association of State Directors of Teacher Education and Certification (NASDTEC), the National Education Association (NEA), the Council of Chief State School Officers (CCSSO), and the National School Boards Association (NSBA). "NCATE accredits schools, colleges, and departments of education (professional education units) in American colleges and universities as well as non-university entities that prepare educators" (Professional Standards, 2008, p. 5).

The organizations do not actually certify teachers; they recommend that an individual receive teacher certification from the state agency because the candidate has met the institutional, state, and national criteria for beginning teachers. American teacher education institutions usually operate under both national accreditation guidelines and state regulations. Not all are required to have national accreditation, but they must meet state regulations for recommending candidates to receive teacher certification.

Any school of education can volunteer for NCATE review and accreditation, but all of them must have state accreditation through a board of examiners. In many states, such as Kentucky, NCATE functions as an educational partner. The state educational review board, or the Board of Examiners, conducts joint review with NCATE of that organization. While the state may have separate standards, it must also satisfy basic NCATE accreditation standards.

In an atmosphere of change fueled by the need for national teacher certification, NCATE is evolving to focus more on content preparation and clinical experiences. Schools of education must prepare teachers to work collaboratively among many levels of professionals rather than as isolated teachers. This changing atmosphere also demands national preparation to ensure that teachers receive rigorous, quality preparation in content, pedagogy, and research analysis.

The school's conceptual framework and continuous assessment plan will set the tone for educational programs. The ways in which the mission and goals of the conceptual framework are actually achieved is of great importance to the NCATE accrediting team. The NCATE standards must be addressed in the conceptual framework and create a full description of all experiences a teacher education candidate will have within a program of study (see Appendix 1: NCATE

Standards). There are six standards governing the following: candidate knowledge, skills and dispositions, assessment system and unit evaluation, field experiences and clinical practice, diversity, faculty qualifications, performance, and development, and unit governance and resources (Professional Standards, 2008, p. 12-13).

ONLINE SITE ARTIFACTS AND ISSUES OF CONFIDENTIALITY

Any NCATE documents used during accreditation require an online presence (Johnston, 2008). Not only are artifacts more streamlined in presentation, it affords institutional clients the access to knowledge of programs, assessments, and communications (Honawar, 2008). As of 2004, NCATE no longer accepts paper documents for its standard review processes. NCATE requires not only online accessible databases, but also online materials up to one year prior to the site visit in an exhibit room format. Educators therefore have to learn simple technologies involved with the Internet (Galan, 2004; Kraft, 2001).

The review will examine whether the school has artifacts that are Section 508 compliant available via the Internet, which can create many questions for educators (Hricko, 2003; Lennex & Flynn, 2009; Reynolds & Lennex, 2009). Does one go with Microsoft Word documents or use portable document files (PDF)? Should it all be coded in hypertext mark-up language (HTML) or extensible markup language (XML) (Rudnick & O'Flavahan, 2000)? A needs analysis for the online accreditation exhibit room must be conducted at least three years prior to the on-site visit date. The needs analysis should be conducted both from an artifacts and constituent perspective. The artifacts must cover all documentation during the previous seven-year cycle for the six NCATE standards. An NCATE site must have documentation or access to the institutional conceptual framework, continuous assessment plan, educational programs course syllabi, field and clinical experiences, faculty curriculum vita, educational programs related committee meeting minutes and associated documents, documentation of attendance to educationally related professional development and shared community planning for institutional planning, inventories of institutional resources, such as computers and their uses, and databases of educational candidate information from which queries can be made about transition points, dispositions, and program completion. If possible, faculty publications should be linked. Teacher education candidate productions including any publications, educational products for courses, or field and clinical materials, such as a teacher productivity assessment, should be included.

What artifacts should be Internet accessible? What should be password-protected for Intranet use? All public meetings should be documented with meeting minutes. *Robert's Rules of Order* (2000) state that all public meetings minutes should record actions of a committee. Open Meetings are required of government agencies. Meeting presence in the United States is governed by Sunshine Laws (n.d.) and the Freedom of Information Act, 5 U.S.C.A. § 552 (1967). Sunshine laws are actually a catch-all phrase for state open records/open meetings statues. They vary widely by state. The educational institution's obligation depends on its home state and its respective law. Its obligation also greatly matters whether it is a private school or a public one. A private school can follow many of its own rules. Following strict procedure to close a public meeting, executive sessions can occur without publicly distributed minutes. Governance records for units, which would include financial statements, placement of field and clinical experience candidates, candidate products, and candidate dispositions are confidential. Such materials must be password protected. Using either an institutional content management system (CMS) or external server, one may assign a guest access. This access should coincide to expire to the accreditation visit.

An example of a candidate product that could be given public access is a teacher productivity assessment (TPA). It completely describes a unit of study from the individual student accommodations per the individualized education program, to the delivery and assessment of the unit, to the analysis of assessment results for each student and the collective class. Recommendations based on current research and theories are given to improve student achievement in future units. The information provided by this assessment should be considered confidential. Names of all participants, schools, and school descriptions should be uniform so as to maintain the confidentiality.

Complete information including curriculum maps, entrance and exit requirements, and goals of the educationally related programs must also be included on the NCATE site. If an institution truly serves its candidates, all documentation, other than the United States Family Education and Rights Privacy Act (FERPA) of 2008 regarding protected materials, will be available to the general public. FERPA prevents disclosure of sensitive information, such as home addresses, course schedules, or grades. Release of personal information, which could result in physical or psychological harm, is prohibited. NCATE reviewers will not violate FERPA in reviewing candidate records through password-protected databases. NCATE reviewers are bound by the NCATE Code of Conduct (2003). Among other areas, this document details actions of members with regard to conflicts of interest and confidentiality. No board member is permitted to discuss the reviewed artifacts outside official channels of the accreditation. The NCATE site itself could display candidate productions, but in order to do so publicly, the candidate must give permission.

The school of education should conduct an artifact needs analysis among the school's actual undergraduates, graduates, faculty, and staff. The NCATE site should not only contain documents for review of the teacher education program, but also any information necessary for current and prospective students' success within the program.

While many colleges of education have a Web presence, this is not enough for prospective candidates. The best Web presence only serves to whet the appetite of prospective staff, students and faculty. One must put forth an effort to include, in a logical fashion, program requirements, course scheduling, curriculum maps (i.e. course requirements), rotation of courses in all locations, and requirements for entrance to, and graduation from, teacher education programs. Without these links, many visitors start looking elsewhere for programs that make their information easier to access.

Web site visitors expect to have information ready for their retrieval. Lennex, Swetnam, and Flynn (2009) conducted a survey to determine perceived needs of undergraduate constituents with respect to NCATE sites. At most institutions, the site is used to educate the populace about the conceptual framework and possibly the transition points of the continuous assessment plan. The survey concludes that more information is obviously needed. This audience consisted of undergraduates from institutions in Alaska, Hawaii, California, Minnesota, Florida, Arizona, and Kentucky. Of those responding, 83 percent were enrolled at a regional college or university and 69 percent had heard of NCATE accreditation. In viewing their institution's NCATE site, respondents stated that they felt too many of the materials required heavy reading to locate information. When searching for program information, a site visitor has to read the entire handbook and locate specific information. A hyperlink directly to information about specific programs was not usually provided. Many respondents stated that sites were difficult to navigate either because of the deluge of documentation or a lack of logical, specific links.

Along with clear navigation, undergraduate clients want information about their professors. Some commented that they were researching their professors. Many of the artifacts related to individual faculty will not be available through the Internet with common hyperlinks (Lennex,

2007). They could be available through a database link, however. The information desired included curriculum vitae, courses taught, contact information and preferred method of contact - the survey respondents clearly indicated that professors did not answer e-mail, even if the address was listed as their primary contact.

AMERICANS WITH DISABILITIES ACT COMPLIANCE FOR WEB PAGES

The Americans with Disabilities Act provides that all Americans, regardless of their physical challenge, shall have equitable access to all aspects of the Internet. Under Section 508 (2006), "agencies must give disabled employees and members of the public access to information that is comparable to the access available to others" (29 U.S.C. ' 794d). Section 508 compliance is not cumbersome. However, if the school does not use a CMS then alternate servers must be located and capabilities assessed. A CMS system will allow automatic updates via cascading style sheets (CSS) to all pages within the system. The use of cascading style sheets allow Web page designers to influence the way browsers interpret pages, for example text attributes and assignment of font families, without altering the basic hypertext markup language (HTML). A style sheet is housed on the Web server and is referenced by the browser to formulate the page's display. It may be necessary to make last minute updates, for which the CSS capabilities would be optimal. When making changes to a Web site, it's incredibly time consuming and tedious to have to constantly correct structural changes. With CSS, the designer can simply upload the altered pages, knowing the overlay of graphics, fonts, and formatting are Section 508, Americans with Disabilities Act, compliant. Using Web site code review is another method to ensure appropriate Section 508, ADA, compliance. One of the most popular is TIDY online. This site provides user-friendly language in detailing the Section 508 compliance of a Web site. A user may see warnings and errors so that they may correct Web markup (Lennex & Flynn, 2009).

However, the primary design must be determined through the cultural views of the institution. In the Unites States, Web site visitors expect to read a page top to bottom, left to right. Many international pages are designed to have right-to-left views and columnar reading. The basic look of the page is obviously very important to the viewer. Taking into account compliance needs, Lennex, Swetnam, and Flynn (2009) found that undergraduate clients ranked readability in Western format as "very important" (57 percent). Van Horn (2003) gives a working definition for Web page accessibility:

The criteria for Web-based technology and information are based on access guidelines developed by the Web Accessibility Initiative of the World Wide Web Consortium (WC3). Many of these provisions ensure access for people with vision impairments who rely on various assistive products to access computer-based information, such as screen readers, which translate what's on a computer screen into automated audible output, and refreshable Braille displays. Certain convention, such as verbal tags or identification of graphics and format devices, like frames, are necessary so that these devices can 'read' them for the user in a sensible way. The standards do not prohibit the use of website graphics or animation. Instead, the standards aim to ensure that such information is also available in an accessible format. Generally, this means use of text labels or descriptors for graphics and certain format elements. HTML code already provides an "Alt Text" tag for graphics that can serve as a verbal descriptor for graphics. This section also addresses the usability of multimedia presentations, image maps, style sheets, scripting language, applets and plug-ins, and electronic forms. (p. 103).

There are several guidelines (see Appendix 2: Guidelines to setting up a Web page) to be followed in meeting requirements for Section 508 (Hudson, 2002) Among the most easily accomplished are using text equivalents for every non-text element, providing alternative pages without color or backgrounds, and using highly contrasted backgrounds and text elements. A strong recommendation is to avoid use of neon colors, such as light green or pink, and all colors in the higher end of the spectrum. The frequency modulation of yellow, red, and orange all increase the probability that one will see "bleeding" or "threading" of color into the text lines. All documents should be readable from the client side. If special applications are needed, provide a hyperlink to the application or program. It is wise to include the browser settings or browser types if a specific item is needed to read documents. Although some would argue that tables should be avoided, tables can be effectively used in compliance with Section 508. A screen reader, such as JAWS, speaks text from top to bottom of the page, right to left. It does not make distinctions for tables. The code is not relevant and thus it will not "see" the need to read top to bottom in columns. However, if one uses identified row and column headers for data tables and markup to associate data cells and header cells for data tables that have two or more logical levels of row or column headers, then it should suffice to give a screen reader and its patron the information necessary to decipher a table (Hudson, 2002, p. 20-21). Arranging the page in a logical format is helpful in all situations. The Web Access Initiative (WAI) (2001) counsels more with visual adjustments. For example, all non-text elements should have alternative text (alt txt) tags so that a screen reader may read the name of the graphic. This makes sense for all Web viewers as scrolling over a graphic for NCATE may reveal university logos or other associated graphics for which text would help give cultural and/or institutional meaning. WAI encourages use of full hypertext links instead of *click here* language. Again, this makes sense for all Web viewers, as hyperlinks may not work properly. If one must view the site source code to determine a hyperlink address, this takes extra technology literacy and requires more time on the part of a viewer. Additionally, consider the modem speed necessary to load the page and the ways in which it will be accessed. While many areas have access to high-speed Internet, it is not universal. Access does not equate to installation. There are serious cost barriers to maintaining high-speed Internet. Clients of NCATE pages are a cross-section of the population. Many of the clients for NCATE pages could be accessing through cell phones, Bluetooth, or wireless devices (Reynolds & Lennex, 2009).

It is recommended to use both standard Word documents (Microsoft Office 2004-2007) and portable document files (Lennex, 2003). Lennex, Swetnam, and Flynn (2009) found that undergraduates requested documents saved as PDF (68 percent) and as Microsoft Word 97-2004 documents (42 percent). Many Internet browsers feature automatic opening of Word documents and PDF files. The more compatible the artifact form, the more likely a NCATE reviewer or prospective student can retrieve the information. Other features on the Web pages can create the sense of being "user-friendly" or very confusing From the same survey (2009), undergraduate clients rated working hyperlinks (90 percent), size of font (38 percent) and actual text font (34 percent) as "very important" Web page features. Color contrasting was "important" (42 percent).

There are certain questions that transcend the basic utility of an online presence, such as to what extent should an online exhibit room be used by the general population of prospective, current, and alumni candidates? It is the author's belief that an NCATE site should be meaningful in providing up-to-date information for candidates on the programs, courses, and college? The site should contain relevant cultural and geographic information for national team members. To this end, the site should be more than a collection of program reviews and syllabi. It should provide a candidate with a clear picture of the faculty and program. Graphics, such as Flash animation and photography, can help with the cultural composition of an NCATE site.

INCORPORATING ADOBE FLASH INTO NCATE ACCREDITATION WEB SITE CONSTRUCTION

Professional Web sites must be constructed and managed in a style that enables the NCATE review team and the state Board of Examiners (BOE) to efficiently browse the supporting materials that show compliance with the standards. However, a Web site must not only be functional and navigable, but also memorable and engaging. One of the most effective ways to accomplish this directive is the inclusion of animated graphics and themes, which can highlight the importance of a topic, draw the user's attention to a particular aspect of the page, provide interactivity with the content, or increase understanding of concepts and institutional methods. When constructing a required Web page for NCATE accreditation, one may add animation, interactive graphics, and media through the use of Adobe Flash software.

Flash, a standard Web graphics and animation software system is a good tool for communicating cultural identity. Flash may prove difficult unless one follows some basic training. Published by Adobe and compiled by the corporation's creative team, Adobe Illustrator CS3 Classroom in a Book (2007) offers a comprehensive tutorial of one of the most recent versions of Flash. With walk-through tutorials and a supplementary CD-ROM, the majority of individuals should have little difficulty mastering the content. In addition to industry endorsed training materials, other independent sources are available.

In addition to being readily accessible, Flash also makes media available across multiple operating systems, which is essential in this age of technology, as many members of a Web audience use different operating systems and varying speeds of Internet connection. This makes Flash an ideal tool for any NCATE Web page preparation committee, as it will enable the largest possible audience to view the material, as well as ensure that the accreditation team is able to examine the content.

With a wide range of tools and options, Flash can insert motion and three-dimensional elements, while being linked to online and metadata support. Interestingly enough, most individuals, though unable to manipulate Flash, are aware of its existence in the form of Flash Player, which enables users to view Web pages and interact with games that have a Flash component.

Flash also provides a method by which a region's unique heritage can be displayed to a virtual audience. Every university, no matter its size, possesses its own legacy of traditions and influences which should not be neglected when preparing for NCATE accreditation, for it is from this heritage that the atmosphere of a university evolves. There are several methods by which Flash can be used to accomplish this goal.

First, Flash can be used to display automated slide shows depicting regional landmarks, university traditions, and any other visuals which are distinctive of the region. For example, universities in Eastern Kentucky might display photos of the countryside during the changing of seasons and local musicians engaged in playing traditional instruments, such as the mandolin, while universities in the Hawaiian islands might include graphics depicting native dances, such as the Hula, and the tropical landscape.

Flash can embed video and audio, by which visitors to the NCATE accreditation site may view students, faculty, and staff partaking in campus activities, such as concerts of regional music, dance, theater, sports, and organizational endeavors, such as Adopt-a-Highway Clean-up. Audio and video may allow the accreditation team the ability to observe students and faculty occupied in academic endeavors, like lecture-based instruction, laboratory experimentation, or practical field experience. In addition to static graphics and live action audiovisual media, Flash may be used to create a glimpse into campus life, by providing virtual campus tours of landmarks, historic buildings, facilities, and classrooms.

THE CULTURAL ASPECT

Michel Foucault defined humans in terms of: (1) the self's relation to knowledge/truth, (2) the self's relation to power, and (3) the self's relation to itself (ethics) (Hofmeyr, 2006, p. 217). Under this philosophy, Web pages, as much as any other outward product of human behavior, are representative of a time, place, and state of mind within a person's, or institution's, psyche (Aycock, 1995; Hofmeyr, 2006; Lennex & Reynolds, 2008; Thoms & Thelwall, 2005). To ignore the cultural aspect of the community would not only create a bland site of solely mandatory information, but would also falsely indicate indifference toward diversity. As it is essential to keep such an attitude from being detected in a college educational program, the designers must carefully observe the site. It is easy to accidentally depict such negative traits in the Web site, thus, as mentioned by Spradlin (2008), it is important to be sensitive to and capable of removing any barrier that could obstruct the intention of celebrating diversity. This would mean constant evaluation of the language used in the Web site (i.e. is it written to the point that the common layman could understand it, or is it loaded with words difficult for some to fully understand?), the images used to depict the campus and the educational program (i.e. is it mainly focused upon the dominant culture, or is it balanced?), and, most importantly, the climate described through the elements of the Web page. Lennex, Swetnam, and Flynn (2009) surveyed undergraduate teacher education respondents who believed that an NCATE site should have cultural elements depicting the demographic nature of the population, geographic region, unique features of the institution, and voice of the teacher education candidates.

These careful design evaluations are well seen through the Web sites of the University of Alabama and the University of Hawaii. Images and information about the campus and region play critical roles in how the school chooses to present the information on the Web site. Using photographs of campus diversity and of the distinctive region, the viewer notices the authorship of the Web pages from more than just a title page or a banner with the name of the university scrolled across it. This also creates an appeal to the viewer, especially to the NCATE reviewers. The process of reviewing Web sites can become quite monotonous, so to see just a graphic banner or animation celebrating the uniqueness of the university may bring new excitement to the viewer as he or she peruses the information in a more unique format.

Authorship and general appeal not only ensure a cultural aspect to the site, but also celebrates differences in the community, while remaining focus upon the university's mindset, or mission statement. A link explaining the ways the university maintains and celebrates diversity can be useful, but words on a Web page are not enough to prove this is actually being done. Images, links, and so forth can assist in affirming the NCATE Standard 4 is present in both the Web site and the university's community.

Schools of education should remember the cultural aspect of the NCATE site when developing a Web site. Sites need graphics, links, and other aspects to improve their efficiency. These design techniques also make the site unique, pointing to its authorship—the university and the surrounding area. NCATE standard 4, Diversity, addresses the degree to which an institution has made an effort to promote traditionally under-represented groups within educational experiences. An analysis of course syllabi and field and clinical experiences will help in assessing this issue, but the actual Web site can have a huge impact on the impressions of the review team and institutional clients.

Thus, cultural climate plays a major factor upon the overall perception of a site. A successful site will create an environment that appears inviting and welcoming of all cultures. The site may also emphasize the campus' own cultural aspects yet it should not be the sole focus of the page. For instance, in Morehead State University's case, the site celebrates the Appalachian heritage of the region.. To destroy the barriers that long-practiced segregation from diversity has caused, one must create an environment that appears as completely accepting and supportive — an institution that treasures the diversity candidates will offer. To accomplish this goal, the site must foster certain perceptions. Spradlin (2008, p. 47) indicates specific inclusions such as classes designed to support cultural diversity. She further suggests communication of high expectations of all students, genuine desire for involvement of outside community, and high levels of community participation.

If such a climate may be established through the structure and information displayed upon the Web pages, the designers may then be able to emphasize the cultural uniqueness of the campus without the belief that one may have undermined other cultures. This positive environment will help instill a perception that the campus is accepting of all groups. Possible acceptance of group collectives is also conveyed. This structure will also demonstrate to the site's visitors that all voices matter to the university and that the faculty and students are an integral part of their own multicultural community, celebrating differences as well as similarities. Undoubtedly, it will help maintain compliance under NCATE Standard 4. However, this is by far not the only factor that needs to be looked to when it comes to the site's appeal. It is also mandatory to examine tone and design when formulating the site's overall appearance and effect.

THE IMPORTANCE OF USING SOCIAL NETWORKING

Students desire an interpersonal connection with the university faculty via the Web site. But what is the appropriate system for that connection? There are many ways to establish contact between the student and the school and make it more appealing through interaction available on the site. Facebook, MySpace, Twitter, SecondLife, and Web logs, commonly referred to as "blogs," have become extremely popular among college students as well as the general population.

Moderated blogging about factors important to the institutional mission, conceptual framework, and continuous assessment plan will always have a place on a university's Web site. Teacher education candidates and faculty need a work space to express their thoughts about the living document. The interaction among varying levels of pre-service, in-service teachers, faculty, and administrators would give meaning to an institutional vision. Some students may be discouraged due to the lack of privacy blogs provide, yet, some are more than willing to explore these new horizons in their educational sites. However, as technology changes so must the way educators use the resources at hand. Thus, blogs become beneficial tools as long as they are used in a professional manner. Blogs may be used to build a community between the students and perhaps give another source to quickly contact the professor when the need arises. If students are interested in their professors' previous research work and honors, then blogs could provide a way to share this information as well as give another source for contact information. It also allows students and teachers to give insights on topics discussed in class or make announcements about upcoming projects.

Some colleges have found uses for alternative interactive sources, like Twitter and Meebo chatrooms. Twitter has been seen as an excellent aide due to its instant messaging service to cell phones, which allows students to quickly get classroom announcements. Young (2008) explains that Blackboard, a program used by many universities, plans to add a Twitter-like messaging tool into its system by acquiring NTI Group, a company that sells text-message notification systems to colleges for use in emergencies (such as to warn of thunderstorms and tornadoes, announcements about classes during snow storms, etc.). Libraries, however, have opted for the Meebo chatroom service so that users may contact the university's education program without the hassle of logging in, downloading software, or even locating the "contact us" link on the Web page. Meebo, a chat program, functions as a textbox embedded into the site for visitors to key in questions and get a quick response from whoever is supervising the chatroom (Matthews, 2009). Therefore, NCATE, as well as many other educational Web sites, should take advantage of the new resources the Web has to offer and include a chatroom and/or a blog function to develop an online community subsequently improving the site's appeal and efficiency.

IMPORTANCE OF TONE AND OTHER DESIGN QUALITIES

Indicating authorship and creativity in the Website not only makes the site more appealing, but also leaves an impression regarding the university. Since one of the main goals of the Web site should be to spark an interest in the campus and its education program, the university should take the opportunity of advertising and celebrating its program through the appearance of the NCATE site. The site's design also facilitates communication in a friendly, welcoming environment that attracts the intended audience's attention, as effective marketing would demand.

Much research on the subjects of organization and accessibility, as mandatory elements of the NCATE site, indicates the following needs for an efficient site: an attractive, yet not too flashy design, that immediately indicates the site's focus and purpose (Goldsborough 2008); accessibility to all information in an organized, easily found manner (such as the use of a site map and ensuring that all links are actually accessible) (Galan 2004); a variety of different sources for content/design such as text, image, sound, audiovisual, etc. as site visitors tend to favor these features in the presentation (Galan 2004); interactivity that is "not only with reference to the contents, but also to interpersonal communication" (Galan 2004, p. 102-3); and, most importantly, relevant information (Vella, 2008).

These needs from an NCATE Web site are also indicated in the opinions of undergraduate teacher education candidates (Lennex, Swetnam, & Flynn, 2009). The majority of the students surveyed found color contrasting (61 percent), text font (65.8 percent), size of font (75 percent), hyperlinks that work (97.5 percent), pictures (55 percent), and site navigation (95.1 percent) as either important or very important to them when viewing the Web page. The survey also noted that, when asked to name one feature that all Web pages must have, 48.6 percent of students indicated a need for some type of navigation system. This may be through a hyperlink to the home page on all descending pages, a search engine, menu, and/or a site map/index. The importance of interactivity was indeed proven as the students indicated a need for interpersonal connection with the university faculty through phone directories, faculty information (general information, brief professional bio of each faculty member, years of experience, certification, office hours, classes the teacher instructs, etc.), and other forms of communication (for example, e-mail, phone, office, etc.).

Tone is indicated to be a major factor in the overall perception of the site. The whole perception of the site is not determined by words alone, but the tone that the site suggests. Hunt (2008) provides marketing clarification of Web writing expectations. These factors are (1) use concise, active voice writing, (2) use an inverted pyramid to front-load important pieces of information, (3) use clear guidelines and headers, (4) consider the users' goals, and (5) establish trust with your audience. Rudnick and O'Flavahan (2000) categorized four common errors in Web writing. The errors are (1) placing excessive print content online, (2) writing too formally, (3) obfuscating the site's message, and (4) delaying placement the site's mission. Striking the appropriate tone for a Web page in public schools can be nebulous. Faculty may impart some of their personality with wording or creative graphics, but the overall design of a page will lend to either a negative or positive tone. While teachers seek to maintain professionalism in their pages, this can be achieved with selected words and reflection.

In response to rules for writing appropriate Web sites, the researchers developed a qualitative schema to determine negative or positive tone for faculty pages. A positive tone should have the following: (1) friendly, respectful English-language words, (2) personal information to give both a professional and personal appeal, (3) effective use of graphic design incorporating non-verbal cues, (4) helpfulness toward either contact, homework, or resources, and, perhaps most importantly, (5) enthusiasm for teaching children. About half of teachers in this study created a positive environment on their pages. A negative tone would have the following: (1) formality in writing giving rise to an unapproachable manner, (2) lack of information on the Web page, (3) grammar or spelling errors unbefitting a professional Web page, (4) brevity without conciseness of thought, (5) stern language used in disciplining a child which may not be appropriate to a Web page, and (6) cues in writing, such as all capital characters, which tend to be interpreted as shouting or aggressive in nature.

Teacher comments about Web pages indicated that they received little or no training for creating Web pages. District Technology Coordinators (DTC) were surveyed about their provision and the nature of technology training for teachers (Lennex & Flynn, 2009). Similar to results from surveys of university Web support personnel (Reynolds & Lennex, 2009), DTC's provide training upon request. The training is minimal and related specifically to uploading pre-formatted Web pages. Trouble-shooting broken links, graphics, and creation of independent pages using industry software is usually dealt with on a case-by-case basis. It is imperative that outside readers view the Web pages with positive and negative connotations in mind. It is unlikely that specific training will be provided to Web designers or support staff in these aspects.

DATABASES

NCATE visits also require database management systems, which provide the most concise way to effectively organize the site. A coordinated database system will improve one's assessment of transition points and provide good data for informed decisions regarding a teacher education program (Johnston, 2008). Most institutions have reasonable databases in place (Richman, 2007). This NCATE requirement mainly concerns the institution's coordination of systems. Whether the designer uses a commercially available product or creates one within the institution depends on the needs of that institution (Richman, 2007). NCATE accreditation requires the conformation to six unit standards, and recommends the use of electronic exhibits, traditionally in an HTML format, to allow supporting reviewer work prior to the visit and facilitate the work of the BOE once they arrive on campus. A database should have a robust query system that allows for myriad uses among faculty as well as accreditation reviewers (NCATE, 2009). Database systems allow universities to analyze patterns in dispositions, transition points in education programs, and the growth of students by retaining work samples and instructor evaluations. As a result, the use of electronic exhibits necessitates the accumulation and organization of a tremendous amount of electronic material.

Universities may use any number of commercial or self-developed databases to organize, manage, and report educational data. Information from teacher education candidates generates the bulk of review data. It is common to track candidates through a program and develop a sense of accomplishment. The degree to which those achievements have resulted from professorial feedback on assignments is essential in understanding whether or not an institution is living its stated conceptual framework mission and continuous assessment plan. In order to verify the quality of the experience, the database must feature an examination of field and clinical experience dispositions. Comments by instructors should be cumulative throughout a candidate's career.

Many universities use Tk20 CampusWide® (2009), a comprehensive assessment and reporting system for collecting and managing data from the program, department, and institution, both academic and non-academic, for the measurement of accountability, institutional effectiveness, and for accreditation, helps businesses and universities collect data systematically, plan assessments, compare the data against specified outcomes/objectives, and generate detailed reports for compliance, analysis, and program improvement.

TrueOutcomes Assessment Manager® (2009) provides a second option to organize data for visiting NCATE accreditation teams, is. This program allows for aggregation and data mining across the institution, as well as the measuring of educational outcomes against student learning. By making use of TrueOutcomes®, institutions may "make evidence-based decisions with the flexibility to support your institutional mission, accreditation, and continuous improvement efforts.

In addition to these commercial database solutions, universities may also construct their own databases, or enlist the assistance of services that construct database systems based upon the individual needs of the institution. However, organizing data effectively is only one crucial facet to building an NCATE-accredited Web site. Faculty 180 (2009) is an independent database built for faculty needs in the tenure and promotion process. It is a needs-driven system that can be individualized to any educational situation. The features of this system are well-suited to NCATE accreditation needs for faculty (see Appendix 3: Faculty 180 Database Features).

In Faculty 180, for example, if a query were built to satisfy NCATE Standard 5, faculty qualifications, an analysis of faculty publications for the last seven years would be generated. A report is available for review without having to scour faculty vitae. More importantly, a reviewer does not have to decipher the institutional code for vita structure in order to interpret scholarly productivity in publications. With coding for a CMS hyperlink, the vitae can be accessed by constituents.

CONCLUSION

Online databases, detailed development of ADA compliant Web (Section 508) sites, technical construction of Web sites for an online exhibit room, special features such as animation and photography, and culturally relevant artifact are specific development features for a successful NCATE online exhibit room.

An NCATE accreditation Web page is not limited in its potential as a simply utilitarian accreditation requirement. After placing the time, effort, and funding into the creation of a unique and honest Web-ready depiction of campus life, universities should be encouraged to make their electronic exhibits highly accessible to the public. Parents, prospective students and faculty, as well as existing students and faculty, stand to benefit from the material available. For prospective students and their parents, these online exhibit rooms can be used to examine various aspects of the universities, which may impact decisions regarding application for admission and enrollment. Universities with the most comprehensive and engaging Web presence may see higher enrollment and have a student body that is better informed on the skills of instructors, campus diversity, as well as the remainder of the information which was provided for NCATE and BOE. Some states, such as Alaska and Montana, where great distances separate the instructors, students, and institutions, may benefit the most from the additional applications of online exhibit rooms. By placing such vast amounts of interactive content on the Internet, students and instructors may remain connected and united for the common goals of their universities.

FUTURE DIRECTIONS

Keeping in mind suggested guidelines for content accessibility, design and variety, interactivity, and tone will greatly assist in creating an interactive NCATE site. For content accessibility, keep words and sentences short and precise. Clearly label where hyperlinks will take the viewer. Make sure all hyperlinks work correctly. Create a site map or some other clearly organized, methodic list of all linked Web pages and sites. Situate a "home" button on every page and a search box for easy access to desired links on the site. The tone of a site is very attuned to the cultural transmission of a site. Pay attention to connotation of the words and of the non-verbal cues being used. Indicate a welcoming, helpful, friendly environment. Establish a desire for a connection with the viewer. Constantly review the site in all factors that may convey a negative tone toward any viewer (Chandler, 1998; Galan, 2004; Goldsborough, 2008; Lennex & Flynn, 2009; Lennex, Swetnam, & Flynn, 2009; Mathews, 2009; Vella, 2008)..

In designing a site, keep in mind that some have slow Internet service; give options to not load certain content or limit the amount of media on each page. Having a text only page is a boon. Think visually rather than verbally and have the multimedia relate to the content. Add some creativity in the design to make the NCATE site your university's site; declare ownership by celebrating the campus' cultural aspects. The design of the site should meet and promote the function of the site at all times. Use contrasting colors, different styles of fonts, etc., but make sure to keep the same theme in all pages. At all costs, avoid site clutter. Keep to an organized, logical format. The interactivity of a site must create a sense of community and immediate accessibility to the staff. If using blogs, allow room for creativity and socialization but make sure to constantly maintain a professional tone in all posts. Adding a chatroom of some sort is beginning to be seen not only as useful, but has become the "norm" of Web sites. Embrace proven technologies such as YouTube, Flicker, Twitter, etc. into the site to provide a certain familiarity for visitors (Chandler, 1998; Galan, 2004; Goldsborough, 2008; Lennex & Flynn, 2009; Lennex, Swetnam, & Flynn, 2009; Mathews, 2009; Vella, 2008).

REFERENCES

Aycock, A. (1995). Technologies of the self: Foucault and internet discourse. *Journal of Computer Mediated Communication, 1*(2). Retrieved November 10, 2006, from http://jcmc.indiana.edu/vol1/issue2/aycock.html

Freedom of Information Act. (1967). Retrieved July 23, 2009, from http://www.answers.com/topic/freedom-of-information-act

Galan, J. (2004). Design of Educational Web Pages. *European Journal of Teacher Education, 27*(1), 99–104. doi:10.1080/0261976042000211793

Goldsborough, R. (2008). Web Design: Balancing Form and Function. [from Academic Search Premier database.]. *Tech Directions, 67*(10), 11. Retrieved April 7, 2009.

Hofmeyr, B. (2006). The power not to be (what we are), the politics and ethics of self-creation in Foucault. *Journal of Moral Philosophy*, *3*(2), 215–230. doi:10.1177/1740468106065493

Honawar, V. (2008, December 14). NCATE commits to streamlining accrediting process. *Education Week*, *28*(14), 6.

Hricko, M. (2003). Understanding section 508 and its implications for distance learning. In Design and Implementation of Web-enabled Teaching Tools (pp. 25-45). Retrieved October 26, 2007, from InfoSci-Online database.

Hunt, B. (2008). *Writing for the Web*. Retrieved October 1, 2008, from http://www.webdesignfromscratch.com/writing_for_the_web.cfm

Illustrator, A. (2007). *CS3 classroom in a book*. Berkeley, CA: Adobe Press.

Johnston, J. (2008). *Piloting NCATE's streamlined system: positive Results*. Retrieved January 1, 2009 from http://www.NCATE. org/documents/news/Johnston_Streamlined.pdf

Kraft, N. (2001*). Standards in teacher education: a critical analysis of NCATE, INTASC, and NBPTS*. Retrieved September 4, 2008, from EBSCOhost database.

Law, S. (n.d.). Retrieved July 23, 2009, from http://www.answers.com/topic/sunshine-laws

Lennex, L. (2003). *College of Education NCATE online exhibit room.* Retrieved May 10, 2004, from http://ed-u-tech.net/msucoe/

Lennex, L. (2007). The faculty Web page: contrivance or continuation? *TechTrends*, *51*(5), 32–37. doi:10.1007/s11528-007-0067-z

Lennex, L., & Flynn, H. (2009). Wisely using cyberspace: needs analysis of P-12 teacher Web pages. In C. Crawford et al. (Eds.), *Proceedings of Society for Information Technology and Teacher Education International Conference 2009* (pp. 3473-3480). Chesapeake, VA: AACE.

Lennex, L., & Reynolds, A. (2008). Whose web page is this? Why faculty create web pages. In C. Crawford et al. (Eds.), *Proceedings of Society for Information Technology and Teacher Education International Conference 2008* (pp. 3840-3842). Chesapeake, VA: AACE.

Lennex, L., Swetnam, B., & Flynn, H. (2009). *Survey of NCATE constituents on Web features*. Unpublished manuscript, Morehead State University.

Mathews, B. (2009). Web design matters. [from Academic Search Premier database.]. *Library Journal*, *134*(3), 24–25. Retrieved April 7, 2009.

NCATE. 2004. *Professional Standards for the Accreditation of Teacher Preparation Institutions* (2008). Washington: National Council for Accreditation of Teacher Education (NCATE). Retrieved September 13, 2008, from http://www.NCATE.org/institutions/process.asp?ch=4.

Professional standards for the accreditation of teacher preparation institutions (2008). Washington: National Council for Accreditation of Teacher Education (NCATE).

Reynolds, A., & Lennex, L. (2009). Can you read this? 508 compliance among Kentucky schools? *TechTrends*, *53*(3), 61–66.

Richman, W. (2007, February). *A psychologist's walk through NCATE: successful creation and implementation of a truly comprehensive database system.* Paper presented at the annual meeting of the American Association of Colleges for Teacher Education, New York, NY.

Robert, H., Evans, W., Honemann, D., Balch, T., & Robert, S. (2000). *Robert's Rules of Order* (10th ed.). New York: New York City.

Rudnick, M., & O'Flavahan, L. (2000). *Four fatal errors of Web writing or how to keep your content from crashing.* Retrieved October 10, 2008 from http://www.powerhomebiz.com/vol8/fourfatal.htm

Section 508. (2006). *General Services Administration*. Retrieved November 20, 2006 from http://www.section508.gov/index.cfm?FuseAction=Content&ID=131

Spradlin, L., & Parsons, R. (2008). *Diversity matters: understanding diversity in schools*. Belmont, CA: Thomson Higher Education.

TK20 Campuswide. (2009). Retrieved April 2, 2009, from http://www.tk20.com/

Thoms, L., & Thelwall, M. (2005). Academic home pages: Reconstruction of the self. *First Monday, 12* 10). Retrieved September 14, 2006. from,http://firstmonday.org/issues/issue10_12/thoms/index.html

TrueOutcomes Assessment Manager. (2009). Retrieved April 2, 2009, from http://www. trueoutcomes.com/

Van Horn, R. (2003). Web page accessibility. [from EBSCOhost database.]. *Phi Delta Kappan, 103*, 173. Retrieved September 26, 2007.

Vella, M. (2008, June 24). The 10 commandments of Web design. *Business Week Online*. Retrieved April 7, 2009, from Academic Search Premier database.

Web Access Initiative. (2001). Retrieved January 21, 2007, from http://www.w3.org/WAI/quicktips

ADDITIONAL READING

America, P. (2009). Retrieved April 2, 2009, from http://www.preserveamerica.gov/overview.html

Auburn University Web site. (2009). Retrieved April 10, 2009, from http://www.auburn.edu.

Clark, J. (2008, October). The Internet connection: Web 2.0, Flickr and Endless Possibilities. *Behavioral & Social Sciences Librarian, 27*(2), 62-64. Retrieved April 10, 2009, from doi:10.1080/01639260802152873.

Faiola, A., & MacDorman, K. (2008). The influence of holistic and analytic cognitive styles on online information design: toward a communication theory of cultural cognitive design. *Information Communication and Society, 11*(3), 348–374. doi:10.1080/13691180802025418

Foster, A. L. (2001, January 26). Colleges focus on making web sites work for people with disabilities. *Chronicle of Higher Education*.

Gevorgyan, G., & Porter, L. (2008). One size does not fit all: culture and perceived importance of Web design features. *Journal of Website Promotion, 3*(1/2), 25–38. doi:10.1080/15533610802052589

History, H. (2009). Retrieved March 18, 2009, from http://www.hawaiihistory.org/

Hudson, L. (2002). Enabling Section 508 Standards. *NetConnect*, 20-21. Retrieved September 26, 2007, from EBSCOhost database.

Hudson, L. (2002). A New Age of Accessibility. [from EBSCOhost database.]. *School Library Journal*, 19–20. Retrieved September 26, 2007.

Kentucky Historical Society. (2009). Retrieved February 20, 2009, from http://history.ky.gov/

Knight, E., Gunawardena, C., & Aydin, C. (2009). Cultural interpretations of the visual meaning of icons and images used in North American Web design. *Educational Media International, 46*(1), 17–35. doi:10.1080/09523980902781279

Li Liew, C. (2005). Online cultural heritage exhibitions: a survey of information retrieval features. *Program: Electronic Library & Information Systems, 39*(1), 4–24. doi:10.1108/00330330510578778

Mcneil, P. (2008). *The Web designer's idea book: the ultimate guide to themes, trends & styles in Website design*. Cincinnati, OH: HOW Books.

NCATE Code of Conduct. (2003.) Retrieved July 23, 2009, from http://www.NCATE.org/ program-review/codeOfconduct.asp?ch=37

Ogbu, J. (2002). Black-American students and the academic achievement gap: what else you need to know. *Journal of Thought*, *37*(4), 9–33.

Ogbu, J. (2003). *Black students in an affluent suburb: a study of academic disengagement*. Mahwah, NJ: Lawrence Erllbaum.

Renfroe, M. (2005). Products You Can Use to Build Your Site. *Knowledge Quest,* 17-18. Retrieved September 26, 2007, from EBSCOhost database.

Savoy, A., & Salvendy, G. (2008). Foundations of content preparation for the Web. *Theoretical Issues in Ergonomics Science*, *9*(6), 501–521. doi:10.1080/14639220701685673

Sawchuk, S. (2009, March 9). *NCATE president outlines plans to update the process*. Retrieved April 9,2009, from http://www.NCATE.org/ public/30509_edweek.asp

Schmetzke, A., & Comeaux, D. (2009). Accessibility trends among academic library and library school Web sites in the USA and Canada. *Journal of Access Services*, *6*(1/2), 137–152. doi:10.1080/15367960802286286

Swanson, T., & Cox, C. (2006). Looking to the future: implementing blogs in a community college library. *Internet Reference Services Quarterly*, *11*(3), 57–67. doi:10.1300/J136v11n03_04

TIDY Library Project. (2005). Retrieved August 13, 2006, from http://tidy.sourceforge.net/

University of Alabama college of education Web site. (2009). Retrieved March 9, 2009, fromhttp:// education.ua.edu/NCATE/index.html

University of Hawaii college of education Web site. (2009). Retrieved March 8, 2009, fromhttp:// www.hawaii.edu/coe

University of Kentucky NCATE Web site. (2009). Retrieved August 12, 2008, fromhttp://www.coe. uky.edu/NCATE/

Web, A. I. M. *(Web Accessibility in Mind)*. (2006). Utah State University. Retrieved August 10, 2006, fromhttp://www.webaim.org/standards/508/ checklist

Web content accessibility and mobile Web. (2008). Retrieved February 2, 2009, fromhttp://www. w3.org/WAI/mobile/

APPENDIX 1: NCATE STANDARDS

(Professional Standards, 2008, p. 12-13):

Standard 1: *Candidate knowledge, skills, and professional dispositions* requires that candidates know and demonstrate the content knowledge, pedagogical content knowledge and skills, pedagogical and professional knowledge and skills, and professional dispositions necessary to help all students learn.

Standard 2: *Assessment system and unit evaluation* determines that an educational unit collects, analyzes data on applicant qualifications, candidate and graduate performance, and unit operations to evaluate and improve the performance of candidates, the unit and its programs.

Standard 3: *Field experiences and clinical practice* reviews the educational unit and its school partners in their design, implementation, and evaluation of field experiences and clinical practice so that teacher education candidates and other school professionals develop and demonstrate the knowledge, skills, and professional dispositions necessary to help all students learn.

Standard 4: *Diversity* determines the extent to which the educational unit designs, implements, and evaluates curriculum and provides diverse experiences for candidates to acquire and demonstrate the knowledge, skills, and professional dispositions necessary to help all students learn. Experiences provided for candidates include working with diverse populations, including higher education and P-12 school faculty, candidates, and students in P-12 schools.

Standard 5: *Faculty qualifications, performance, and development* provides that faculty are qualified and model best professional practices in scholarship, service, and teaching, including the assessment of their effectiveness as related to candidate performance. They also collaborate with colleagues in the disciplines and schools.

Standard 6: *Unit governance and resources* analyzes the unit leadership, authority, budget, personnel, facilities, and resources, including information technology resources, for the preparation of candidates to meet professional, state, and institutional standards.

APPENDIX 2: GUIDELINES TO SETTING UP A WEB PAGE

(Hudson, 2002, p. 20-21):

1. A text equivalent for every non-text element shall be provided.

2. Equivalent alternatives for any multimedia presentation shall be synchronized with the presentation.

3. Web pages shall be designed so that all information conveyed with color is also available without color, for example from context or markup.

4. Documents shall be organized so they are readable without requiring an associated style sheet.

5. Redundant text links shall be provided for each active region of a server-side image map.

6. Client-side image maps shall be provided instead of server-side image maps except where the regions cannot be defined with an available geometric shape.

7. Row and column headers shall be identified for data tables.

8. Markup shall be used to associate data cells and header cells for data tables that have two or more logical levels of row or column headers.

9. Frames shall be titled with text that facilitates from identification and navigation.

10. Pages shall be designed to avoid causing the screen to flicker with a frequency greater than 2 Hz and lower than 55Hz.

11. A text-only page, with equivalent information or functionality, shall be provided to make a web site comply of this part when compliance cannot be accomplished in the other way. The content of the text-only page shall be updated whenever the primary page changes.

12. When pages utilize scripting languages to display content or to create interface elements, the information provided by the script shall be identified with functional text that can be read by assistive technology.

13. When a Web page requires that an applet, plug-in, or other application be present on the client system to interpret page content, the page must provide a link to a plug-in or applet that complies with 1194.21 (a) through (l).

14. When electronic forms are designed to be completed on-line, the form shall allow people using assistive technology to access the information, field elements, and functionality required for completion and submission of the form, including all directions and cues.

15. A method shall be provided that permits users to skip repetitive navigation links.

16. When a timed response is required, the user shall be altered and given sufficient time to indicate more time is required

The Web Access Initiative (2001):

1. Images & animations: Use the alt attribute to describe the function of each visual.

2. Image maps. Use the client-side map and text for hotspots.

3. Multimedia. Provide captioning and transcripts of audio, and descriptions of video.

4. Hypertext links. Use text that makes sense when read out of context. For example, avoid "click here" page organization. Use headings, lists, and consistent structure. Use CSS for layout and style where possible.

5. Summarize or use the longdesc attribute for graphs and charts.

6. Scripts, applets, & plug-ins. Provide alternative content in case active features are inaccessible or unsupported.

7. Use the no frames element and meaningful titles.

8. Make line-by-line reading sensible for tables. Summarize tables if at all possible.

9. Check your work, validate. Use tools, checklist, and guidelines at http://www.w3.org/TR/WCAG.

APPENDIX 3: FACULTY 180 DATABASE FEATURES

(Williams, L., personal communication, April 7, 2009)

1. Collect profile data in profile sections (e.g., contact information, employment history, degrees) and activity sections (e.g., teaching, research, professional development, consulting and service).

2. Activity tags: Tag faculty activities (e.g., tag a published journal article by: basic, applied and pedagogical).

3. Faculty tags: Tag faculty members (e.g., tag a faculty member by: tenured, tenure-tracked, non-tenure-tracked).

4. Reports for faculty members: Allows access to personal vitae for annual reviews and tenure/promotion processes, and to activity trend reports for a faculty member's self-evaluation.

5. Reports to administrators: Provides profile and activity reports filterable by activity tags and faculty tags (mentioned in b and c above), and provides faculty reports for regional and professional accrediting bodies (e.g., SACS, AACSB, NCATE).

6. Web-based hosting of stored files: Provides a web-based application that allows faculty to attach and store supporting files (e.g., an electronic copy of a journal article to support the activity entry). Attached files can be images, videos, audio clips and more (e.g.,.DOC,.XLS,.PDF,.ZIP,.JPG,.TXT,.WAV). Attached files are accessible from within a faculty member's vita by clicking on the blue link.

7. Customizable: Provides dynamic customizability--allowing tailoring of profile and activity data sections, activity tags and faculty tags within minutes

8. Workload Process: Provides procedures for inputting faculty data and making sure the data are accurate and complete.

9. Reporting: Provides output for all profile and activity sections, with filtering by activity tags and faculty tags. Allows drilldown within reports from aggregated levels to disaggregated levels, along with the ability to review and edit specific activity entries.

Chapter 12
Electronic Portfolios in Teacher Education:
Practical Reflections and Insights from a Systemic Implementation

Howard Coleman
UNC Wilmington, USA

Jeremy Dickerson
East Carolina University, USA

Dennis Kubasko
UNC Wilmington, USA

ABSTRACT

Electronic portfolios serve a variety of needs within the field of education as the information technology age collides with the age of educational accountability. This chapter discusses the successes and challenges of an electronic portfolio integration process over five years in a large teacher education program. Specific details for selecting an electronic portfolio system are explained at length. Issues concerning student products, teacher standards, evaluation and accreditation are addressed through the lens of reflective experiences and practice.

INTRODUCTION

Electronic Portfolios in the Age of Educational Accountability

National and international educational standards have made both teacher and student assessment a priority for the field of education (US Department of Education, 2009). Legislative mandates such as the 2001 No Child Left Behind Act (NCLB) have increased the demands for accountability in our nation's schools and made documenting and ensuring teacher competencies an even higher priority for institutions of higher education. Portfolios have been a common process to attain more meaningful and holistic perspectives of teacher and student performance standards for many years. Advancements in information technology have made electronic portfolio systems popular because of the improved economic feasibility, web ubiquity and increased

DOI: 10.4018/978-1-61520-899-9.ch012

efficiency they provide. Electronic (E) portfolios consist of work that the learner has collected, selected, reflected on and desires to present in order to demonstrate growth and capabilities (Barrett, 2007). E-portfolios are flexible, digital tools for teaching, learning, assessment and evaluation which provide organizations and students with innovative ways to understand experiences and achievements (Chambers and Wickersham, 2007; Goldsmith, 2007). E-portfolios have been successfully used in universities to track student progress and to document learning (Wilhelm et al. 2006; Cambridge, 2008) in many diverse areas of academics, including medicine (Dornan, Carroll and Parboosingh, 2002), physical education (Hastie and Sinelnikov, 2007) and athletic training and therapy (Delmont, 2003). E-portfolios can be important components of student evaluation and assessment in online courses in higher education due to their ability to enhance reflection using advanced technologies (Bauer and Anderson, 2000). E-portfolios have been used to teach college students how to assess and evaluate their work (Heath, 2002) as well as the work of their peers in structured, technology-rich environments (Brandes and Boskic, 2008). Beishuizen, Van Boxel, Banyard, Twiner, Vermeij and Underwood (2006) state that the structure of e-portfolios assists in archiving work for reflection, analysis and presentation for college students. Beck, Livine and Bear (2005) suggest that formative electronic portfolios support the development and evaluation of professional teaching standards and outcomes.

The International Society for Technology in Education (ISTE, 2009) has established technology standards that teachers should meet as they design, implement, and assess educational experiences to engage students and improve learning. ISTE's National Educational Technology Standards (NETS) have served as guidelines for improving teaching and learning through the use of technology in the areas of students, teachers and administrators (NETS-S, NETS-T, and NETS-A). The NETS were designed to guide educators as they increase and improve their knowledge, skills, and attitudes with technology. The National Council for Accreditation of Teacher Education (NCATE) incorporated the ISTE NETS technology standards for colleges of education to ensure that all teacher candidates would be able to use educational technology to help students learn (2009). NCATE's commitment to technology standards has prompted colleges of teacher education to provide opportunities to develop knowledge, skills and dispositions related to education and information technology. These standards encourage teacher candidates to learn how technology is integrated throughout planning, curriculum, instruction, field experiences, clinical practice, assessments, and evaluations. This effort of aligning teacher preparation with technology standards has been used to prepare pre-service teachers to work in the digital age. E-portfolios have advanced in capacity, function and form during the last five years and have now become a means for reflection and assessment. E-portfolios play a major role in the integration of technology in education today.

E-portfolios are becoming more common in various educational settings due to their range of uses and because of the increased amount of technology on many campuses (Capraro, 2003; Chambers and Wickersham, 2007). The use of e-portfolios allows pre-service teachers to use technology to support effective instructional practices in K-12 schools after graduation. Advanced, high-quality e-portfolio systems provide a means for teachers and students to digitally display what they have learned and to connect their work products to standards. Bartlett (2002) states that teacher preparation programs are increasingly using electronic portfolio assessment tools to document students' development of instructional dispositions and standards. In addition, portfolios provide a comprehensive collection of materials and work products to document students' accomplishments and give them the opportunity to reflect on their instructional dispositions. Ring and

Foti (2003) state that portfolios allow students to engage in instructional tasks in authentic contexts and situations. Campbell, Cignetti, Melenyzer, Nettles and Wyman (2001) describe e-portfolios in teacher education programs as having the following useful characteristics:

- Encourages students to understand the teaching profession by reflecting on the practice of aligning work products with the teaching standards
- Encourages students to better understand themselves and their work, then reflect upon the evaluation & assessment process
- Promotes growth by identifying students' strengths and weaknesses
- Provides a holistic or authentic assessment to capture the complexities of teaching that can be viewed and assessed by others.

Strudel and Wetzel (2008) investigated the benefits and costs of using electronic portfolios in pre-service teacher education programs. Their study examined the perspectives of faculty members in six programs in which electronic portfolios had been used on a large scale over time. They identified the following benefits;

- Increased opportunities for students to reflect and learn
- Better student understanding of teaching standards
- Better faculty access for student work assessment
- Increased faculty communication with students; and improved tracking of student performance for purposes of accreditation and program improvement.

Some of the disadvantages included the amount of time and effort expended to set up and monitor the e-portfolios and the lack of compatibility with faculty members' beliefs, values, and needs. Overall, Strudel and Wetzel concluded that faculty satisfaction with electronic portfolios appears to be strongly related to their views on student-centered teacher education and their willingness to balance individual preferences to accomplish the program goals.

Derham (2003) investigated the reliability and validity of an electronic portfolio that was designed to assess the instructional competencies of pre-service teachers. This study examined evidence of the electronic portfolio's psychometric properties based on test content (measured by expert opinion), relations with other variables (other pre-service teacher assessments) and reliability estimates (internal consistency and inter-rater reliability). The results indicated that it is feasible to develop and implement an electronic portfolio that adequately assesses a majority of widely adopted standards for beginning teachers. The study also encouraged further analysis and exploration of the advantages and shortcomings of electronic portfolios to determine the most appropriate uses of this technological innovation in educational settings.

Chambers and Wickersham (2007) used descriptive data collected over two semesters to track and articulate the advantages and disadvantages of e-portfolio implementation in a teacher education program from a teacher candidate's viewpoint. In practice, student technology self-efficacy was cited as the primary barrier to successful integration. Conversely, increased student awareness that e-portfolios can assist with the organization of their learning and the reflection or their work products were viewed as primary advantages to integration. Peer review, increased communication patterns, and reliable and efficient feedback were favorably viewed. Wilhelm et al. (2006) described the implementation of e-portfolios at three different teacher education universities. Faculty resistance to implementation was highlighted as a potential barrier. The paper encouraged establishing a shared vision, well-articulated conceptual framework and agreement on underlying philosophies prior to engaging and selecting a vendor for integration.

Wilhelm et al. outlines the following factors to be considered prior to selection: local context, cost, template design flexibility and technical support. Overall, such studies have shaped the conversation around e-portfolios and prompted the investigation of possible adoption across the educational landscape.

Reflective Experiences & Insights from an E-Portfolio Implementation

This section describes a specific real-world scenario of e-portfolio integration within teacher and school administration education programs at a university with approximately 1200 students majoring in education. The consideration of e-portfolios for assessment and documentation of student performance standards in this institution coincided with the need to collect and display evidence for national and state accreditation. Barrett (2006) suggests that e-portfolio integration should have a clear intended purpose within an educational organization. In this case, e-portfolios had the clear, intended purpose of providing a technological solution to the need for organization and display of accreditation evidences. Student performance evidences/artifacts are required to support and verify the effectiveness of the teacher education and school administration programs. A need to improve the documentation process was one of the driving forces behind the selection of an e-portfolio system approach. Effective information technology was needed to organize and collect the large amount of evidence for teacher and administrator candidates and to prepare data and records for national and state accrediting agencies.

A group of university administrators, technology specialists and university faculty led the e-portfolio implementation process. This included product selection, program integration and consideration of stakeholders at all levels of the organization. Identification and adoption of a unit-wide solution should involve all stakeholders from the outset (Wilhelm et al. 2006). The following is an overview of the organizational stakeholders' and relevant conceptual questions utilized in adopting and implementing e-portfolios in this scenario:

Figure 1.

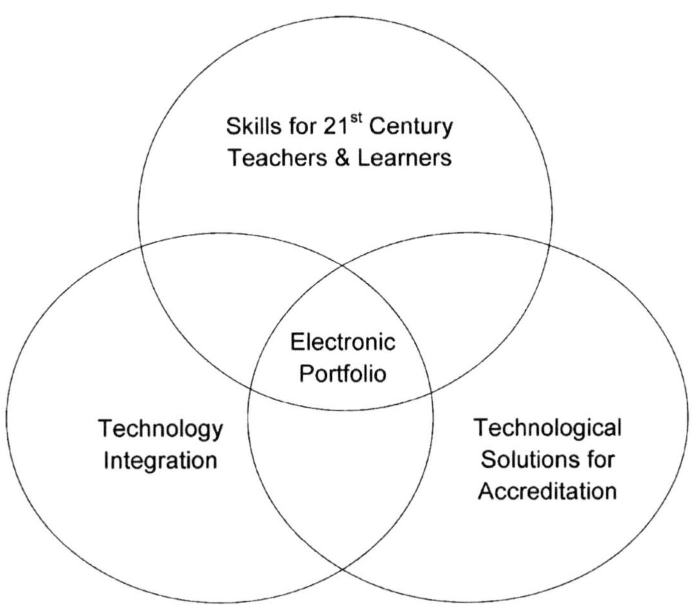

1. University administrators (*top-down support*). Would the need for technological change be led and/or supported by university administrators? This process would have to be supported from the "top down" because of the obvious requirements for additional resources (funding, time) and unit-wide (personnel) efforts.
2. Technology support staff (*Middle-level support*). Would technology support personnel have buy-in and understand the need for technical support and training or would this be perceived as "another technology fad" concocted by administration or faculty?
3. University faculty (*Middle-level support*). The entire faculty would have to be engaged in this process to be successful. What were faculty members' limitations relative to technological skills, abilities, knowledge, and dispositions and would all faculty members be willing to acquire the knowledge and skills to implement and electronic portfolio system?
4. Students (*bottom-up support*). How would students respond to the use of an e-portfolio system? How would the cost, technical assistance and technical skills required to integrate an e-portfolio impact students?

These stakeholder issues needed to be acknowledged and addressed. Table 1 lists each primary stakeholder groups' perspectives on issues which affected the e-portfolio implementation process.

These issues helped guide the process of reviewing and discussing both in-sourcing and outsourcing solutions for e-portfolio design and development. Gibson and Barrett (2003) examined the use of generic tools (static files made with word processors, etc.) in comparison with customized system approaches (databases, servers and advanced technologies). While it was believed that developing an "in-house" e-portfolio product via campus technology staff might have provided many benefits, it was determined that technicians would need too much time to develop an in-house e-portfolio solution. Therefore, an external e-portfolio product approach was selected to accomplish the task of serving the emerging needs of the teacher and administrator education programs. The decision to choose an outsourced electronic portfolio product was also based on the need for immediate programmatic integration and advanced technological capabilities. Once it was agreed that outsourcing was the best option, a number of products were considered and reviewed. The following organizational characteristics later proved to be invaluable to the identification, adoption and integration of a viable, external e-portfolio system.

- **Shared Vision.** Faculty and staff members had a clear understanding of the need and purpose for system integration
- **Risk Taking.** Faculty and staff members were willing to work in an unfamiliar, virtual environment with their students

Table 1. Synopsis of stakeholders and issues to consider

Stakeholder	Issues to Consider
University Administrators	Providing personnel support and project funding, establishing buy-in across programs without authoritative pressure
Technology Staff	Changes in training needs, questions of infrastructure adequacy and systemic approach to technology integration
University Faculty	Limitations of technology literacy, questions of support and investment/balance of time
Students	Questions/concerns of cost feasibility and value added relative to changing from three-ring binder hard copies to e-portfolio system

- **Collaboration.** Faculty and staff members had experience working together on a team
- **Technology Literacy.** Faculty and staff members participating in the e-portfolio pilot project possessed high-level technology skills.

The faculty and staff associated with the e-portfolio pilot implementation possessed characteristics, experiences and skills that were critical to promoting and ensuring a successful integration process.

A study of the current literature on selecting, developing and implementing portfolios in education (Barrett & Wilkerson, 2004) emphasized a conceptual framework that could balance the needs of the institution for an assessment management system with the needs of learners for a reflective portfolio that would support meaningful learning. The faculty and staff were interested in selecting an electronic portfolio system that could meet the needs of 21st century learners. The team considered emerging and adaptable new technologies to be important components of electronic portfolio functionality. A system was needed that could incorporate advanced communication and collaboration technologies given the increasing use of these tools by students. These "Web 2.0 tools" include email, instant messaging, video clips, audio clips, online collaboration and sharing of resources. Such built-in functions could enhance student work as well as the overall integration of emerging technologies into the organization. Based on all of these factors and a review of several products, the Taskstream© electronic portfolio system was recommended. Table 2 displays the timeline for adoption and implementation.

Taskstream© refers to a suite of products that are an "electronic toolset" with combinations of communication tools, standards integration capabilities and other advanced features and options. Beginning in year 2, Taskstream© was adopted and integrated with a small group of faculty and students prior to a full systemic integration. During year two, the e-portfolio toolset was piloted with two secondary teacher education methods classes. Each faculty member implemented the toolset during the student teaching semester was responsible for leading a small group of secondary teacher candidates through the training, adoption and use of the technology. Secondary science and social studies students were selected because of the manageable size of students and the willingness of the faculty to experiment with new technology.

During this pilot period, the e-portfolio toolset was used as an electronic repository system for students to submit unit plans, lesson plans and rubrics and to provide students with access to lesson plan templates. National and state standards were integrated into the toolset interface for lesson alignment. In addition, the toolset was used for the sharing of work products between university instructors and students (teacher candidates) and for peer reviews between students. Secondary interns were trained during a face-to-face seminar in the use of the electronic toolset. University technology trainers supported students using the toolset on the first day of training and provided

Table 2. Timeline for electronic portfolio implementation

Time	Action
Year 1	Interest Group Formed; Discovery and Exploration of Products, Processes and Issues
Year 2	Pilot Program-Level Implementation
Year 3	Large-Scale Implementation
Year 4	Accreditation Review with Use of Electronic Portfolio Toolset Evidences
Year 5 and Beyond	Management, Maintenance, Expansion of Uses in other Programs and Ongoing Reflection

ongoing assistance throughout the semester. The interns' use of the online toolset was recorded electronically through the toolset function during their placements at area high schools. Each intern was surveyed at the end of the internship.

Data was collected from the internship and analyzed in the summer following the first year of implementation. Based upon the positive feedback and results of the pilot project, the implementation team decided that a comprehensive plan for integration was needed. This information was used identify what worked, what did not work, and what need to be done to improve the e-portfolio integration process on a large scale. For example, the pilot implementation group lacked a clear understanding of the students' technology learning curve. While many the science students were able to attach documents and post content to the lesson plan templates, their organization of materials and ideas were disjointed. Some social studies students questioned the relevancy and use of the toolset. These students felt encumbered by the structure of the toolset and complained about a lack of flexibility as they developed their materials. As a result, training and support mechanisms were discussed and examined which could support large-scale implementation.

A large number of students indicated that the toolset had redeeming qualities and felt strongly that it represented a more modern approach to documenting and reflecting on their internship experiences. Several students indicated that they preferred the electronic system over traditional internship approaches that relied on paper products, three ring binders and 100% synchronous communication. Students stated that they quickly gained an appreciation for the internal communication functions such as instant messaging and the e-mail components. They also said the immediate access to the teaching standards allowed them to attach assignments such as lesson and unit plans to the standards. The pilot implementation process was critical in providing a means to review the e-portfolio toolset's capabilities and to identify potential problems before a large-scale adoption of the product. If substantial technical difficulties and other major problems had occurred during a systemic adoption of the product, this would have led to a decision to end the implementation testing and the use of the e-portfolio technology.

The experiences and knowledge gained from the pilot implementation process allowed the Taskstream© electronic toolset to be easily adopted for full integration across all departments. The pilot process for reviewing the Taskstream© product served the department well and exposed important issues and potential barriers prior to the larger systemic implementation of the product. This information allowed university leaders to establish specific action plans to ensure successful implementation. Table 3 displays how the knowledge gained from the pilot implementation provided solutions to the stakeholder issues.

The comprehensive implementation of Taskstream© across other departmental areas occurred in year three. The lessons learned and the adjustments made during the pilot process proved to be invaluable. Taskstream© was readily accepted throughout the school of education as the teacher candidates and administrators began using the toolset. A series of adjustments and actions by the university leaders made for a smooth and effective transition process. These adjustments and actions (see Table 3) provided a support structure which enabled the toolset to be successfully used across all programs. The leadership provided by the university administrators was characterized by proactive visioning, teambuilding, careful analysis and the enabling of faculty and staff to learn and to grow. The problems experienced in year three were minimized due to the lessons learned during the pilot process and the actions taken by the university administration to support a smooth implementation process. The technical, logistical and policy issues usually associated with a large number of users were easily resolved. The remaining problems were typically individual rather than systemic issues. Students with low-

Table 3. Stakeholders, issues and actions taken

Stakeholder	Issues	Actions Taken
University Administrators	Providing technical personnel support and project funding issues; establishing buy-in across programs without authoritative pressure	• Openly supported the project as a substantial and worthwhile endeavor • Conversations held with faculty to discuss implications • Exploring grants to support associated research • Led cost negotiations with technology vendor
Technology Support Staff	Changes in training needs, questions of infrastructure adequacy and systemic approach to technology integration	• Conducted professional development training which was key to overcoming faculty learning curve • Comprehensive approach to training all stakeholders • Immediate support for faculty and students • Relationship building with technology vendor
University Faculty	Limitations of technology literacy, questions of support, purpose and investment/balance of time	• Learning curve was addressed with professional development training & technical support • Programmatic approach used, facilitating faculty-to-faculty support & interaction • Clear connections to electronic documentation for future reviews (accreditation, etc.)
Students	Questions/concerns of cost feasibility and value added	• Reasonable cost for students was negotiated with vendor by university • Technical support and training was provided by university and vendor • Value became evident through improved feedback, organization and communication

level technology skills and/or poor dispositions towards technology had barriers which were overcome with the help of the technical support staff.

Year four was the accreditation year conducted by national and state review teams. The electronic portfolio toolset provided a means to streamline and organize the accreditation process. The Taskstream© system provided electronic documentation and display of student materials from the previous year. These materials complemented the other years of student work. The electronic format also demonstrated a transition from the paper-age to the digital age. While some reviewers were tech-savvy and impressed with the electronic format, others were encumbered by the interface and the navigation process of the electronic materials. Technical staff personnel were available for assistance and paper copies were prepared in the event that the electronic portfolios were unacceptable by any reviewers. This process established an efficient and effective data management system for future accreditation visits and provided the organization with the momentum needed to move towards institutionalizing a sound, reliable and useful the electronic documentation process. Year five (and beyond) has become a process of continual expansion, refinement and improvement. The electronic toolset continues to become embedded in the activities and actions of the faculty and students each year. The electronic portfolio and toolset has been integrated into graduate programs such as the Master of School Administration program. Technical support and training for new students and faculty are always necessary, but the majority of faculty members are well versed and capable of using the Taskstream© e-portfolio toolset on a variety of meaningful levels.

The relationships developed between the Taskstream© company and the university during years one and two proved to be a solid investment of time. These relationships have allowed for continuous dialogue to occur, resulting in open and responsive discussions of technical problems, capabilities and business related issues. Through five years of work, the university has been able to establish an effective process for e-portfolio integration across all program areas. The results of this process have improved the organization's preparation for accreditation, enhanced the effectiveness of electronic communication tools, increased the quality of student work products and provided an electronic work environment for preparing teachers and students to have 21st century skills that are necessary for the digital age.

Figure 2 displays screenshots from the Taskstream© interface. Both screenshots show the static TaskStream "Learning Achievement Tools" on the far left and different templates for student entries on the right of the page. The first screenshot represents a Masters of Arts in Teaching student's teaching portfolio. The second screenshot represents another student's 10-day unit plan.

Reflective Practice: Selecting an Electronic Portfolio System for Your Organization

The process discussed in this chapter allowed the organization to learn many lessons about how to efficiently and effectively implement e-portfolios in teacher education and school administration programs. This process of e-portfolio implementation and integration revealed many factors to consider and discuss before moving forward

Figure 2. Basic student e-portfolio interface examples

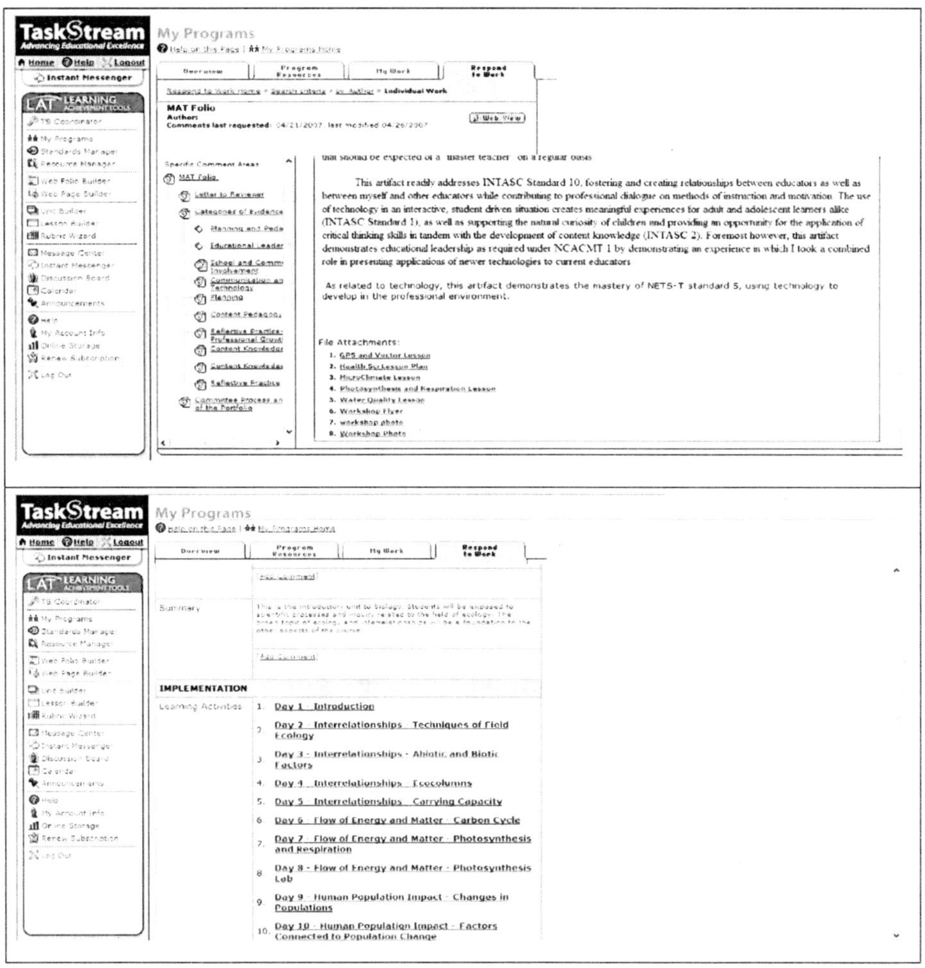

with the adoption of a particular product. Once a decision is made to adopt an external technological solution, perhaps the most critical step for any organization is the selection of the right electronic portfolio system (Strudler and Wetzel, 2005). If organizational participants are not willing to commit sufficient time and effort at the beginning of this process, then large amounts of time and effort will be unnecessarily expended during implementation. Worst still, the lack of commitment can damage the perception of the value of e-portfolios for many of the stakeholders in the organization. Selecting a specific technology product or system for any e-portfolio endeavor can be complicated and confusing. There are many companies that offer software, hardware, web-based interfaces and applications for creating electronic portfolios for educational organizations. The educational technologies market is abundant with products which have an array of capabilities and functions.

E-portfolios can be used for many reasons, including collecting student work, presenting longitudinal data and creating paperless learning environments. The implementation of electronic portfolios requires the selection of products and methods that are a good fit for the needs and goals of the organization. There are numerous e-portfolio companies or service providers in the marketplace. These private companies specialize in developing, maintaining and upgrading complex web-based hardware and software systems. This approach is commonly referred to as "out-sourcing." The wide array of available products can sometimes make the selection process cumbersome and confusing. The technology selection process is often overlooked or taken too lightly by many organizations. If the wrong product is chosen, the results can lead to frustration, disappointment and a loss of time, money and/or data. Selecting an ineffective or inappropriate electronic portfolio technology is the result of misunderstandings, haste, a lack of research, fiscal restraints and overly zealous sales pitches by software companies. These mistakes and errors may be avoided thorough systemic analysis of the factors that are critical to meeting an organization's needs and goals. Before selecting an electronic portfolio system, leaders and stakeholders must have an accurate understanding of present and future needs, goals and conditions in their organization. Further, leaders charged with making decisions about electronic portfolios technologies must also be able to clearly identify and communicate the potential problems that could affect and/or limit successful implementation. Organizations that do consider all of the issues in the electronic portfolio adoption process may have mixed results and/or be disappointed with their efforts. The following list presents factors to consider when selecting an electronic portfolio system:

1. Organizational Needs
2. Cost
3. User Skills and Capabilities
4. Training & Technical Support
5. Technological Infrastructure

Although there may be additional factors, analyzing these areas will provide a solid foundation for making the best e-portfolio decision for an organization. The following sections provide specific questions, answers and explanations to assist decision-makers in the selection process.

Organizational Needs

One of the most critical components in strategic planning is to identify what is needed to meet the organization's needs for students and faculty members. The gap between an organization's current conditions and their desired conditions represents their needs. Needs should be a shared reality and all stakeholders should believe that addressing their needs will improve the organization. Clearly identified organizational needs are essential for productive decision making regardless of the scenario. If appropriately integrated, electronic portfolios can help educational organizations to meet a variety of needs. Some examples include improving communication, blending information technologies into the curriculum, providing students with more timely feedback and collecting data to meet accreditation standards. Conversely, if inappropriately selected, adopted and integrated, electronic portfolios can be perceived as "add-ons" or superfluous tasks that are characteristic of many technological applications in schools and universities today.

The electronic portfolio system needs to be viewed as a productive, helpful, useful and purposeful tool that is aligned with the goals of the organization. More importantly, an electronic portfolio system should serve and meet the needs of students, faculty and administrators. If any of these primary groups believe that electronic portfolios are a waste of time, then the communication and articulation of how electronic portfolios assist the achievement of needs should be revisited. The following are questions to consider regarding electronic portfolios and organizational needs:

1. Are electronic portfolios the best option for the organizational needs?
2. Specifically, what organizational needs will the adoption of electronic portfolios supposedly fulfill?
3. Are these long term or short term needs? Since electronic portfolios are a long term investment, is this decision based on simply meeting short term needs?
4. Will the adoption of electronic portfolios create more needs within the organization?

Cost

The rising cost of education coupled with a volatile global economy makes the addition of anything with an associated cost a tenuous topic. E-portfolios are no exception and cost is a significant factor for stakeholders to consider. Every e-portfolio technology has some form of cost, whether in the form of commercial vendor costs, in-house technician/programmer development, or installation and training for a freeware solution. It is common practice in many educational organizations to select professional, commercial software with web-based interfaces for electronic portfolio solutions. Such applications usually offer a high-quality product and require some form of monetary transaction either between the company/vendor and the institution or the company/vendor and the individual user. In higher education, this issue means either the college and/or the student will be paying for the right to use the product. This is often referred to as a "subscription" and comes with an agreement and terms of use, including the length of time for the subscription.

Cost is an issue which must be determined before adoption of an e-portfolio system. When leaders make a decision to go forward with an electronic system, they must carefully consider who will pay for the monetary costs and strive to ensure that these costs are necessary and will be as reasonable as possible. Costs may often be negotiated with vendors based on the number of subscribers who will be using the product. Most importantly, faculty or students who are "required" to purchase subscriptions need to know all the facts about the transaction before being forced into making any payments. Faculty and students also need to know that the organization's leaders selected the electronic portfolio system after in-depth research, assessment and analysis and that this product will have positive impact on their learning environments. In addition, all stakeholders also need to know that the leaders did their best to negotiate the price they are paying and understand why a particular product was selected. Subscription costs aside, the organization must also consider how much it will cost in terms of human resources and time.

Questions to Ask about e-Portfolio Costs

1. How much will an electronic portfolio system cost each category of stakeholder

(faculty, staff, leadership, organization) in terms of time and money and how does this cost compare to the existing methods and practices?
2. What additional human resources will be needed and what is the cost associated with these human resources in terms of time and money?
3. If there are special software or hardware needed, what is the cost of these items and who will install and maintain any necessary hardware and software?
4. How much time will it take users of the electronic portfolio system to learn how to use the product and does that time translate into lost hours of wages or time off existing tasks?

User Skills and Capabilities

Information technologies have come a long way in the last decade in terms of user design interface. In addition, it is commonly believed that end-user capabilities and computer ownership/access have also increased. However, the organization's end-user must be carefully considered before adopting any electronic portfolio product. It is a mistake to assume that everyone within an organization has the technological skills and capabilities to use any new technology-based system. In educational organization there are a variety of individuals with various experiences, knowledge, skills and limitations. In planning for the adoption of an electronic portfolio system, leaders need some form of user skills and capabilities inventory to compare with the skills and capabilities necessary for successfully using a new technology. Once leaders and decision makers understand what skills and capabilities are necessary for using the new technology, then they may compare those skills and capabilities with what they know and understand about the end users who will be using the newly adopted product. Analyzing the skills needed for successful use of the product as well as the capabilities of the end users can provide an organization with an idea of potential problems that may be encountered, as well as training or special accommodations that may be needed after product adoption. Technical support personnel who service the end user group can be a rich source to gain informal information about users.

Questions to ask about electronic portfolios user skills and capabilities:

1. Who are the end users of this product (faculty, staff, administrators, students)?
2. What information exists about the computer skills of the end users?
3. Are there any known limitations of the end users which could be a barrier to success?
4. Does the electronic portfolio system require unique skills or capabilities which are not typically performed by the end users in the organization?

Training and Technical Support

Training and technical support are necessary for any new technology. E-portfolio products often include new tool sets with unique interfaces for users to understand and to develop proficiency level skills. New log-on screens, new ways to upload files and advanced printing and file sharing techniques are common in most electronic portfolio systems. Some packages and products require certain web browsers, plug-ins and setting adjustments to perform certain tasks. All of these things can be a source of frustration for many end users and are often seen as "one more problem" for them to work through - especially if buy-in hasn't been effectively established. Because of these issues, training and technical support needs to be in place *before* an electronic portfolio system is introduced to an end user group.

Training and technical support may be provided in many different ways. The company which supplies the product usually provides both in varying degrees with some limitations and conditions.

Company-based training can sometimes be negotiated when purchasing the product and often occurs early in the adoption process. In the past, face-to-face trainers representing the company would make site visits to conduct training. However, it is currently becoming more commonplace to have training provided from a distance via the Internet in the form of webinars, virtual reality, streaming video and audio technologies. Many educational organizations have in-house staff members who replace and/or supplement the initial training sessions. These individuals usually become the "in-house experts" who provide formal training sessions and just-in-time training for end users who need help to accomplish particular tasks.

Technical support is often supplied with a subscription or active license for an electronic portfolio product. Phone and online technical support personnel from the company that sells or develops the product are typically very knowledgeable and provide problem-solving databases to assist users. Technical support can be limited and/or become problematic for several reasons. Response delays, limited hours of availability, a lack of personal interaction and irritating automated response systems are all common complaints of technical support systems. In-house technical support staff often become proficient trouble shooters for general problems and can complement the technical support services provided by the company.

Questions to Ask about Electronic Portfolio Training and Technical Support

1. Who will provide initial training and technical support?
2. Who will provide long-term training and technical support?
3. How will training and technical support be evaluated?
4. If training and technical support are ineffective or inefficient, what are the options?
5. Are in-house support staff available to assist end users?
6. How much time will be allotted for the in-house staff to assist end users?

Technological Infrastructure

Technological infrastructure has become a diminishing issue for electronic portfolio systems in recent years. In the past, many electronic portfolio systems were built on-site using local computers running specialized software and stored on a local network server. This type of scenario required designated software licenses to be renewed and server space to be provided, backed-up and secured. Most electronic portfolio systems are now contracted through outside companies and are accessible via a web-based interface. Software is usually not necessary because of the design and tools of the web interface. Storage, security and file back-ups are often included in the business agreements between the organizations and the electronic portfolio company.

Questions to Consider Concerning Electronic Portfolios and Technological Infrastructure

1. Is any special hardware or software necessary to use the electronic portfolio system?
2. If so, how much does the hardware and software cost?
3. If student files are stored by a third party, are these files secured from being hacked?
4. If student files are stored by a third party, are these files properly and redundantly stored in case of file server catastrophe?
5. What written policies are in place guaranteeing file security?
6. Will users be informed if there are technical difficulties?

These are critical issues to consider when selecting an electronic portfolio system. The questions provide a starting point for decision-making and support a logical adoption process. From the authors' experiences, the questions listed above should be answered before making decisions about which product will work best for an educational organization. Failure to address these issues decreases the likelihood of selecting an e-portfolio system that will be a good fit for the organization. The overarching idea is to take the selection of an e-portfolio product seriously and to thoroughly analyze all of factors that are relevant to meeting stakeholders' needs and organizational goals.

FUTURE RESEARCH DIRECTIONS

There are several future research directions that should be pursued to continue gaining knowledge about the effectiveness of electronic portfolios in education. Based on the review of the literature for this chapter and the longitudinal implementation process previously discussed, the authors present the following for future research:

1. Compare the Tools Barrett and Gibson (2003) discuss the use of generic tools vs. customized, high-tech tools such as servers, databases and advanced programming to create e-portfolios. Questions for future research in comparing e-portfolio tools include: What is gained and what is lost from the development of e-portfolios created using these two very different methods? Which of these methods represent the most modern and contemporary skill set? As more university and public school environments move towards e-portfolios, who should make the decisions about how the e-portfolios are created? Administrators? Teachers? Students? What should be the reasons or justifications for choosing either method?
2. Examine the Immediate and Long Term Implications for Faculty and Supervisors Penny & Kinslow (2006) examined a series of factors associated with faculty interaction with e-portfolios and questioned how professors conceptualize their roles with e-portfolios. Questions for further research on the impact of electronic portfolios on faculty members include: What should university faculty members be able to do with e-portfolios? Should e-portfolio technology be as common as office productivity software? Should faculty members be required to integrate e-portfolios in all classes? Should e-portfolio instruction occur in non-technology based classes or just technology-centric classes? Should faculty members be expected or required to attend professional development on emerging trends and issues concerning e-portfolios?
3. Implementing and Monitoring E-portfolios Throughout an Educators' Career Educators using electronic portfolios assume responsibility for their own progress and play an active part in setting goals for themselves and in shaping their personal learning process while developing their professional development plans (Foote, 2001). Questions for further research on monitoring educators electronic portfolios throughout their careers include: Should e-portfolios be kept and monitored throughout a teacher's career? If e-portfolios improve the ability to effectively assess teacher candidates through reflection, should this also be the case for practicing teachers? What could be learned from integrating e-portfolios at the district, state and federal levels? Could other forms of teacher assessments be replaced with an effective electronic portfolio methodology?

CONCLUSION

How will Electronic Portfolio Implementation Change in the Future?

The uses of e-portfolios will continue to grow as teachers, students and administrators find new ways to use student work for assessment, evaluation, accreditation, record keeping and longitudinal research. It is hard to imagine electronic portfolio systems leaving the educational landscape since their use complements and supports other assessment methods. Hawkins and Black (2004) recommend a layered electronic portfolio system consisting of archived and current information that can be developed into a presentation portfolio for different applications and situations. Some major organizations and state education systems are calling for a longitudinal electronic portfolio process that chronicles all the work and achievements from the time teachers begin college throughout their entire careers.

The continuing development of new technologies serves as a catalyst for implementing electronic portfolios systems that can be considered to be a beacon for what is to come in educational organizations. With so many companies offering e-portfolio solutions at reasonable prices, the argument of outsourcing vs. in-sourcing will probably begin to subside. The web-ubiquity, multimedia capabilities, privacy and overall "turn-key" advantages that outsourced technology solutions offer makes developing an in-house e-portfolio product an unrealistic option. As technologically sophisticated, aesthetically pleasing e-portfolio packages evolve and become the standard, Conrad (2008) asks if form over content in e-portfolios is becoming an issue. There are very few similarities between advanced, web-based e-portfolio technologies of today and the tools which were being used ten years ago. This progression of technologies will continue and as e-portfolios become increasingly more main stream, they will likely be used more frequently in K-12 settings and take on many of the qualities found in K-12 technology environments. As younger students begin to interact in e-portfolio environments, there will be an emphasis for more privacy and security of student work that is housed on the Internet. In addition, the e-portfolio companies will need to begin looking at tools that will automatically integrate with online course delivery systems such as Blackboard©, WebCT© and Moodle© so that there will be seamless transitions between online course systems and e-portfolio systems – regardless of the platforms that are being used.

Technology is advancing rapidly, getting faster and smaller with each generation. It is unknown what e-portfolio systems will look like in the future. It isn't too far fetched to imagine e-portfolios that will be accessible via smart-phones with built-in real-time video conferencing features and many of the qualities found in Facebook©, Second Life© or YouTube©. These technologies, along with current Web 2.0 (and presumably Web 3.0) tools will almost certainly be a part of electronic portfolios. Regardless of the hardware or software involved, educators must continue to strive to understand these technologies to enhance and improve assessment, evaluation, accountability and communication in educational organizations.

REFERENCES

Barrett, H. (2006). Using electronic portfolios for formative/classroom based assessment: The reflect initiative. *Connected Newsletter*, June 2006.

Barrett, H. (2007). Researching electronic portfolios and learner engagement: The Reflect Initiative. *Journal of Adolescent & Adult Literacy, 50*(6), 436–449. doi:10.1598/JAAL.50.6.2

Barrett, H., & Wilkerson, J. (2004). *Conflicting paradigms in electronic portfolio approaches*. Retrieved March 20, 2009, from http://electronicportfolios.org/systems/paradigms.html

Bartlett, A. (2002). Preparing preservice teachers to implement performance assessment and technology through electronic portfolios. *Action in Teacher Education, 24*(1), 90–97.

Bauer, J., & Anderson, R. (2000). Evaluating students' written performance in the online classroom. *New Directions for Teaching and Learning, 84*(4), 65–71. doi:10.1002/tl.849

Beck, R., Livine, N., & Bear, S. (2005). Teachers' self assessment of the effects of formative and summative electronic portfolios on professional development. *European Journal of Teacher Education, 28*(3), 221–244. doi:10.1080/02619760500268733

Beishuizen, J., Van Boxel, P., Banyard, P., Twiner, A., Vermeij, H., & Underwood, J. (2006). The introduction of portfolios in higher education: a comparative study in the UK and the Netherlands. *European Journal of Education, 41*(3), 491–508. doi:10.1111/j.1465-3435.2006.00278.x

Brandes, G., & Boskic, N. (2008). E portfolios: From description to analysis. *International Review of Research in Open and Distance Learning, 9*(2), 1–17.

Cambridge, D. (2008). Universities as responsive learning organizations through competency-based assessment with electronic portfolios. *JGE: The Journal of General Education, 57*(1), 51–64. doi:10.1353/jge.0.0007

Campbell, D., Cignetti, P., Melenyzer, B., Nettles, D., & Wyman, R. (2001). *How to develop a professional portfolio: A manual for teachers*. Boston, MA: Allyn & Bacon.

Capraro, M. (2003). *Electronic teaching portfolios: technology skills + portfolio development = powerful pre-service teachers*. ERIC Number ED476367. Retrieved from ERIC database on April 1, 2009.

Chambers, S., & Wickersham, L. (2007). The electronic portfolio journal: A year later. *Education, 127*(3), 351–360.

Conrad, D. (2008). Building knowledge through portfolio learning in prior learning assessment and recognition. *Quarterly Review of Distance Education, 9*(2), 139–150.

Delmont, G. (2003). Using electronic portfolios to document learning. *Athletic Therapy Today, 8*(4), 22–23.

Dornan, T., Carroll, C., & Parboosingh, J. (2002). An electronic learning portfolio for reflective continuing professional development. *Medical Education, 36*(1), 767–769. doi:10.1046/j.1365-2923.2002.01278.x

Foote, C. J. (2001). Teaching Portfolio 101: Implementing the Teaching Portfolio in Introductory Courses. *Journal of Instructional Psychology, 28*(1).

Gibson, D., & Barrett, H. (2003). Directions in electronic portfolio development. *Contemporary Issues in Technology & Teacher Education, 2*(4), 559–576.

Goldsmith, D. (2007). Enhancing learning and assessment through e-portfolios: A collaborative effort in Connecticut. *New Directions for Student Services, 119*(1), 31–42. doi:10.1002/ss.247

Hawkins, C., & Black, S. (2004). Developing electronic portfolios across the state of Utah: Breaks, Breakdowns, and Breakthroughs. *Computers in Schools, 21*(1-2), 95-113.

Hastie, P., & Sinelnikov, O. (2007). The use of web-based portfolios in college physical education activity courses. *Physical Educator, 64*(1), 21–28.

Heath, M. (2002). Electronic portfolios for reflective self-assessment. *Teacher Librarian, 30*(1), 19–24.

International Society for Technology in Education. (2009). *The ISTE National Educational Technology Standards and Performance Indicators for Teachers*. Retrieved February 11, 2009, from http://www.iste.org

National Council for Accreditation of Teacher Education. (2009). Retrieved February 16, 2009, from http://www.ncate.org/public/faqaboutNCATE

Penny, C., & Kinslow, J. (2006). Faculty perceptions of electronic portfolios in a teacher education program. *Contemporary Issues in Technology & Teacher Education*, *6*(4), 418–435.

Ring, G. L., & Foti, S. L. (2003). Addressing standards at the program level with electronic portfolios. *TechTrends*, *47*(2), 28–32. doi:10.1007/BF02763422

Strudler, N., & Wetzel, K. (2005). The diffusion of electronic portfolios in teacher education: Issues of initiation and implementation. *Journal of Research on Technology in Teacher Education*, *37*(4), 411–433.

Strudler, N., & Wetzel, K. (2008). Costs and benefits of electronic portfolios in teacher education: faculty perspectives. *Journal of Computing in Teacher Education*, *24*(4), 135–142.

US Department of Education. (2009). Retrieved April 7, 2009 from http://www.ed.gov

Wilhelm, L., Puckett, K., Beisser, S., Wishart, W., Merideth, E., & Sivakumaran, T. (2006). Lessons Learned from the Implementation of Electronic Portfolios at Three Universities. *Curriculum Journal*, *17*(4), 397–411.

Section 5
Web 2.0

Chapter 13
Web 2.0 in the Classroom

Ron Lombard
Chatham University, USA

Stella C. Porto
University of Maryland, USA

ABSTRACT

The suitability of Web 2.0 technologies for learning has been widely discussed in the literature. The Web 2.0 term refers to what is understood as a change to a second version or generation of the web, with a distinct model for application development and design. This new model is based on enhanced communication and collaboration tools and services, information sharing, and interoperability. This trend has enabled the creation and development web-based communities, web-hosted services, and a diverse set of web applications. Some of the most known examples include social-networking sites, video-sharing sites, wikis, and blogs. This chapter reviews some of the major web 2.0-based tools and provides examples of their use in an educational setting. The goal of the chapter to expose readers to such tools, describe and exemplify their potential use in the classroom. We introduce Web 2.0 fundamental concepts, discuss its importance for educators, and suggest means for effective integration into the classroom. Readers in the field of education will find information and tools that can be applied in classrooms at the elementary school level to graduate- level classes. The chapter includes major challenges and key issues in the use of web 2.0 tools for learning, and serve as preview of the current trends in this environment.

INTRODUCTION

The Horizon Report: K-12 Edition (NMC, 2009) presents a thorough analysis of emerging technologies that are "likely to have a large impact on teaching, learning, research, or creative expression within education around the globe" (p.3), focusing on the pre-college sector. The report adopts three distinct horizons of adoption, namely one year, two to three years and five years. In all studied timeframes, the identified topics include prominently web 2.0 technologies. Moreover, the report also identifies key trends that affect K-12 education. These trends are profoundly influenced by web 2.0 technolo-

DOI: 10.4018/978-1-61520-899-9.ch013

gies, because they are directly related to the way we collaborate and communicate in all settings. Technology Skills have become essential to success. The web has become a personal experience, provided that emerging tools allow users to customize their virtual experiences. The ubiquitous availability of technology has thus placed high stakes in acquiring these skills through education. Through the use of technology for learning we are not only able to facilitate the learning process, but also provide learners with critical skills for any of the evolving occupations and multiple careers they might face throughout their lives. Thus, as in businesses, there is a pivotal need to embrace technology in schools, and "learning experiences must reflect the growing importance of innovation and creativity" (p.6).

The suitability of Web 2.0 technologies for learning has been widely discussed in the literature (Alexander, 2006). The Web 2.0 term refers to what is understood as a change to a second version or generation of the web, with a distinct model for application development and design. This new model is based on enhanced communication and collaboration tools and services, information sharing, and interoperability. This trend has enabled the creation and development web-based communities, web-hosted services, and a diverse set of web applications. Some of the most known examples include social-networking sites, video-sharing sites, wikis, and blogs.

This chapter reviews some of the major web 2.0-based tools and provides examples of their use in an educational setting. The goal of the chapter to expose readers to such tools, describe and exemplify their potential use in the classroom. In what follows, we introduce Web 2.0 fundamental concepts, discuss its importance for educators, and suggest means for effective integration into the classroom. Readers in the field of education will find information and tools that can be applied in classrooms at the elementary school level to graduate- level classes. The chapter also includes an overview of challenges and concerns from educators and parents, which have been a major cause for the frequently significant lack of support for a sustained adoption of such tools in the teaching and learning process. For the most part, concerns are related to student security, exposure to questionable materials, and access from individuals outside of the schools' control. This lack of support for Web 2.0 applications by traditional educational establishments promises to widen the gap between students' information technology literacy and the needs of a 21st century workforce.

Following this introduction, the chapter also provides a review of different educational areas for effective deployment of Web 2.0 tools:

- Digital storytelling and presentations
- Collaboration and Network Building
- Storing and Sharing Information
- Online Synchronous Communication tools

Under each area, the chapter provides a review of various tools and applications that can be utilized in by teachers and students for learning. Recommendations as to effective uses, challenges, critical issues and guidelines to find additional information are provided.

Finally, in the conclusions, major challenges and key issues in the use of web 2.0 tools for learning are discussed, and serve as preview of the current trends in this environment.

BACKGROUND: REVIEW OF THE LITERATURE

It is said that O'Reilly (2005) coined the term 'Web 2.0' when referring to practices and technologies emerging on the web after the fall 2001 dot.com shake up. The term in a sense is still debated and there seems little rigor in its usage. However, it is undeniable that there is an essential new way of capitalizing on the use of web-technologies. Web 2.0 is a generalizing term that centers on a major shift in the way the web is utilized. While the original Web 1.0 centered on a passive review of content and information by students, Web 2.0 allows and calls for active participation and interaction with materials. Web 2.0 is sometimes referred to as the "read/write web" since it centers on a non-passive approach calling for active sharing of information and creation of new materials and content.

The diffusion of the term has relied on a community-based 'intuitive recognition', since the term serves as a label for a trend and a set of new paradigms of web usage, which is increasingly recognized by its users. Users at growing numbers have found in such services a resonance with their personal expectations.

The principle of "the web as a platform" sheds light on the fact that the value-added moved from web-applications (such as browsers, which became mere commodities) to 'services' over the web platform. As stated by Roush (2005), the Internet has moved from "collection of static pages into a vehicle for software services". The database is where the power of the tools resides, but the tools allow the data to be managed and produce usable information: "the value of the software is proportional to the scale and dynamism of the data it helps to manage" (O'Reilly, 2005, p.3)

The inherent nature of the web based on hyperlinking generates a continuous organic growth of the "collective activity of all web users" (O'Reilly, 2005, p.4). Most of the organizations, including many start-up companies (e.g. eBay and Amazon) have capitalized on this principle, reaching out to all sorts of groups, including those smaller niches, reaching out to the entire web, not just the majorities at the center (i.e. 'The Long Tail'). The collective intelligence has been embraced also through innovative approaches, such as Wikipedia, del.ici.ous, Flickr, Technorati, etc. Although, there might be a resistance based on the fact that these initiatives are rooted primarily in new business models, they are definitely becoming part of everyday practice of all those with access to computers and mobile devices.

Web 2.0 tools provide the means to communicate, share, and present materials within the classroom and to the outside world. These tools are known to be effective for open-ended tasks (Cook & Harrison, 2008), and their ubiquitous availability encourages extended and enhanced learning. In a Web 2.0 world, there are continuous opportunities to share ideas, get feedback from others, expand on existing information, socialize, and collaborate. Thus, the use of these Web 2.0 applications reflects efforts to enhance the level of meaningfulness of information and content in the context of expanding students' insights (Plough, 2008).

Web 2.0 applications are open to all platforms. They hold and manipulate a variety of types of information. There are also a vast amount of similar tools, or applications that aggregate multiple functions. In the search for web 2.0 tools, it is common that one will encounter a significant volume of irrelevant information. Thus, in order to select an appropriate application, there is a critical need for assessment of relevancy and meaning from the part of the user. This is one more reason to be informed about Web 2.0 existing resources. Becoming aware of what is available is the first step to effective use of such resources.

Web 2.0 has promoted users to assume the role of collaborators in the presentation, manipulation and storage of information (Brown and Adler, 2008). For the most part, software developers and providers offer web 2.0 tools in basic versions free of charge (added features or storage space usually require extra fees.) This has made possible the inclusion of a significant number of users (individuals and institutions), who in the past may not have had the necessary financial precondition to utilize such tools. The possibilities of networking and developing content with different media through the support of Web 2.0 tools open a whole new world to teachers and students alike.

If schools are to meet the skills and knowledge needs of teachers and students for success in the twenty-first century, guided efforts must be made to utilize the tools that will become commonplace for the learning processes and tools that will dominate this new approach to learning. Change in both the teaching and learning process will become the norm rather than the exception in the future and the schools need to prepare students for this (Solomon and Schrum, 2007). The use of web 2.0 applications provides opportunities that allow students to be active participants in the learning process. This increases the value students place not only on content, but also on the manipulation and creation of new knowledge and artifacts (Conrad, 2008). When teenagers are quizzed about their expectations from the Internet, not only do they mention their desire for new information, but also seventy-five percent respond "to learn more or to learn better" (Oblinger, 2009; McNeely, 2009). A recent survey dealing with groups calling for the utilization of Web 2.0 applications in the schools, identified students as one of top three groups driving for Web 2.0 adoption. Those that feel comfortable with new technology appear to also see a place for such applications in the learning processes (IESD Research Report, 2008). The student centered learning process and the application of new skills and tools to widening and dynamic set of needs and wants demonstrate the power of Web 2.0. It is not an end in itself, but the means through which interaction channels an ever growing use of technologies to communicate, share and present information (Brown and Adler, 2008).

Teachers feel an obligation to provide students with the skills and knowledge they need for the future and these include skills in technology. Technology fluency and informational literacy are key educational elements that educators understand must be included as part of the educational process. Social software (aka Web 2.0) is viewed as critical to learning (Kirkland, 2007). Educators perceive the participatory aspects of Web 2.0 as crucial to academic success, since many students frequently consider school a source of boredom. Many educators express the belief that the use of Web 2.0 could meet curricular objectives, while at the same time boost motivation as a result of soaring levels of interactivity in an environment with which students feel at ease (Boyd and Ellison, 2007; Prensky, 2005).

Web 2.0 applications also reveal a good deal of positive aspects to school administrators. First on the list is an examination of the cost factor. The use of applications like blogs and wikis can hopefully elevate the quality of vital skills like writing - an area of major mandated assessment. The decision to adopt these tools in class can often be made without budgetary constraints (Huang and Behara, 2007). Research also provides insights on positive changes in student behaviors. Use of interactive web tools has demonstrated that students are more engaged and on task. The quality of student work remained constant or demonstrates improvement overall. Students also become actively involved in the learning process prompting administrators to note that potentially less time needs to be devoted to classroom management. As an example, according to Murphy and Lebans (2008), in the context of ESL students, many administrators are evidently satisfied with the positive impact that the adoption of Web 2.0 tool on literacy skills and students' attitudes to language use.

The literature reveals many counts of positives and negatives when it comes to Web 2.0 tools. Positives include the potential ability of Web 2.0 to diminish the effects of the digital divide. There is a clear possibility of improving processes that are no longer bound by continuous upgrading of expensive proprietary software or large investments in hardware. Due to the open-source nature of Web 2.0, problems and improvements can be made without as much monetary investment. Significantly higher levels of networking and communication can be achieved as a result of open architecture, cross-functionality, and integrated platforms for schools and classrooms that are less than state of the art. Another positive aspect, as previously discussed, is the change of old processes of education and learning with the use technology into student-centered approaches. The process of reviewing, selecting, and applying Web 2.0 tools allows students to become real creators and collaborators, who have greater ownership of their knowledge and have acquired power to deciding how it should be applied (Bruce & Levin, 1997). A more constructivist approach to learning will gain dominance based on the recognition of the significance of collaborative activities. More recently, Siemens (2004) has added an additional term to explain this approach, which to him is beyond the principles of constructivism. He coins it 'connectivism'. In a 'connectivist' approach, learning is based on the fact that "new information is continually being acquired." (p.4) Filtering and assessing the relevancy of information are key skills in such an environment. Making connections and recognizing the impact of such new information are also vital to learning in this dynamic model. Learners understand and value the ability to reconfigure, reconnect past information with new information, and changing decisions based on this new landscape.

The digital natives (Prensky, 2001) have experienced informal learning through media like YouTube and blogging tools and look for such interactive learning experiences in formal education situations. Student have expectations that interactive technologies will be applied as learning tools and further expect that other technological innovations as they arise can seamlessly also be introduced to learning situations. The potential of using such innovations serves as a positive factor is promoting student engagement in the learning process and in supporting the creation of learning communities of teachers and students. Access to technology, however, does not guarantee the existence of a learning community. A learning community develops when the participants recognize their shared goals and responsibilities and commit to working toward realization of those goals. A true learning community is one in which active interaction involving content and personal communication between students and the instructor takes place (Pallof and Pratt, 1999). The role of the educator in this environment is to provide support and model the use of such technology to aid in the creation of an effective learning community (Pallof and Pratt, 2003).

Thus, it is critical that users of such Web 2.0 tools learn how to effectively employ them in student-centered learning activities. This will depend greatly on effective instructional design techniques and on appropriate and continuous teacher training.

On the other side of the spectrum, there are also a number of groups that perceive Web 2.0 with a potential for a more negative than positive impact. These groups include parents, educators, and institutional traditionalists who fear there are threats coming from the use Web 2.0 as a major tool for teaching and learning. Educators and parents express major concerns when it comes to students' extensive use of the Internet as a learning tool. A lack of understanding of the possible effective uses of the Internet and Web 2.0 tools in many cases gives rise to an over-reaction to the threats of cyber-bullying, exposure to pornography, questionable media sites, and sharing of too much personal data and information on social networking sites. While such threats do exist, pitfalls can be avoided by educating individuals about Internet safety and proper use. In the long run, understanding the potential threats is more important than over-reacting and finally limiting or even banning the use of these types of technologies. For institutional traditionalists the core issue becomes providing adequate security opposed to individual choice. In many cases the decision comes down on the side of security (Palfrey and Gasser, 2008). Such decisions impose the use of filters on Internet access, controlling what students can see and utilize, at the expense of encouraging self-learning activities that provide the skills students will need for the future (O'Neal, 2007). Some educators also become uncomfortable with the new roles for students and teachers in a constructivist approach, where teachers step aside from the position of owners and distributors of knowledge. The question arises if students in fact can assume the role of active learners and will educators be able to accept the role of coaching rather than relying on primarily direct instruction in the classroom (Bates, 2009). Substantial future administrative decisions will center on the effective application of Web 2.0 tools in the schools weighted against roadblocks resulting from overreacting fears, which will diminish the potential of such tools to bring valuable change to current rigid educational structures.

In summary, in the K-12 realm, two important aspects are shaping the adoption of emerging technologies, namely 'filtering' (reducing access to selected information determined as inappropriate) and 'assessment' (determining if students have achieved specific learning goals) (NMC, 2009). These particular aspects have worked as barriers to the adoption of some of the technologies already under way in the higher-education environment. In the K-12, collaborative environments and online communication tools have had their adoption somewhat delayed due to restrictive policies concerning Internet access in schools. However, it has been observed that there is an "erosion of some of these barriers as mobile devices become more capable and as the value of these tools for collaborative work becomes more evident" (p. 4). The same is true because of difficulties in assessing students' learning in a standardized way.

Assessment "continues to present a challenge to educators at all levels, particularly in the context of new media and collaborative work" (NMC, 2009, p.4) Evaluating students while using these new tools is still difficult and there aren't yet any best practices that can be readily adopted. Beyond assessment, schools also need to be able to translate them into metrics, which can further be standardized. Thus, assessment is still a hot spot when discussing the adoption of all innovative technologies.

AN OVERVIEW OF USEFUL WEB 2.0 TOOLS FOR THE CLASSROOM

Since there is such a wealth of tools and materials available in the context of Web 2.0, we present an overview of some web 2.0 tools organized in basic educational areas, namely:

1. Digital storytelling and presentations
2. Collaboration and Network Building
3. Storing and sharing Information
4. Online Synchronous Communication tools

This is not a comprehensive or exhaustive overview since new tools are added daily. Also the specific tools discussed in the context of one area can easily fall into more than one of the four areas. This overlap is in fact a characteristic of web 2.0 apps, a trend that is reinforced with the use of 'mash-ups' (the term 'mash-up', in a web development context, represents simple and quick integration of other web-based applications and data sources, generating a new functionality for the user). An example of this overlap is blogging, which could easily be placed into collaboration, network building, or collecting information. The power of Web 2.0 is that the individual chooses how to use a particular tool. The specific tools and applications have been selected based on present use in classrooms and the low learning curve for their adoption and implementation in formal learning situations.

Digital Storytelling and Presentation

According to Helen Barrett (2006), "a digital story is a personal narrative that may show the author's identity: strengths, weaknesses, achievements, disappointments, learning experiences, passions, and hopes for the future; in other words: reflection". Barrett also refers to commentary by Catherine Howell, where she "emphasizes the writing (and media-savvy) skills that are acquired/investigated as part of the process of creating digital stories".

The value of storytelling is that it has the potential to encourage students to explore different styles, and what are the most effective ways that we can model good practice for them, as they learn the skills they need in order to communicate compelling personal narratives".

The tools discussed below are helpful in generating such digital stories and creating generic visual presentations, individually or collaboratively. They also allow for seamless sharing of these artifacts seamlessly on the web.

Animoto (http://animoto.com/): Animoto is a web application that produces videos using images and music selected by the user resulting in a professional quality video. Users choose which images and a music background they prefer, and then customize it into a unique video in a widescreen format. The resulting video has the potential for a high emotional impact, through the combination of effective visuals and music. Such presentations are excellent in getting attention while introducing new topics. Animoto is technology that mimics the role of the movie director and editor by combining music and video functions and relates to the digital camera revolution by giving the story creator the ability to capture an entire experience, not just individual moments. The videos are maintained onsite with 30-second videos made and stored for free. Animoto charges for the production and storage of longer videos. One possible example of the use of Animoto in an educational setting is a project that involved matching pictures from American history to the lyrics of Billy Joel's "We Didn't Start the Fire." (http://www.emsc.nysed.gov/nysatl/SocStudies/fire/html/proce.html). This student project explored the events mentioned in the songs, adding related visuals, exploring students' understanding and engagement with American history.

Animoto provides the necessary functions that allow students to explore topics through the use of multimedia in an easy way. They can practice skills of presenting critical information in limited time. Thus, it requires students to utilize critical thinking skills into the process of effectively selecting meaningful images to be placed in a coherent sequence in order to convey a clear message.

Podcasting: Podcasting is the process of creating podcasts. A podcast is a series of audio or video files (in many cases a series of video files are called similarly vodcasts) accessible online for download or via web syndication. Web syndication is syndication done over the web, where web content is made available through several sites. The common form, and the one we refer to here, is the one called 'feeds' from a specific website. By signing-up to receive such feeds (new information made available on these sites), the user is relieved from the need to visit the sites to gather updated information. Common forms of web syndication are RSS and Atoms. Differently than just audio files sitting on a website for download, syndication gives podcasting a distinct functionality. The series of media files (podcast), generated by the content provider usually with a certain frequency in time, are automatically identified and retrieved as they become available by special software, called 'podcatchers'. Podcatchers are also responsible for delivering these files to users, who have signed up for such feeds. These files, associated to a particular podcast, are then automatically downloaded to the users' machines. Thus, in simple terms podcasts are audio files that are delivered via RSS.

Podcasting has become popular among educators since it gives learners the opportunity to listen to presentations by experts and also to create audio broadcasts demonstrating their knowledge of topics being covered in their class. Podcast use includes:

- Sharing audio information with anyone at any time. An absent student can download the podcast of the recorded lesson.
- Communicating curriculum, assignments and other information to parents and the community in an audio format.
- Recording book discussions, vocabulary or foreign language lessons, music performances, interviews, and debates.

- Serving as a publishing tool for students' oral presentations.

An example of the use of podcasts in education is the incorporation of podcasts from National Public Radio (http://www.npr.org/podcasts). NPR has a wealth of podcast programs available. NPR partners with many of the NPR stations and other public radio organizations nation-wide to provide quality podcasting service to the public. In an on-line course in technology and education, the use of podcasts was able to provide to students the recorded interview with Thomas Friedman concerning his text "*The World is Flat*." This podcast communicates ideas as to the impact of technology in both a cultural and global contexts. Students have an opportunity to listen to the author rather than reading summaries of the text. Podcasts also can serve as an introduction to on-line courses, providing an opportunity for students to listen to instructions rather than read them. This format also allows for a more personal touch than a written introduction.

For educational purposes, there are two main uses of podcasts: the production of podcasts by teachers and/or students, and the use of existing podcasts from a variety of content providers as additional instructional resources. When discussing the production of podcasts, there are two main processes involved. One is the generation of the audio file, which includes recording and editing. And second, there is the distribution of the produced audio files through web syndication (as mentioned above).

We discuss a few tools that can be helpful in the production of podcasts, as well as a few podcasting providers, whose content can be useful to educators. A recording program such as Audacity (http://audacity.sourceforge.net/), which is freeware (open source), can be used to record and edit sounds. It is available for multiple computer platforms.

For storage and broadcast of podcasts, there are also several available free software versions on the web. These software applications do a few things: convert the recording to appropriate format for podcasting (if necessary, depending on the kind of original recording), create the necessary RSS feed and upload the podcast to the specific website. RSS is in fact a file with an extension.rss, which contains XML code, and one can actually write such file from scratch (http://radio.about.com/od/podcastin1/a/aa030805a_3.htm). However, this can be somewhat complicated. There are other easier options, which do not require the user to generate any code. These include applications such as MyRSSCreator.com (http://www.myrsscreator.com/) or LibSyn (http://www.libsyn.com/). Another option is to use RSS file generators, such as Podcast RSS feed generator (http://www.tdscripts.com/webmaster_utilities/podcast-generator.php), ListGarden RSS Feed (http://www.softwaregarden.com/products/listgarden/index.html), and Generator Program and Simple RSS File Generator (http://www.nightskyobserver.com/RSSGen/).

When it comes to using existing podcasts in education, the web has a wealth of possibilities. As an example, consider Open Culture (http://www.openculture.org). It offers cultural and educational media, including a long list of podcasts and videos. These are all available for free. Open Culture is also a blog, thus it serves multiple functions for education and information. Open Culture, different that simple engines for search of content, sifts through what is available and shares it with the public for cultural and educational purposes. Podcasts can also be searched through Google (http://www.google.com or Yahoo (http://www.yahoo.com). iTunes also contains an outstanding number of podcasts, many of them through channels of content generated by universities (iTunes U) and other educational institutions, such as Stanford on iTunes (http://itunes.stanford.edu/), UC Berkeley on iTunes (http://itunes.berkeley.edu/) or Penn State on iTunes (https://itunes.psu.edu/).

One interesting initiative is this arena is The Education Podcast Network (http://epnweb.org/). It is, as Open Culture, a site that aggregates a wide range of podcasts, in this case aimed at supporting teachers. Most of the podcasts are produced by educators, who are willing to share "their knowledge, insights, and passions for teaching and learning and for the stories that they relish and teach" (paragraph 1).

Podcasts can include videos when the correct software is applied. These podcasts, sometimes referred to as vidcast or vodcast, are attached to blogs and other postings and advertised to others through RSS. From a web server, a video podcast can be distributed as a file or as a stream. Both methods have their advantages and disadvantages. Downloading complete video podcasts in advance gives the user the ability to play the video podcasts offline on, for example, a portable media player. A downloaded version can be watched many times with only one download, reducing bandwidth costs in this case. Streaming allows seeking (skipping portions of the file) without downloading the full video podcast, better calling for lower bandwidth costs for the servers.

Most students have different learning styles and podcasting provides teachers with a way of expanding the way in which information can be presented. The opportunity is provided to listen, go back over particular passages, as many times as necessary and to hear information via a different source is a useful addition to the approaches to support students. In terms of the most effective learning time for students, the podcast allows you to be able to capture this information, enabling students to listen when they are in a more receptive learning state. This use of podcasts also provides more of an opportunity for students to reflect a major element in effective learning (Ashwin, 2006).

Collaboration and Network Building

Collaboration, more than ever before, is a focal point in education. This is a consequence of the same trend in the workplace, where due to globalization, "professionals are expected to work across geographic and cultural boundaries more and more frequently" (NMC, 2009, p.5) There is recognition that online tools supporting collaboration have the potential to maximize "opportunities to work creatively, develop teamwork skills, and tap into the perspectives of people around the world" (p.5), increasing diversity and expanding knowledge. Moreover, "the 'spaces' where students learn are becoming more community-driven, interdisciplinary, and supported by technologies that engage virtual communication and collaboration" (NMC, 2009, p.6).

Web 2.0 tools offer many tools that support collaboration and networking. These two activities are probably the main drivers of the web 2.0 trend, which more frequently than not is called interchangeably as 'social software', given its potential of boosting socialization in the cyberworld. In this section we focus on blogs, wikis and document sharing (Google docs and Microsoft Office Live Workplace) as collaboration applications; and we discuss a few existing applications under the umbrella of social networking as well.

Blogs: A blog is a shortened version of the term weblog and represents a specific type of website, in which its core part is a linear sequence of posts (entries), presented in the reverse chronological order in which they were created. Blogs are easily created and updated, and are written about any subject. In many cases, blogs contain reflections, ideas, conversations, and links to other web resources. Blogs also provide opportunities for posting multimedia. Since readers can comment on individual blog entries, blogs also serve the purpose of generating online conversations between the 'blogger' and the readers. Blogs can frequently be searched, and have functions that allow older posts to be archived and accessed through specific links referring to the period of time in which they were created. Posts can be 'tagged', which allow searches based on keywords, as well as the aggregation of posts under specific keywords. According to Wikipedia (http://en.wikipedia.org/wiki/Tag_(metadata) "A tag is a non-hierarchical keyword or term assigned to a piece of information (such as an internet bookmark, digital image, or computer file). This kind of metadata helps describe an item and allows it to be found again by browsing or searching." Tagging has gained enormous importance with the advent of Web 2.0 applications and services. A few positive aspects of blogs are:

- Takes very little time or technical knowledge to set up;
- Allows students an opportunity to interact with information with posting of individual comments;
- Keeps teachers informed with the latest developments in their field;
- Creates collaborative learning space for teachers and students, allowing for discoveries, sharing ideas and discussing important topics; and
- Provides excellent means of collaboration with minimum or no cost.

A list of uses of blog in the classroom certainly includes:

- Gathering and organizing Internet resources for a specific course;
- Providing links to appropriate sites and annotating the links as to what is relevant about them;
- Creating a dynamic teaching site;
- Posting not only class-related information, but also activities, discussion topics, links to additional information about topics studied in class
- Have students create blogs as learning journals; and
- Share current events related to the discipline.

Some concerns about the use of blogs in the classroom are again related to the possibility of access to inappropriate or indecent content. As mentioned before, this is a current theme when discussing the use of the Internet and web resources. Teachers should discuss with their students the school's Acceptable Use Policy, as well as issues of cyber-ethics and self-management. Teachers can also locate some useful blogs to be used by students. Users must also be made aware that not all information on the Internet is reliable or even true and this certainly includes blogs, which are the most popular way people have found to express their opinions about current issues. Teaching student's skills in critical literacy will help them distinguish the opinionated and frequently misleading materials from good and helpful resources.

Thus, as in podcasts, blogs can be developed as part of the instructional activities in the classroom, or the access to existing blogs can serve as extra resources for learning. In order to create a blog, there are many blogging tools (blog hosting sites) available for free on the web. Below are a few common ones.

- **Edublogs** (http://www.edublogs.org): Edublogs is a blog hosting service, which hosts hundreds of thousands of educational blogs developed by "teachers, students, researchers, professors, librarians, administrators and anyone and everyone else involved in education". In its basic version, "Edublogs are completely free, and come with 20MB of free upload space". For a fee, there are supporter version with up to 5 GB and some extra features. There is also the possibility of supporting institutional blogging services, called Edublogs Campus (http://edublogs.org/campus/). In this case, the institution has its own domain of blogs after installing the necessary software in their own servers. This will give full control of creation and management of all blogs under this institutional domain.
- **Class Blogmeister** (http://www.classblogmeister.com/): this blogging engine has been developed specifically for classroom

use. One can create an account and start using their blog immediately for free, or browse through thousands of blogs created by teachers in the K-12 setting. One will need a school pass code to create an account.

- **Blogger** (https://www.blogger.com/start): Blogger was one of the first companies to offer blogging service for free. In 2002 it was bought by Google. It is very easy to set-up and offers many good features in an easy to use form.
- **Live Journal** (http://www.livejournal.com): Live Journal is both a blogging engine and a social networking site. It has offered free blogging services since 1999, so it is one of the oldest providers of such kind of tool on the web. LiveJournal offers a user-friendly interface, which allows users to develop a highly customizable journal. With an account in LiveJournal, one is automatically a part of a social networking environment with other users, who also have accounts through the site. The union of these two functions is becoming commonplace in the web 2.0 world.

As mentioned earlier, blogs can also serve as a resource of teaching materials. The 'blogsphere' is swarming with blogs covering a whole variety of topics. In order to make it easier on blog readers, there are also a variety of sites specialized in searching and aggregating blog posts. Services like Technorati (http://www.technorati.com) and Bloglines (http://www.bloglines.com). These aggregators allow users to search, subscribe, create and share news feeds, blogs and rich web content.

There are many blogs with useful information to teachers, including on the use of technology in the classroom, such as:

- 2 cents Worth (http://davidwarlick.com/2cents/)
- The Tech Savvy Educator (http://www.techsavvyed.net/)
- Edutopia blogs (http://www.edutopia.org/spiralnotebook)
- EdTech Solutions: Teaching every student (http://teachingeverystudent.blogspot.com/) - by Karen Janowski, who is an Assistive & Educational Technology Consultant
- Ed Tech Review (http://www.edtechreview.net/)

A long list of educational bloggers can be found here: http://supportblogging.com/Links+to+School+Bloggers

It is also rather easy to find blogs that are used by teachers to support classroom activities:

- Learning about Greece using a blog (http://my-ecoach.com/blogs.php?blog=1451) - a teacher share with her students her travel journal through Greece and other European sites.
- Mr. C's Class Blog (http://mrcsclassblog.blogspot.com/) - a blog kept by a 5th grade teacher, reporting on students' activities, suggesting books, and other information.
- An AP Calculus class blog 2006-2007 (http://apcalc06.blogspot.com/) - A blog used between the years 2006-2007 for an AP calculus class, with information for students and parents.
- Mrs. Cassidy's blog (http://classblogmeister.com/blog.php?blogger_id=1337) - a blog done by a Canadian 1st grade teacher. She reports on students' activities and invites the world to see.

Wikis: A wiki is a website enabled by a special software (wiki software), which provides a friendly and easy to use interface, allowing users to create and edit quickly any number of interlinked web pages. Frequently, wikis are used in a collaborative way, where several authors contribute in the editing of the pages that compose the wiki. Wikis serve very well as knowledge bases for projects or studies, where a group of collaborators work as a team. Wikis allow also readers, who will not have the ability to edit the wiki, but can read all its content. Changes made to a wiki are recorded and can be easily undone, if the administrator of the wiki so decides. One of the most famous wikis on the web is Wikipedia, which exists in many languages. It is an example of an active wiki that allows anyone with a Wikipedia account to create and improve its content. The Wikipedia contains catalogued pages that are cross-reference, covering an unimaginable number of topics in all fields of study and interest.

Teachers can use wikis to communicate and collaborate with students. Classes can have a wiki with detailed information resources on many academic topics. Since wikis are in fact a structured collection of interlinked web pages, wikis can include text, pictures, links to other resources and multimedia. In a collaborative manner, students share knowledge and learning with each other. The classroom is expanded giving students both access to a global web of information and a worldwide audience. The power of the wiki lies in students having ownership for their work, since they have sought the knowledge to create it. The format also allows excellent opportunities for higher level thinking skills through collaboration with others.

The http://www.education-world.com/a_tech/sites/sites079.shtml site offers other suggestions for use of wikis in the classroom include:

- "Provide a space for free writing"
- "Debate course topics, including assigned readings"
- "Share resources such as annotated bibliographies, websites, effective writing samples, conferences, calls for manuscripts"
- "Require students to collaborate on documents, such as an essay written by the entire class"
- "Discuss curricular and instructional innovations"
- "Encourage students to revise Wikipedia pages or take on new wikipedia assignments"
- "Inspire students to write a Wikibook"

There are many Wiki providers that can be used by teachers in creating their own classroom wikis, such as: Wetpaint (http://www.wetpaint.com), PbWiki (http://www.pbwiki.com) or Wikispaces (http://www.wikispaces.com). These and many others offer ad free limited storage space for free for educational purposes.

The groups involved in the development of a wiki vary from small groups, such as a group working in a class project, and a worldwide community like Wikipedia, including wikis that include a large set of high-schools like the ones that signed up in http://schools.wikia.com/wiki/High_School_Online_Collaborative_Writing focused on collaborative writing. Smart Teaching.org (http://www.smartteaching.org/blog/2008/08/50-ways-to-use-wikis-for-a-more-collaborative-and-interactive-classroom/) lists several other uses of wikis, including development of study guides, creating a glossary or class encyclopedia, vocabulary lists, collection of information, creating classroom scrapbook or a newspaper. There are also wikis discussing ways of using wikis in the classroom, with a variety of options for teachers, such as Wikis in Education wiki (http://wikisin-education.wetpaint.com/) or EduWikis (http://educationalwikis.wikispaces.com/).

One interesting example in the use of wikis is the set of activities involved in the pedagogical approach labeled as "Just in Time Learning." The instructor posts question and assignments in the wiki. Students then share information and collaborate on the answers. This is done before covering class materials in greater depth. The objective of the exercise is for instructors to capture the levels of understanding displayed by student responses. (Higdon & Topaz, 2009).

Existing wikis on the web are also, like blogs, a wealth of information that can be used in the classroom. Besides Wikipedia, there are many other wikis worth considering as further class material. Some examples to be considered include: Wikibooks (http://en.wikibooks.org/wiki/Main_Page) - a community of free educational textbooks that anyone can edit; Wikijunior (http://en.wikibooks.org/wiki/Wikijunior) is a subset of the previous project, with books for children of different age groups; or K-12 OpenSource wiki (http://wiki.k12opensource.com/) which is a project that collects and shares the wealth of open source resources available on the web today for a K-12 audience.

Other schools have been active at creating useful wikis as well. One example is the Westwood School wiki (http://westwood.wikispaces.com/), containing links to both public and private resources for students.

As in other web 2.0 tools, user-developed content is exposed on the net, which might create opportunities for sabotage and/or vandalism, despite the usual password protections and available functionalities for setting specific rights to different users. However, in the case of wikis, one extra characteristic is advantageous in such situations. A history of all changes is recorded, and previous versions can be easily restored. This is what frequently happens in Wikipedia, when watchful users quickly restore content when any such outside damage occurs. A second concern deals with misinformation and untruths being published as fact in wikis. The very strength of a wiki is that this information can quickly be corrected. Such misinformation usually is corrected by those that recognize the value of the wiki and make efforts to support its continued use and growth as a learning tool. A wiki can be set up to allow only authorized users to have editing rights. Wikis can also be created that only selected people can edit, providing protection for student work. A caution to keep in mind concerning wikis is that since the materials are public, last names and details on students should not be published.

In summary, an effective use of Wikis includes (Duffy & Bruns, 2006):

- The Wiki can be effective in allowing participants separated by time and space an opportunity to work in collaborative manner;
- Has the potential to provide opportunities for students from different content areas to work in collaborative manner on common themes of an interdisciplinary unit.
- The flexibility of the Wiki can deal with scheduling problems for the students allowing for ongoing collaboration when it is difficult for all participants working on the unit to meet at particular place at a particular time.
- Informational Wikis can be utilized to provide background information for student review of materials.

Goggle Docs application: Google Docs is a free, Web-based application that functions as word processor and generator of Office compatible spreadsheets, presentations, and forms offered by Google. It allows users to create and edit documents online while collaborating in real-time with other users. Teachers can upload existing files since Google Docs accepts most popular file formats.

The following aspects of the Google Docs make it a very effective tool for collaborative work, developing class documents:

- By clicking common editing toolbar buttons (similar to the ones used in other PC-based applications), the user can make changes and additions after a document has been uploaded.
- Documents can be edited and presented to others in real time and multiple people can view and make changes in real-time.
- There is an on-screen chat window for spreadsheets, and document revisions show exactly who changed what, and

when. Viewing a presentation together is very effective since anyone who joined in a presentation can automatically follow along with the presenter.

- The user has the power to choose who can access documents by entering the email addresses of the people with whom the document can be shared and sending them an invitation. Documents, spreadsheets, and presentations can be created within the application itself, imported through the web interface, or sent via email. They can also be saved to the user's computer in a variety of formats. Open documents are automatically saved to prevent data loss, and a revision history is automatically kept, documents can be tagged and archived for organizational purposes.
- Google Docs helps promote group work and peer editing skills and that it helps to fulfill the stated goals for effective writing by approaching writing as a process and encouraging multiple revisions and peer editing.
- Teachers are using Google Docs both to publish announcements about upcoming assignments and to monitor student progress interactively, which allows the teacher to give guidance when it might be of maximum benefit, while the student is still working on an assignment. Through the revisions history, the teacher can see clearly who contributed to what assignment and when.

An example of the application of Google Docs in the classroom occurred in one of the author's teaching methods class. A group of students from differing curriculum areas created interdisciplinary units through the use of Google Docs. Students were assigned specific themes for the unit and asked to work in a collaborative manner through Google Docs to combine their independent work into an organized module that crossed curricular lines. Discussions and collaboration took place using the Google Docs tool, since the students met a differing time for face-to-face class work. Once students became familiar with the process they were able to work in a cooperative manner towards the completion of their assigned task.

Another example is offered through Tech& Learning Blog (http://www.techlearning.com/article/8214), where a Californian high-school teacher has her students in her "Journalism class keep their entire writing portfolio on Google Docs. That way she is able to check and verify which assignments have been turned in on a daily basis. Everything is centrally located. Students are able to manage the entire writing process: share ideas, create revisions, and publish their final work. The teacher can track development of each writing assignment."

Google provides a wealth of information on how to use Google docs in education, including real-life examples in their own site at http://www.google.com/educators/p_docs.html. Another informational site for data on Google Docs can be found at http://communication.howstuffworks.com/google-docs.htm/

Social Networking: "A social networking site is generally focused on building online communities of people who share interests and/or activities, or who are interested in exploring the interests and activities of others." (Jones, 2009) Most social networks on the web offer a variety of tools for users to interact. Sites such as MySpace (http://www.myspace.com) and Facebook (http://www.facebook.com), with minor adaptations or guidance, can become tools for learning not just socialization. Schools could endorse a format of social networking similar to MySpace or Facebook, and all students in a school could then have an account in such a site that was controlled by the school. Teachers would be able to communicate through blogs, message boards, video, and audio to students who are members of such a school-supported site. Recent research supports the use of such social networks in classes and expresses beliefs that this could be a future approach to instruction or extended instruction time beyond the school. The research demonstrates that networking sites have functionality, such as the ability for users to link and group themselves, which is not available in other common web-facilitated learning environments such as course management systems. In this research project each student was assigned the role of a unique mineral and rock. They were required to create a separate web page for each, with a photograph and description, on MySpace.com. After reviewing materials students were required to join groups based on the classification of the rock or mineral. Finally, they were required to link to the minerals that constitute each rock by becoming "friends". A post-exercise questionnaire showed that all students found this a useful and enjoyable exercise, and most believed it helped them to learn and remember information (Kennelly, 2009).

Thus, social networking has great potential for enhancing teaching and learning as evidenced by the comments listed here:

- Teachers would be able to share and collaborate on lesson plans and curriculum
- Teachers would be able to enlist aid and support for projects that could be collaborated upon by other classes in and out of the same building
- Students could be exposed to contact with other students working on similar projects
- Students could exchange information and insights with other students from all over the world
- Students and teachers would be kept informed as to possible collaborative projects

Despite the potential, there are many critical concerns, as mentioned earlier, including:

- The issue of how much control the school district should have over social networking begs the question as to free exchange of ideas and what is and what is not deemed as acceptable.
- The issues that arise are acceptable use policies, free speech in the face of school security and public image of schools
- Over-exposure of personal student information
- Possible needs for filtering systems to protect the schools and teacher's sites as well as student information. These are issues that must be discussed, but teachers do need to consider the potential of such innovation weighted against the problems that could arise.

There are many social networking tools available today that allow the creation of online communities. A few of those, which could possibly catapult the educational potential, while addressing the concerns above are presented below.

Curriki (http://www.curriki.org/xwiki/bin/view/Main/): This tool eliminates the fears of the social network being too open and a possible threat to school security. Curriki is a socially entrepreneurial organization that supports the development and free distribution of open source educational materials to improve education worldwide. The online community gives teachers, students and parents universal access to peer-reviewed K–12 curricula, and powerful online collaboration tools. Curriki is building a community that will share lesson plans, curriculum, and projects. It also supports collaboration on a number of different projects.

E-pals (http://www.epals.com/): This organization provides ongoing networking to keep teachers and students informed as to collaborative projects that they can take part in with students from all over the world. Photos and videos can also be exchanged and shared with network members. The school and teachers can build communities, using school-safe email and blog tools. Teachers can set different levels of monitoring, even for individual students, make pages public, or limit blog views to particular audiences, including workgroups within a class.

Ning(http://www.ning.com): Ning is an online platform for users to create their own social websites and social networks. The unique feature of Ning is that users can create their own custom social network for a particular topic or need, catering to specific audiences. What is good about the Ning setup is that it is highly connected to other social networking sites like MySpace and Facebook, making student connections easy to carry out. This allows students to move in and out of their common use of social networks to another social network used for educational purposes and supposedly controlled by the teacher. To help educators benefit from Ning's unique social networking environment, Ning in Education has offered to remove the ads from educational networks which are geared toward students between the ages of 13 and 18. The network is easy to set up and allows message posts, images, and staying in contact with students in an environment in which they feel comfortable. Ning is one example of a growing number of sites that allow one to create a social network for a specific audience around practically any interest, group, or activity. Ning has great potential value as an educational tool, especially for professional development and building professional connections (Rosenfeld, 2008).

In summary, some of the advantages of using a Ning for both teachers and students include:

- The control of membership and topic of Ning site is more closely controlled by the school
- Promoting student reflection using collaborative tools to reveal and clarify students' conceptual understanding
- Engaging students in exploring real-world issues and solving authentic problems using digital tools and resources
- Creating class environments for interaction and media sharing
- Opening up opportunities for students to write for larger authentic audiences and creating class environments for interaction and media sharing
- Promoting creative and innovative thinking and inventiveness, while personalizing learning activities to address students' diverse learning styles

Some concerns related to the use of social networks such as Ning, center on the functions available in these sites and the powers that are given to the students and others. Thus there are some aspects that need to be carefully considered, such as:

- A decision needs to be made as to how the blog of the social network will be used within the social network.
- The teacher needs to provide some level of privacy for students, by defining privacy settings.
- A decision needs to be made concerning the contact with the rest of the world. Will the public outside of the school group see the created social network? Will it be open for others to join?
- Enabling other applications as part of the social network is also a concern to be considered. What will the teacher let your students contribute and change? Will they be able to change the themes and colors of their My Page? If too many options are allowed, students may be more distracted by personalizing their site rather than responding effectively to assignments, and such pedagogical effects need to be addressed.

There are many existing online communities concerned with these and other issues. Two of these are listed below as a source of information of these and other related issues.

Classroom 2.0 (http://classroom20.ning.com/): This Ning is for educators using Web 2.0 technologies, recently won a 2007 Edublog Award for best educational use of a social networking service, providing constantly updated information related Web 2.0 in the classroom.

Ning in Education (http://education.ning.com/): This is a Ning that which groups educators online using Ning, offering excellent resources and materials for effective use of Ning in the classroom

Another good source of information related to Ning can be found here http://wardsworld.pbworks.com/Nings

Finally, another worthwhile use of the Ning is that it can be very helpful in keeping contact with students after graduation. Since graduates, frequently lose access to the institution's Web site after graduation, the Ning provides a means of staying in touch with the school's network. The school can keep students informed about employment opportunities and share insights with others who are Ning members.

ONLINE SYNCHRONOUS COMMUNICATION TOOLS

Many of the web 2.0 applications mentioned earlier, especially social networking ones, offer means for users to communication online, including via synchronous interaction. In most cases, chat environments are available. The New Horizon Report 2009: K-12 Edition (2009) gives a special highlight to online communication tools within K-12 environments. The workforce has become mobile, and companies are not working in a global environment. Communication is at a premium. With the advent of VoIP (Voice over IP), which has enabled the development of cheap and easy to use communication over the Internet has created the possibility of an entire new set of tools that are becoming rapidly as commonplace as the regular phone. VoIP is a common term when we refer to voice over the Internet. Other terms frequently encountered and synonymous with VoIP are IP telephony, Internet telephony, Voice over broadband (VoBB), broadband telephony, and broadband phone (http://en.wikipedia.org/wiki/VoIP). These tools, like others such as instant messaging and 'microblogging' platforms, "facilitate connections and the dissemination of information between and among students and teachers, keeping classroom communities in touch with each other on a more extensive basis than ever before" (http://wp.nmc.org/horizon-k12-2009/chapters/online-communication-tools/#0).

We discuss a few online synchronous tools below, which have been massively adopted and are becoming mainstream in terms of synchronous communication over the Internet:

Skype (http://www.skype-freedownload.com/index.htm): Skype is a voice over Internet protocol (VoIP) application that lets users conduct free phone calls between Skype-equipped computers and inexpensive calls between Skype computers and landline or cell phones. Skype functions on a P2P model rather than as a centralized application, and it offers features such as voicemail, call forwarding, conference calling, and video chat. In most circumstances, Skype provides access to voice and video communication for a fraction of what other options cost. It allows more frequent contact between colleagues, collaborators, and friends and permits connections with those not likely to be in touch through conventional phone systems (Educause Learning Initiative, Dec. 2007).

The value of Skype is found in its ability to:

- Add a new dimension to meeting new people. The meetings could also take place in a chat room, but Skype adds a new dimension by allowing real-time audio conversations at little or no cost. For example, a teacher has a class question about education in Australia and the teachable time for answering that question is now. The teacher could make an arranged phone call to a colleague in Australia, call up online for the whole class to hear, and perhaps even utilize video for the teachable moment.

- Serve as an excellent tool for use in foreign language classes. Dr. Richard Robin, a language teacher at George Washington University sees the use of Skype as a real breakthrough for effective teaching of foreign languages. Dr. Robin expresses his view based on three years of using Skype in this observation:

"In a classroom setting, a lot of the Russian that students hear will be from teacher-talk or student-to-student conversation, which is basically fake." said Robin, who began using Skype as a classroom tool almost two years ago. "This enables (students) to make their Russian communications and conversational skills better [through exchanges with other Russian students]. Right now Skype is a very hot commodity, almost exotic, so a lot of (professors) don't use it. Twenty years from now when I retire, it won't be so exotic, so I'm sure it will be in use like this in many more classrooms" (Prerna, 2007, p.6).

The potential use for Skype as a format for online courses and lectures at a lower cost than most other presentation formats presents possibilities for the future. It is also suggested that Skype can bring about a higher level of engagement for class assignments, since a Skypecast not only presents insights and discussions in your class, but from others throughout the world, which might have something else to say about the topic and can also enter the discussion and add insights (Foote, 2008).

Storing and Sharing Information

One major concern when dealing with large amounts of information and media is storage space. There are also considerations with security as well. Audio and media files can take up a great amount of space on personal computers and Web 2.0 may provide a solution to this problem. The use of sites that will provide, store and share - pictures, photos, videos, and other materials in an organized manner is an extraordinary aid in helping students carry out research and construct presentations. Some of the applications place major emphasis on aspects of providing effective storage; some provide areas where the collection of materials is the most important function. In most cases the applications are capable to carry out both functions, but for the sake of the information presented here, the applications and tools are listed under a specific area, in most cases for which the applications are best noted.

Collecting and Sharing Tools

Some tools that can be utilized to aid in the collection and sharing of information are presented here for review

SlideShare (http://www.slideshare.net/): This free online application lets users upload PowerPoint or Open Office presentation files and share them online. Power Point documents, or any office document, stored on the web with a permanent URL are a valuable resource. No need to email the file to recipients, or carry a copy around on a USB drive. The presentation can easily be shared and, with permission controls, kept relatively secure. The potential uses of online Power Point documents are numerous and allow for making lectures and presentations much easier. The process also provides a permanent record of these and other presentations available on the Internet for easy access and reference. This provides an excellent resource for students seeking to locate specific visual information for projects and also provides a place for organization of the materials to take place.

When students or teachers are searching for photos and videos, they can locate them on sites by topics and in most cases the photos can be copied and used for class projects. SlideShare is a great place to share presentations as well as documents with others and to find some of the best presentations on the web on topics of interest. The uses of applications like SlideShare are recognized as examples of best practices for social software and need to be supported as effective educational tools. The presentation of available materials under specific topic saves time and effort in searching the web (Stephens, 2007).

Flickr (http://www.flickr.net/): This application is an image and video hosting website that provides other web services, including that of an online community, where images and videos can be both stored and shared. The service is widely used by bloggers as a photo repository. In an article dealing with social networking and education, Flickr is recognized as one of the most successful and useful tools for schools (Stephens, 2007). This same use of organizing pictures of school activities and projects can go a long way in keeping the community informed as to what the schools are doing and are capable of accomplishing. The tagging system utilized for various types of images provide excellent control over a review of what is available and specific ongoing projects.

Photobucket (http://photobucket.com/): This application is an image hosting, video hosting, slideshow creation and photo sharing website. Like Flickr, this is a web-base application to store, manipulate and share visual media. One can store 10,000 photos and hours of video for free, create slideshows, working with special effects, captions, and much more. One can keep all their media in one place and share it with others. This material can also be linked to selected blogs and other sites. Multiple views from thumbnails to slideshows can be tagged for identification and organization.

Many of the new camera phones can also send their photos and images to Photobucket automatically, allowing students to see images from outside the classroom in real-time. Virtual field trips could be created by a small group of students from a class to be shared with the entire class. If students are at a specific location, students in the classroom could request specific shots and images that can be forwarded to Photobucket, where the photos could be organized into a presentation and stored for future use.

Social Bookmarking: Social bookmarking is the practice of creating a user-generated collection of bookmarks to different Web-content in an organized form. To put it more simply, users can bookmark any kind of web content, and generate tags, or keywords, associated with the selected content. The result is that users have their own pages of bookmarks sorted by the keywords they have assigned. Social bookmarking websites are becoming a popular way to categorize and search for information on the Web. This is important because tags are user-generated rather than developed by search engine robots. Users are also able to do searches and find information from other users with similar tags. You can search through popular tags generated by other users and can even browse over the bookmarks generated by fellow bookmark site users. This allows networking with others over similar topical interest and one is able to keep track of other users' recently added bookmarks. Del.icio.us (http://del.icio.us) allows users to discover sets of tags developed by other users, who interpret Web content in a similar way. All of this makes a wide body of Web information easy to search and access (Jolly, 2007).

The major value of social bookmarking lies in the ability to share and collaborate in finding collected information related to specific topics. It is difficult for one individual to find all the information related to a topic, but when individuals can share what they have bookmarked, the work of the crowd can save one individual a great deal of time searching for information (Eastment, 2008).

The value of this social bookmarking system can be summed up through a review of the following points (Maxymuk, 2007):

- Sites can be reviewed from other computers when required since it is stored online

- You will not be filling up your own computers bookmarks and favorites allowing less clutter on your personal computer
- You are able to share your discoveries with others with similar interests in an effective manner
- A group of searchers can locate more information than one individual alone, and the search for new materials can continue over time and one can see what new information areas have been found as the process evolves.
- The tagging system is broad enough in scope to allow for related areas related to the topic

Examples of tools that can be utilized for social bookmarking work can be examined below:

- **Del.icio.us** (http://delicious.com/): Del.icio.us is a social bookmarking website and its primary use is to store bookmarks online, allowing access to the same bookmarks from any computer and adding bookmarks from anywhere. Tags (keyword descriptors) are used to organize and remember bookmarks. It also allows one to see the interesting links that friends and other people bookmark, and share links with them in return. The tagging system is user-centered and natural than the use of folders. One site might be associated to different tags, and this site might have aspects in common with different groups of websites. It allows for more complex relationships, which are more authentic to what the content represents to a particular user.
- **Digg** (http://www.digg.com/): Digg is website that offers special services for sharing web content among Digg users. The sharing, however, is based on a special voting system. Users as they use the web they can vote on certain (URLs). These votes serve as accumulating scores, which are then displayed in their website, allowing users get to see the most popular destinations selected by other users. Web sites are also organized by categories, which aids in research. One of the major functions is to provide a place where people can collectively determine the value of content, by what is reviewed.
- **RSS tools**: As discussed earlier, web syndication is an important function on the web, which in fact brings real meaning to the use of other services such as blogs and podcasts. Through RSS (Really Simple Syndication), one can sign-up for updates of numerous sites. Before RSS, web viewers had to visit individual websites to see if any new content had been added. For a teacher who regularly likes to visit a few particular blogs or websites, this can become time consuming. Now web viewers can subscribe to the feeds of their favorite websites. Basically this means content from these blogs and websites is delivered to the reader in one convenient location. Instead of visiting many different websites regularly, a viewer can now visit the RSS reader and instantly receive the updates of all of the syndicated websites. A teacher can visit one website to get the updates of all favorite sites. RSS provides an efficient way to stay in touch with colleagues and to receive updates about class assignments and activities. Faculty can utilize RSS to stay up to date with educational resources from sites like Open Course-Ware (http://ocwfinder.com/) and MERLOT (http://www.merlot.org/merlot/index.htm) or other selections. This tool is one of the greatest time savers as the site collects updates and notifies the user.

As distance educators seek to improve the quality of online courses, they face the challenge of meeting the needs of a diverse population that is more mobile and technology-savvy than any previous generation. The 21st-century learner requires educational opportunities not bound by time or place; yet allow interaction with the instructor and peers. The utilization of RSS meets these requirements well and has become a common practice for updating materials and research. Students can take advantage of the application by using it to keep them updated on new materials as they become available and in particular in science and social studies current events where change is an ongoing process (Beldarrain, 2006).

Benefits of RSS for teachers and students include (Educause Learning Initiative, 2008):

- Students can share their sites with each other creating a collaborative research environment
- Students can become globally aware by subscribing to news and current affairs sites
- Students can subscribe to Podcasts
- Students can track activities on blogs and wikis
- Teachers can utilize RSS as a powerful research tool
- Teachers can subscribe to educational blogs in their field of study
- Teachers can make announcements students after class
- Most important, teachers and students alike are exposed to new expressions and ideas and the restricting walls of the classroom are lowered to enhance connections with the outside world.

One important RSS tool is one called an RSS aggregator (http://en.wikipedia.org/wiki/RSS_aggregator) feed reader or feed aggregators. These tools serve to aggregate syndicated web content, including news, blog posts, and podcasts. These are then displayed in one single place for the user. Users can usually organize these locations by folder, or areas of interest. Many browsers or email tools carry such ability as an embedded functionality, such as Mozilla Firefox, Flock, Safari (Mac's default browser), Internet Explorer, Microsoft Outlook, etc. There are, however, specific software applications that can be used for this purpose, such as NewsFire (http://www.newsfirerss.com/) or NetNewsWire (http://www.newsgator.com/NetNewsWire) - both developed for the Mac OS X, Snarfer (http://www.Snarfware.com) - standalone free downloadable application), and FeedReader (http://www.feedreader.com) - for Windows. There are also website-based feed aggregators. These are aggregators that generate a page of feed aggregates for the reader to access online. Thus, one can access them from anywhere. One good example of this service is Google Reader (http://reader.google.com). It is able to read Atoms feeds and RSS feeds, and can be accessed online and offline.

Storage for Materials and Data

Areas to store data and information are useful for three reasons: it can free up space on your personal computer; it can aid in the organization of data and materials; and materials become accessible from anywhere. Listed here are some free or low cost sites that can serve this purpose.

Jungle disk (http://jungledisk.com) - Jungle Disk Desktop Edition automatically stores files and creates a backup file easily and securely to Amazon's S3 Storage Service. The process works just like another hard drive in the computer for storage. The user simply drags and drops, copies and deletes. To backup files, the user follows the same steps as in creating a backup. This format keeps valuable data safe and secure since data is encrypted using a personal key known only to the user. No one else can access the data. The application supports multiple platforms. Jungle Disk gives the user access to all of the data in

Windows, Mac and Linux, with unlimited storage at 15¢ per GB with no minimum or maximum. The user only gets charged for the space used. This is a great deal cheaper than purchasing an additional hard drive.

The application offers backup reporting to keep the user informed with reporting via web, email or RSS. The application also facilitates worry-free, automatic backups since selected data is continually monitored to ensure all files are backed up automatically. Also important since so many students and teachers have computers both at home and in school is the fact that the application provides online backup and storage for every computer the user owns.

Some free storage sites on the Web that might meet your needs and are listed below:

- With **Digital Bucket** (http://www.digital-bucket.net): you can store and access your important data and organize your files. Your information can be shared with anyone allowing for collaboration on-line and allowing for editing of documents.
- **Gmail Drive**: Gmail drive is developed by a third-party (not offered through Google) for people who have Gmail email accounts. Ever since Google started to offer users a Gmail e-mail account, which includes storage space of 2 GB, users have had plenty of storage space, but not a lot to fill it up with. With Gmail Drive the user can easily copy files to a Gmail account as if it were a separate drive and retrieve them again. The software exists only for Windows users. Many sites offer the option of downloading this software, such as the Cnet download site (http://download.cnet.com).
- **Box.net** (http://www.box/net): Box.net offers storage and several features that facilitate sharing and collaboration online. It offers a 'lite' account version for free with a total of 1 GB of total space, 25MB maximum for upload, and a maximum of 5 collaboration folders. There is a fee-based individual account and also a business account, with several other features, including email and more storage space.
- **Orbitfiles** (http://www.orbitfiles.com): Orbitfiles can save time and money with the easiest way to back up and access files online and shares them with friends and colleagues. The user gets 6GB of space for free. There are also fee-based solutions for more storage space.
- **Yahoo! Briefcase** (http://www.yahoo.com): Yahoo! Briefcase is a tool that offers 30MB of online storage.
- **Ripway** (http://www.ripway.com): Ripway provides web hosting and online storage services. Ripway offers users 30 MB for free. More storage comes with fee-based accounts.
- **Screencast** (http://www.screencast.com): Screencast gives the user storage space and tools for managing and sharing videos, documents and presentations. The free account version offers 2GB of space and a 2GB monthly bandwidth.

Manipulation of Data

Jing Project (http://www.jingproject.com/): Jing combines many of the features of Camtasia and SnagIt which have fees attached. It allows for both screen capture and also for video capture and provides a place to store what is captured with opportunities to edit. The user has options as to where to send captured materials. It could be saved at Screencast.com, a local folder, a network drive, Flickr, an FTP server, or if only an image to the clipboard. It's still free and also including a complimentary Screencast.com account (free version). This storage option is one of the best assets that Jing offers. Also a big advantage is that Jing offers technical support and is constantly available for use from the desktop. Jing is sometimes referred to as a stripped down version of SnagIt or Camtasia Studio. The key difference is about workflow. Jing is designed to be fast-visual communication shared with others in a variety of locations.

Jing is an excellent and easy way to create videos through the computer using a simple webcam that can be utilized in face-to-face classes or by allowing student access to the video on-line. It is a great tool for visual instruction for on-line class presentations. It saves a great deal of time in teaching on-line technology classes, since the teacher can use screen captures of the computer screen, edit the capture with comments and the use of a marking process. Complex topics can use visual format to enhance explanations shared with students (Anonymous, 2009).

FINAL REMARKS

For years educators have acknowledged the importance of individual skills and learning styles of students in the context of effective learning. Utilization of aspects of new technology, like Web 2.0, can provide the tools allowing for diverse approaches to education. And even more important the role of the teacher can change from the role of a disseminator of knowledge to a position where the teacher guides student learning rather than merely controlling it. As stated at the beginning of the chapter these new technological tools make a constructivist approach to learning possible as never before experienced in the educational field (Levin, Arafeh and Raine, 2002).

There is evidence that a more learner-centered approach has greater potential to achieve "deeper and more sustained learning across the curriculum" (NMC, 2009, p. 7). However, this approach requires new teaching practices and new tools. Including in such practices is assessment, which has shown to suffer from greater inertia when compared to new teaching methods, tools and materials.

The emergence of Web 2.0 has had a vast impact on the nature of literacy and the aspects of informational literacy. Teacher that employ this technology in their classrooms provide opportunities to prepare students to assume a place in this new world of informational literacy. Its use in the classroom must be more than attempting to capture students' attention with new flashes of technology (Borsheim, Merritt and Reed, 2008).

If schools do not assume the responsibility of modeling and providing effective instruction in the use of technology like Web 2.0, then the schools will be helping widen the gap between socioeconomic groups. Literature points to an expanding distance between home-use of such tools and what is available in schools. Those that can afford the hardware and share the technological knowledge with their own socioeconomic group from their home will have a greater advantage over those that do not have the opportunity to employ such skills and use such technology within the school setting. By not attempting to incorporate such knowledge and skills in the schools for all students, schools could be indirectly contributing to the digital divide (Jenkins and et al., 2006). Critical issues must be considered if change is to take place. Teachers need to be trained in order to effectively utilize new tools and services. The review of a study of pre-service teachers reveals that while technology training can be carried out, it is the inability of the pre-service teachers to recognize the usefulness of technology in the educational environment that needs to be urgently addressed. Classroom application of technology to serve as an effective teaching tool needs to be supported as a major thrust to push teachers to utilize new technology. To foster a belief in the power of applications like Web 2.0, more efforts must be made for teacher training programs to assume the role of modeling how such technical knowledge can enhance the educational process (*Lambert*, *Gong* and *Cuper*, 2008).

The sustained adoption of new technologies

is a difficult process. Many of these tools are part of students' life outside the school and are part of many professionals in their workplace. Thus, these should also be consistently incorporated in the teaching and learning process. However, it has been hard for teachers to make the necessary shift, acquiring mastery of these tools in order to effectively use them in the classroom. This will require a profound change in a well-established system. There is an urgent need for "professional development, intellectual interactions with peers, adequate training and preparation time" (NMC, 2009, p.7). These resources are at a premium in most teachers' work schedule. Moreover, there is a clear resistance from an organizational standpoint, due to the focus on "maintaining the basic elements of the existing system" (p.7) Learners, more than ever before, have many more educational options at their reach, including home schooling and on-line learning. Thus, there will be a natural push for change if institutions are to remain relevant.

REFERENCES

Alexander, B. (2006, March/April). Web 2.0: A new innovation for teaching and learning? *Educause review*. Retrieved on January 20, 2008, from http://www.educause.edu/ir/library/pdf/ERM0621.pdf

Anonymous,. (2009). The 2.0 tech I can't live without. *Knowledge Quest*, *37*(4), 34–36.

Ashwin, A. (2006). GCSE business studies: The essentials. *Teaching Business & Economics*, *10*(2), 42–44.

Barrett, H. (2006). *Digital Stories in e-Portfolios: Multiple Purposes and Tools*. Retrieved June 2009, from http://electronicportfolios.org/digistory/purposesmac.html

Beldarrain, Y. (2006). Distance Education Trends: Integrating new technologies to foster student interaction and collaboration. *Distance Education, 27*(2), 139-154. Retrieved from Proquest databases on September 2008.

Borsheim, C., Merrit, K., & Reed, D. (2008). Beyond technology for technology's take: Advancing multiliteracies in the twenty-first century. *Clearing House (Menasha, Wis.)*, *82*(2), 87–91. doi:10.3200/TCHS.82.2.87-90

Boyd, D., & Ellison, N. (2007). Social network sites: definition, history, and scholarship. *Journal of Computer-Mediated Communication, 13*(1), 210-230. Retrieved April 2009, from http://plcmcl2-things.blogspot.com/

Brown, J., & Adler, R. (2008). Minds on fire: Open education, the long tail, and learning 2.0. *EDUCAUSE Review*, *43*(1), 16–32.

Conrad, D. (2008). Reflecting on strategies for a new learning culture: Can we do it? *Journal of Distance Education*, *2*(3), 157–162.

Crook, C., & Harrison, C. (2008). *Web 2.0 technologies for learning at key stages 3 and 4: Summary report*. Retrieved April 2009, from http://schools.becta.org.uk/upload-dir/downloads/page_documents/research/web2_ks34_summary.pdf

Duffy, P., & Bruns, A. (2006). The use of blogs, wikis and RSS in education: a conversation of possibilities. In *Proceedings Online Learning and Teaching Conference 2006*, Brisbane (pp. 31–38). Retrieved September 2008, from http://www.scu.edu.au/twt/wiki01.html

Eastment, D. (2008). Social networking. *ELT Journal*, *62*(2), 217–221. doi:10.1093/elt/ccn007

Educause Learning Initiative. (Dec. 2007). 7 things you should know about Skype. Retrieved December 18, 2008 http://net.educause.edu/ir/library/pdf/ELI7032.pdf

Foote, C. (2008). See me, hear Me: Skype in the classroom. *School Library Journal, 1*(1), 4–8.

Higdon, J., & Topaz, C. (2009). Blogs and wikis as Instructional tools: A Social software adaptation of just-in-time teaching. *College Teaching, 57*(2), 105-110. Retrieved May 2009, from http://web.mac.com/chad.topaz/ChadTopaz/Blogging_files/ht2009.pdf

Huang, D., & Behara, R. (2007). Outcome-driven experiential learning with Web 2.0. *Journal of Information Systems Education, 18*(3), 329–337.

IESD Research Report. (2008). *Safe schools in a web 2.0 world initiative: National online survey of district technology directors exploring district use of Web 2.0 technologies.* Retrieved from http://www.prweb.com/releases/Web20/schools/prweb2300494.htm

Jenkins, H., Purushotma, R., Clinton, K., Weigel, M., & Robison, A. J. (2006). *Confronting the challenges of participatory culture: Media Education for the 21st Century.* Chicago, IL: John D. & Catherine T. MacArthur Foundation.

Jolly, G. (2007). *An overview of some of the social network web sites.* Retrieved May 15, 2009, from http://www.associatedcontent.com/article/465599/an_overview_of_some_of_the_social_network.html?cat=35

Jones, M. (2009). *What is social networking?* Retrieved June 2009 from http://tech.blorge.com/Structure:%20/2009/05/30/what-is-social-networking/

Kennelly, P. (2009). An online social networking approach to reinforce learning of rocks and minerals. *Journal of Geo-science Education, 57*(1), 33–35.

Kirkland, A. (2007). Becoming librarian 2.0. partnership. *Canadian Journal of Library and Information Practice and Research, 2*(1), 25–31.

Lambert, J., Yi, G., & Cuper, P. (2008). Technology, transfer, and teaching: The impact of a single technology course on pre-service teachers' computer attitudes and ability. *Journal of Technology and Teacher Education, 16*(4), 385–411.

Levin, D., Arafeh, S., Lenhart, A., & Rainie, L. (2002). The digital disconnect: The widening gap between internet-savvy students and their Schools. *Pew Internet & American Life Project.* Retrieved April 2009 from http://epsl.asu.edu/epru/articles/EPRU-0208-36-OWI.pdf

Maxymuk, J. (2007). Whose space? *The Bottom, 20*(1), 54–57. doi:10.1108/08880450710747461

McNeely, B. (2009). Using technology as a learning tool, not just the cool new thing. *Educause.* Retrieved May 2009, from http://www.educause.edu/Resources/EducatingtheNetGeneration/UsingTechnologyasaLearningTool/6060

Murphy, J., & Lebans, R. (2008). Unexpected outcomes: Web 2.0 in the secondary school classroom. *International Journal of Technology in Teaching and Learning, 4*(2), 134-147. Retrieved April 2009, from http://www.sad61.k12.me.us/Web2.0/

New Media Consortium. (2009). Horizon report: 2009 K-12 Ed. *The New Media Consortium.* Retrieved on March 30, 2009, from http://www.nmc.org/pdf/2009-Horizon-Report-K12.pdf

O'Reilly, T. (2005, September 30). *What Is Web 2.0 Design Patterns and Business Models for the Next Generation of Software.* Retrieved January 31, 2007, from http://www.oreillynet.com/lpt/a/6228

Oblinger, D., & Oblinger, J. (2009). Is it age or IT: First steps toward understanding the net generation. *Educause.* Retrieved May 2009, from http://www.educause.edu/Resources/EducatingtheNetGeneration/IsItAgeorITFirstStepsTowardUnd/6058

Palfrey, J., & Gasser, U. (2008). *Born Digital.* New York: Basic Books.

Pallof, R., & Pratt, K. (2003). *The virtual student: A profile and guide to working with online learners*. San Francisco, CA: Jossey-Bass Publishers.

Palloff, R., & Pratt, K. (1999). *Building learning communities in cyberspace*. San Francisco: Jossey-Bass Publishers.

Plough, C. (2008). Web 2.0 tools motivate student creativity. *Tech and Learning.* Retrieved April 2009, from http://www.techlearning.com/article/8534

Prensky, M. (2001). Digital natives, digital immigrants. *On the Horizon. NCB University Press*, *9*(5), 5–10.

Prensky, M. (2005). Engage me or enrage me: What today's learners demand. *Educause Review*. Retrieved January 2009 from http://net.educause.edu/ir/library/pdf/ERM0553.pdf

Prerna, R. (2007). Skype as a language-learning tool. *Student Newspaper: The Hatchet*. George Washington University. Retrieved December 2008, from http://media.www.gwhatchet.com/media/storage/paper332/news/2007/01/29/Life/Skype.As.A.LanguageLearning.Tool-2682418.shtml?sourcedomain=www.gwhatchet.com&MIIHost=media.collegepublisher.com

Rosenfeld, E. (2008). Expanding your professional network with Nings. *Teacher Librarian*, *35*(3), 60–65.

Roush, W. (2005, October 7). 'Web 2.0' has arrived. *Technology Review – MIT*. Retrieved on January 10, 2008, from http://www.techreview.com/Infotech/14869/?a=f

Siemens, G. (2004). Connectivism: A learning theory for the digital age. *Elearnspace*. Retrieved February 2008, from http://www.elearnspace.org/Articles/connectivism.htm

Solomon, G., & Schrum, L. (2007). *Web 2.0: New Tools, New Schools*. Eugene, OR: International Society for Technology in Education.

Stephens, M. (2007). Tools from web 2.0 & libraries: Best practices for social software revisited. *Library Technology Reports*, *43*(5), 15–32.

ADDITIONAL READING

Atwell, G. (2007). Personal learning environments—The future of eLearning? *Elearning Papers, 2*(1), 1-8. Retrieved from http://www.elearningeuropa.info/files/media/media11561.pdf

Belz, J. (2003). Linguistic perspectives on the development of intercultural competence in telecollaboration. *Language Learning & Technology*, *7*(2), 68–99. Retrieved from http://llt.msu.edu/vol7num2/belz.

Blake, R. (2008). *Brave new digital classroom: Technology and foreign language learning*. Washington, DC: Georgetown University Press.

Duffy, P., & Bruns, A. (2006, September 26). *The use of blogs, wikis and RSS in education: A conversation of possibilities*. Paper presented at the Online Learning and Teaching Conference, Brisbane, Australia. Retrieved from https://olt.qut.edu.au/udf/OLT2006/gen/static/papers/Duffy_OLT2006_paper.pdf

Jones, B. L. (2008). *Web 2.0 heroes*. Indianapolis, IN: Wiley Publishing Inc.

Lund, A. (2008). Wikis: A collective approach to language production. *ReCALL*, *20*, 35–54. doi:10.1017/S0958344008000414

Parry, D. (2008, February). Teaching with Twitter. *The Chronicle of Higher Education, Chronicle Multimedia*. Retrieved from http://chronicle.com/media/video/v54/i25/twitter

Sathe, N., & Waltje, J. (2008). The iPod project: A mobile mini-lab. *Journal of the Research Centre for Educational Technology*, *4*, 32–56.

Stanley, G. (2006). Podcasting: Audio on the internet comes of age. *TESL-EJ, 9*(4), 1-7. Retrieved from http://tesl-ej.org/ej36/int.html

Warschauer, M., Knobel, & Stone, L. (2004). Technology and equity in schooling: Deconstructing the digital divide. *Educational Policy, 18*, 562–588. doi:10.1177/0895904804266469

Yan, J. (2008). Social technology as a new medium in the classroom. *New England Journal of Higher Education, 22*(4), 27–30.

Young, A., & Norgard, C. (2006). Assessing the quality of online courses from the students' perspective. *The Internet and Higher Education, 9*, 107–115. doi:10.1016/j.iheduc.2006.03.001

Young, J. R. (2008, January 28). Professor's tips for using Twitter in the classroom. *The Chronicle of Higher Education*. Retrieved from http://chronicle.com/wiredcampus/article/2699/a-professors-tips-for-using-twitter-in-the-classroom

Chapter 14
One Plus One Doesn't Always Equal Two

Terry L. Herman
Bowling Green State University, USA

ABSTRACT

Web 2.0 applications have exploded onto the scene in the past 2 years resulting in an impressive number of interactive tools and Web services. These online Web services and applications can be integrated into the pedagogical mix to energize student learning and provide participatory learning experiences. Educators can pick and choose favorite applications and online Web services, include user created data, and combine them in unique ways through data mashups. Mashups involve the reuse, or remixing, of works of art, music, content, or data for purposes that usually were not planned or anticipated by the original creators. This chapter will explore the concept, techniques, and strategies of data Web mashups. Educational data mashups are in their infancy. Several significant ethical issues of concern to educators and students are explored including possible mitigating strategies to allow educators to leverage the teaching and learning potential of data mashups in the classroom.

INTRODUCTION

Business Week proclaimed 2007 the Year of the Mashup. Mashups involve the reuse, or remixing, of works of art, music, video, content, or data for purposes that usually were not intended or even imagined by the original creators (EDUCAUSE Learning Initiative [ELI], 2006; Johnson, Levine, & Smith, 2008; Lamb, 2007). In the New Media Consortium's (NMC) 2008 Horizon Report, mashups were reported to be 2 to 3 years from ideal time-to-adoption by the masses (Johnson et al., 2008). Even so, Web 2.0 applications have exploded onto the educational scene in the past 2 years resulting in an impressive cadre of learning tools and Web services including data mashups. This may be the time to explore the integration of these online Web services and applications into the pedagogical mix. With data mashups educators can pick and choose favorite applications and online Web services, in-

DOI: 10.4018/978-1-61520-899-9.ch014

clude their own data, and combine them in unique ways to energize student learning and provide an integrated learning experience for students.

At the heart of the data mashup are characteristics that make the Internet a compelling educational resource: collaboration, participation, aggregation, innovation, visualization, participation, and representation. The mashup creation process accentuates the pedagogical flexibility and potential learning opportunities possible through the remixing, repurposing, and reimagining of the plethora of online resources available. In this chapter the concepts, techniques, and strategies of data or content data mashups will be explored.

Through this chapter the reader will explore the following:

- Characteristics of today's student to discover some of the reasons teaching strategies such as data mashups may be compelling pedagogical tools;
- Mashup history;
- Mashup technology and processes to provide a basis for understanding this powerful tool and provide a conceptual framework;
- Types, characteristics, educational uses, and examples of data mashups and where they might be integrated into teaching and learning further underscoring the potential of mashups to personalize learning experiences for students;
- A discussion of scholarly mashups and examples of integrating data mashups into learning experiences;
- Several popular and accessible mashup editors that allow educators to seamlessly remix existing online Web services, application programming interfaces, tools, and widgets for new and unique applications relevant to the learners' needs and goals;
- A discussion of the potential drawbacks to the promising educational inclusion of data mashups including intellectual property rights, copyright, the dynamic nature of resources on the Web, assessing new Web technologies, and cultural and ethical considerations;
- And finally, future research concerns and questions.

LEARNER AND DATA MASHUP BACKGROUND

Today's Learner

As a society, we spend countless hours engaged in classes, training, workshops, seminars, and other educational venues that fall short of providing a truly enriching, engaging, and efficient learning experience or don't result in meaningful changes in behavior. Students tune out if they find the learning environment or experience irrelevant, boring, or frustrating (Prensky, 2005). Often, this ineffective learning experience is not a result of boring or inconsequential content or a reflection of the knowledge of the instructor but of the delivery, collaborative, and instructional design strategies employed for that particular student. Adapting to a student's prior experience, personal learning goals, and other student characteristics within the framework of the course content can make a compelling difference in the overall impact of the learning experience (Bransford, Brown, & Cocking, 2000).

The way our students prefer to learn has fundamentally changed. The singular difference between the Digital Natives' (DNs) and Digital Immigrants' (DIs) relationship with current and emerging digital technology profoundly influences the teaching and learning process. DNs are used to accessing and receiving data at what Prensky (2001) calls "twitch speed" (p. 3). Digital Native students expect a certain level of interactivity, instant feedback, and parallel processing or multitasking. DNs have grown up with hypertext and non-linear access to information. The DNs give new meaning to Barabasi's (2003) notion of being linked or networked. DNs are likely the most connected segment of the population on the planet (Draves, 2002; Palloff & Pratt, 2003; Prensky, 2001). DIs, on the other hand, grew up with the factory-like industrial model of education that focused on the structured, linear nature of content delivery in a traditional classroom setting (Draves, 2002; Prensky, 2001). The organization of education has changed little in light of the technological advancements and advent of the information age.

Implicit in a sincere plea for transformation is an awareness that a current situation needs improvement. When we advocate institutional change for learning institutions, we are making assumptions about the deep structure of learning, about cognition, about the way youth today learn (about) their world in informal settings, and about a mismatch between the excitement generated by informal learning and the routinization of learning so common to many of our institutions of formal education. We advocate institutional change because we believe our current formal educational institutions are not taking enough advantage of the modes of digital and participatory learning available to students today. (Davidson & Goldberg, 2009, p. 20)

The skills so prized by the DNs are not easily assimilated, or necessarily understood, by the DIs who are responsible for the instructional design and teaching of the DNs, whether in a traditional or online classroom environment. The salient point is that these students are dramatically different from the people charged with teaching them, almost all of whom are Prensky's (2001) Digital Immigrants. The implications for education and for those engaged in teaching the DNs are immeasurable and almost unimaginable. The individuals charged with organizing, leading, and teaching the DNs, the DIs, are fundamentally different in their use and consumption of technology. Education stands at a cross roads which requires the express and concerted efforts of DI teacher educators to reassess organizational policies, teaching strategies, delivery models, and content creation and presentation (Prensky, 2001; Prensky, 2005; Senge, Cambron-McCabe, Lucas, Smith, Dutton, & Kleiner, 2000).

Many students are entering the educational system with technology experiences including computer usage (Brown, 2005; Prensky, 2008a; Prensky, 2008b). Due in large part to the National Educational Technology Standards that are part of today's K-12 curriculum, students enter higher education with more advanced skills and knowledge in the use of technology (McGee & Diaz, 2007). Students of all ages also have much higher expectations about what and how they will learn (McGee & Diaz; Prensky, 2005). According to Prensky (2008b), "students universally tell us they prefer dealing with questions rather than answers, sharing their opinions, participating in group projects, working with real-world issues and people, and having teachers who talk to them as equals rather than as inferiors" (p. 4). Data mashups provide an innovative pedagogical strategy to foster what our students long for, content creation and knowledge building opportunities dealing with real-world issues. Data mashups allow teachers and students to work together on the explorative end of the learning continuum as illustrated in Figure 1.

Web 2.0 Applications

Web 2.0 applications are everywhere on the Internet. But what are they exactly? And what role do they play in data mashups?

Web 2.0 represents a broad collection of recent trends in Internet technologies and business models. Particular focus has been given to user-created content, lightweight technology, service-based access, and shared revenue models. (Gartner, Inc., 2007)

Figure 1. Learning continuum

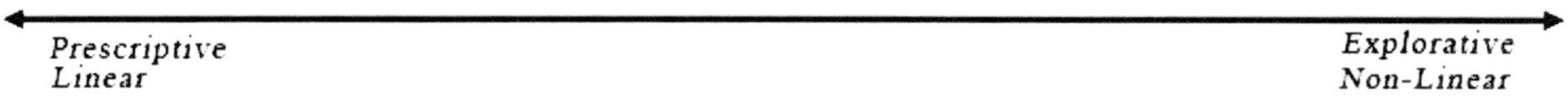

Another definition asserts that Web 2.0 is not a thing but rather a set of ideas and technologies that enable people to engage and interact with services, applications, and data found on the Internet (Alexander, 2006; O'Reilly & Battelle, 2009; Slater, 2009). According to O'Reilly and Battelle, "Web 2.0 is all about harnessing collective intelligence" (p. 1). Wikis, blogs, syndication, tagging, and social bookmarking, just to name a few, exemplify the read/write nature of Web 2.0 technologies (Franklin & van Harmelen, 2007). Web 2.0 characteristics can be found in sites including Flickr, Google Maps, My Yahoo, Facebook, Digg, Delicious, Twitter, and YouTube, among others. As Internet services, applications, and data have become more accessible and sophisticated, the allure of being able to manipulate these technologies in new and interesting ways has encouraged the growth of data mashups. "The emergence of Web 2.0 introduced us to the ideas of user generated content, collaborative information creation, crowd sourcing, and mashups" (Schmelzer, 2008, ¶ 2).

Mashup History and Technology

Mashups involve the re-purposing, re-mixing, or combining of a genre of media to develop a new work with results not expected or intended by the creators of the original works (Hodgins, 2008; Karch, 2009; Lamb, 2007). While mashups are frequently also referred to as remixes, Lamb makes a distinction between a remix and a mashup. "Remix is the reworking or adaptation of an existing work" (p. 14). As with many new technologies, different buzzwords are applied to the new or emerging technology. Online learning, eLearning, distance learning, distance education, and virtual education are terms applied to the same concept, teaching, and learning processes supported by technology. Each of these terms may imply subtle differences in the inherent characteristics of the technology. Mashups may be referred to as data mashups, content mashups, Web mashups, and digital data mashups among others. For the purposes of this chapter, the term data mashup will be defined as the unique combination of the data and functionality of two or more Web applications to create a new application. For example, data from Flickr and Google Maps could be combined to illustrate the location and images of specific mountains of the world (http://www.rapidmonkey.com/mountainsoftheworld/index.php).

Though they are popularly called mashups today, mashups as a concept have a long and interesting history. They have also been known as smashups, blends, cut-ups, bootlegs, bastard pop, and remixes depending upon the genre of the mashup (Berlind, 2006; Hodgins, 2008; Lamb, 2007). Mashups predate the Internet. The first mashups were a combination of two or more songs or sound tracks blended to form a new work from the original works. In 1956 two musicians, Bill Buchanan and Dickie Goodman, released *The Flying Saucer*, perhaps the first musical mashup combining Orson Welles *War of the Worlds* fictitious emergency broadcast and various musical snippets to comically punctuate key points within the Welles broadcast (http://www.mashupshub.com/music/). This foray into musical mashups was short lived, fading in less than a year. However, as technology has evolved so have the genres and uses of the mashups created from resources on the Web. From a Web development perspective, a mashup is a web application that combines data from multiple sources into a single integrated application (Berlind, 2006; Lamb, 2007; Novak & Voigt, 2008).

Data mashups, as defined earlier, are better defined as a combination of two or more digital media sources that are very different from each other to form a unique work (Hodgins, 2008; Lamb, 2007). The fact that mashups are often designed, created, and used by the same person is a defining characteristic of the mashup (Hodgins). The following excerpt from the NMC 2008 Horizon Report highlights the unique nature and use of data mashups.

Overlay the location of every Flickr photo tagged with "bluejay" [sic] on a map of the United States and see where people are finding blue jays (http://www.flickr.com/map). See Twitter updates from your geographical area (http://www.twittermap.com) or follow the global progress of the public stream (http://www.twittervision.com). Each of these applications is a mashup: a combination of data from multiple sources in a single tool. Mashups have been around for several years, but in recent months they have captured greater interest, due in part to a broader exposure from their integration with social networking systems like Facebook. While most current examples are focused on the integration of maps with a variety of data, it is not difficult to picture broad educational and scholarly applications for mashups. (Johnson et al., 2008, p. 20)

Data mashups are made possible through the open nature of the Internet. "A variety of open access sources provides access to information such as geographic data, pictures, videos, news or taxonomies" (Novak & Voigt, 2008, p. 1). Source sites expose key pieces of data and function through their application programming interfaces (API). An API is a set of rules that make it easier to extract data from a website. Application programming interfaces facilitate communication between the technologies without user modification of the source code (ELI, 2006).

Other types of web services such as Really Simple Syndication (RSS) and the Atom syndication format can also be leveraged in mashups. Other lightweight development applications including JavaScript, Ajax, and Extensible Markup Language (XML) are also a part of the data mashup development toolkit. The creation of a mashup requires multiple input sources which usually have an XML based output stream. The mashup uses the XML outputs and inputs and consolidates them or mashes them together (Merrill, 2006).

MASHUPS ILLUMINATED

Inherent in the data mashup process is the promise of student engagement. At the core of mashup technology is collaboration, sharing, creating, innovating, and opportunities for the student to pursue personal learning goals within the framework of a learning environment. In Figure 2, the mashup tag cloud highlights the themes of personalization, learning, learners, and innovation that engage today's students.

An exploration of the teaching and learning strategies and processes possible through the use of the technology of educational data mashups will provide a possible roadmap for integrating data mashups into the learning experience. The ways in which different services and applications can be uniquely combined to form powerful, relevant new educational learning applications underscores the participatory nature of data mashups. "At the conceptual level, mashups can provide a multiplying effect for learning, education, and training, since mashups are effective for both those who use them and those who design and create them" (Hodgins, 2008, p. 6). Mashups allow students to actively engage in the learning process through the creation and construction of knowledge (Hodgins; Lamb, 2007).

Figure 2. Mashup cloud

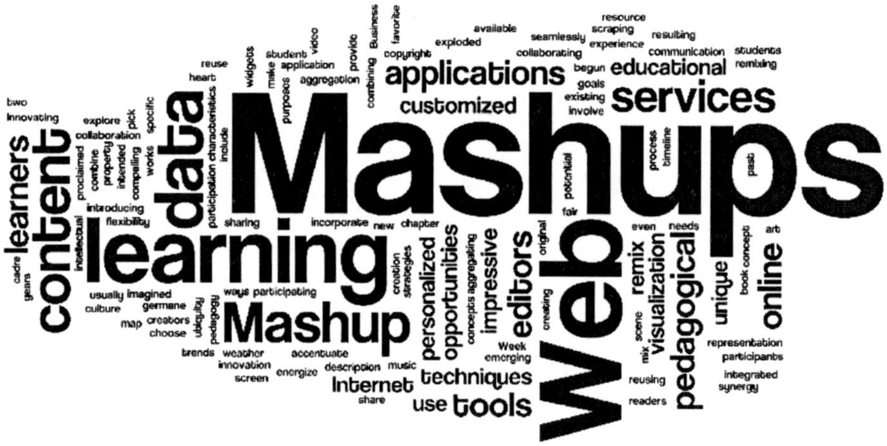

Data mashups can be integrated into the pedagogical mix as both a teaching strategy and a student assessment strategy. The pedagogical significance of data mashups includes the following (ELI, 2006; Hodgins, 2008; Johnson et al., 2008; Lamb, 2007):

- Mashups incorporate technology students already understand;
- The interactive nature of mashups are ideal for students who increasingly seek opportunities to take an active role in their learning;
- Mashups provide instant feedback through the connection of content with its physical place in the world;
- Mashups can address a variety of learning styles; for example, visual representations of data through mashups benefit visual learners;
- Learners construct and better understand content and content relationships.

The number, sophistication, and users of data mashups have grown exponentially over the past 2 years as the cost of essential hardware and software has become more powerful and affordable (Hodgins, 2008; Lamb, 2007; Merrill, 2006). Another driving factor is the wide spread availability of high speed connectivity. The educational use of Web 2.0 applications such as wikis and blogs has encouraged the desire for even more do it yourself, participatory learning experiences.

The primary types, characteristics, educational uses, and examples of data mashups follows in Table 1.

The pedagogical significance of these data mashup examples is evidenced by the sweeping educational applications that allow student and teacher to actively construct knowledge together. For instance, if a learning outcome of a particular class was to convey advanced programming principles to students, data mashup and mashup creation could be used to explore algorithmic thinking (Batson, 2008). Students could also visually interact with the mashup editor interface to experience programming sequencing, filtering, and repetition and to a lesser degree building the user interface. The graphical user interface of many of the mashup editors makes concepts such as input, output, and processing more obvious.

Another interesting example is a use of a mapping mashup to visually display major events leading up to and during World War II. In this

Table 1. Data Mashup types and examples

Type of Mashup	Characteristics	Educational Uses	Examples
Mapping	Cartographic services Map with Crime Statistics Map with impact of sea level rise	Social studies; Geography Criminal Justice Ecology	**Find the Landmark** http://landmark.mapsgame.com/ This versatile mashup includes categories as diverse as planets, mountains, volcanoes, bridges, monuments, and many others. Teachers can customize the map to include their own landmarks for students to locate. **CrimeReports** http://crimereports.com/ Law enforcement officers file crime reports each time they respond to a call. This data is updated daily and could be used to study crime trends over time. **The Globe is Warming** http://www.mibazaar.com/nationundersiege/index.html This mashup provides a compelling visual representation of locations, such as Honolulu, Hawaii, as they appear today and how they would appear if, through global warming, we experienced a 1.75m sea level rise. This would make a powerful discussion starter.
Photo	Flickr and mapping Flickr and color Flickr and News Feeds	Economy Print; Web Design; Design Research; Social Studies; Business	**The Five Dollar Comparison** http://fivedollarcomparison.org/ The Five Dollar Comparison mashup explores the relative nature of five dollars and what that amount of money can buy around the world. This is an eye-opening experience for both teachers and students. **Multicolr Search Lab** http://labs.ideeinc.com/multicolr/ With this mashup, a user can choose from over 10 million Creative Commons images that match the particular color palette chosen. **Visual Headlines** http://visualheadlines.com/ For current events and cultural studies, the Visual Headlines mashup is a visual powerhouse displaying today's headlines in clickable images that transport the user to the full story behind the headline.
Search	Employment Google; Yahoo; Live Amazon book search	Research; Economy Data Search Research; Books under 200 pages	**Joblighted** http://joblighted.com/ The Joblighted mashup could be used in any course that focuses on careers, career development, or forecasting. The mashup draws from 26 job sites and can be filtered by location, date of posting, and keyword. **Triplify** http://www.triplify.com/ Enter a search term, click on the Search button, and in seconds a list of top results appears complete with the asset title, description, URL, and the Search Engine from which the item was retrieved (Google, Yahoo, or Live Search). **Lazy Library** http://lazylibrary.com/ The Lazy Library mashup focuses on helping users find concise and effective books on any topic that are 200 pages or less in length.

continued on the following page

Table 1. continued

Type of Mashup	Characteristics	Educational Uses	Examples
Timeline	Flickr; YouTube Flickr; Google Maps; Flickr; Google	Geography; Politics; Research Geography; Meteorology History; Archaeology; Geography; Geology	**TimeTube** http://www.dipity.com/mashups/timetube Educators and students can type in a single keyword or a combination of keywords to produce a visual timeline (images and videos) of the chosen topic(s). Each item on the timeline is clickable for additional information. **Tickr** http://www.dipity.com/mashups/tickr/Sunsets/World The Tickr mashup provides a visual timeline for topics such as glaciers over time, Roman architecture, and Alcatraz just to name a few. **Dinosaur Timeline** http://simile.mit.edu/timeline/examples/dinosaurs/dinosaurs2.html A fascinating timeline mashup that includes dinosaurs from various periods such as the Jurassic. Each dinosaur is clickable and provides additional information in a pop-up window format.
Visualization	Visual Search Icons and cloud tags for kids Google Maps and time zones	Research on any subject Research especially for kids Social Studies; Research	**Search Cube** http://www.search-cube.com/ The Search-Cube mashup displays search results in an interactive three-dimensional cube displaying up to 96 websites. Floating the cursor over any pane of the cube displays additional information. Clicking the pane opens the Web site in a new window. **Quintura for Kids** http://quinturakids.com/ Quintura for Kids is a visual search engine mashup providing younger students with images and word clouds to conduct their searches. **World Time Engine** http://worldtimeengine.com/ This mashup displays the current time anywhere in the world, provides a map displaying the location, and time differences between two locations.
Weather	Google Maps; Weather.com Yahoo; Flickr; Wikipedia WeatherBug; Flickr; Wikipedia; Google News	Research; Geography; Meteorology Research; Geography; Meteorology Travel; Geography; Meteorology	**Woozor** http://woozor.us/free-10-days-weather-forecast/weather-forecast-of-los-angeles-ca-in-usa-united-states_214_7200_us.html The Woozor mashup provides much more than weather information. A clickable map with weather data, moon phases, pollen reports, airport information and rush hour traffic information can be explored. **Yahoo-Flickr-Wikipedia-Weather Map** http://www.allapis.com/Yahoo_Flickr_Weather_Maps.aspx The Yahoo-Flickr-Wikipedia-Weather map mashup provides for targeted weather searches through a dialog box to enter city, address, and / or zip code. The visual display includes a map, images, current conditions and forecast. **Mapdango** http://mapdango.com/ The highlight of the Mapdango mashup is the global location listings which facilitates retrieving the information sought.

mashup, learners could zoom in different areas of the world to find flags scattered around the location of specific events. When clicked, the flag opens a pop-up box naming the location and what happened there and when it happened complete with a photograph of the site at or near the date in question. Data mashups represent a compelling new pedagogical resource that focuses on the attributes of today's learners and their desire to actively engage in their learning process.

Scholarly Data Mashups

Scholarly data mashups are expressly created for educational purposes. The New Media Consortium and the EDUCAUSE Learning Initiative's (2008) *The 2008 Horizon Report* projects data mashups time-to-adoption as 2 to 3 years. "While most current examples are focused on the integration of maps with a variety of data, it is not difficult to picture broad educational and scholarly applications for mashups" (Johnson et al., 2008, p. 20).

The visual representation of data and relationships produced by data mashups provides a method to assist educators, students, and researchers in drawing conclusions and identifying trends. The research findings can be displayed as interactive charts, maps, or graphs.

Mashups of geotagged data have obvious applications for education; researchers can use public, tagged media to create mashup maps with embedded annotations. These "hyperlocal" annotations—minute details about a specific location in the form of everyday photographs, blog entries, and video clips—offer opportunities for research that were previously only available by actually living in the location in question" (Johnson et al., 2008, p. 21).

From a pedagogical perspective, data mashups could be used to visually represent course concepts. Further, educators could use data mashups in assessing student learning through student created data mashup projects and assignments. Visual representations of data through mashups can also provide a powerful springboard for discussion.

For students studying current events, aviation studies, geography, geology, as well as other subjects, the Havaria Information Services Alert Map displays data including severe weather conditions, epidemic alerts, seismic incidents, and other disasters and emergencies in North America. The user can choose both Disaster and Emergency AlertMap by region or Pandemic Monitoring System by region. This data mashup created by the National Association of Radio-Distress Signalling and Infocommunications (RSOE) draws from over 200 news sources. The data mashup map in Figure 3 displays airplane incidents and accidents, hazardous materials incidents, and seismic activity on the west coast including the dates and times of the occurrences. This visual representation could provide a context for discussion, research, or various assignments.

A research assignment in a Weather and Climate class on volcanoes could be facilitated by having students use the Search-Cube data mashup as seen in Figure 4. The Search-Cube mashup presents search results in a three-dimensional cube displaying up to 96 websites, videos, and images. The cube can be manipulated to see all sides, top, and bottom with either the arrow keys or the combination of the mouse and SHIFT key. Clicking on a particular resource opens the website in a new browser window. The Search-Cube could be used for virtually any subject matter.

Data Mashup Editors

Another driving force behind the phenomenal growth of mashups is that less and less technical skill is required to develop media rich, visual educational data mashups (Johnson et. al., 2008; Lamb, 2007). New mashups are being created daily. New APIs including Pings, YouTube, Twit-

Figure 3. North America Disaster and Emergency AlertMap

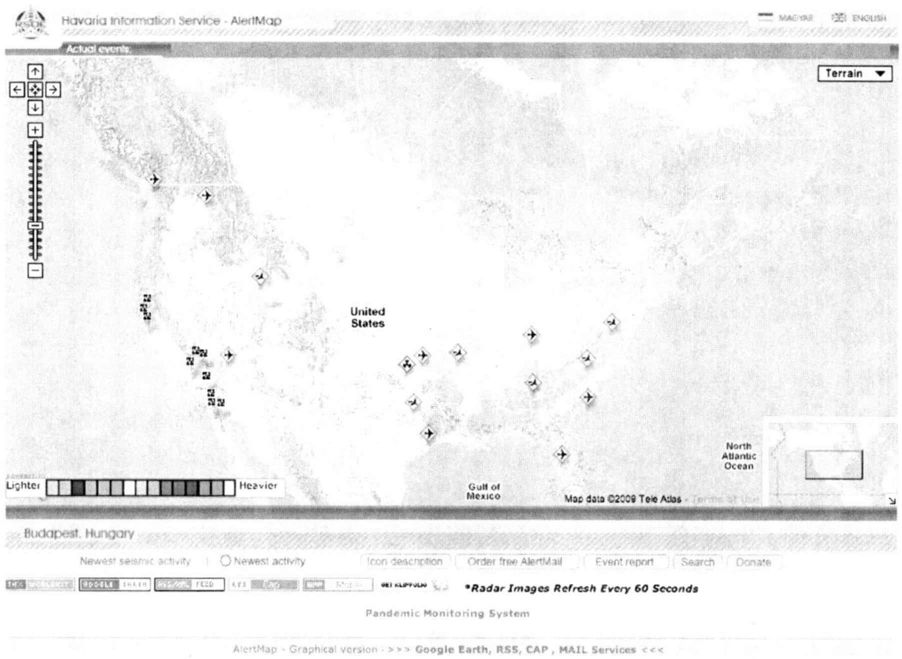

ter, and Google Maps are also being added at a record pace to participate in the data mashup culture.

The following matrix of current and emerging mashup tools presents the strengths and weaknesses of each. Please note that the Google Mashup Editor which was in beta for a little over a year is no longer available. Google plans to replace the Google Mashup Editor (GME) with an updated application called App Engine based on feedback from beta testers of the GME.

The Building of a Data Mashup

The following data mashup was built using the Yahoo! Pipes editor to explain the process of building a mashup. The mashup in Figure 5 represents a data output of 10 current events news items drawn from the CNN International Edition and displays the latitude and longitude through Google Maps.

Step 1. Fetch Feed: Gets the basic feed from CNN International Edition. Next Google News was used to create a custom feed. So if we are studying alternative fuels, it will only show items for that topic. Pipes would also let us merge feeds from general news and specialization sites.

Steps 2 and 3. Organize (Sort): the feed by publication date and only take the first 10 results (Truncate). This is mostly to cut down on processing time in the next step.

Step 4. Used the web service Calais. This takes any input data, analyzes it, and appends meta-data of any locations, people, and companies from the text.

Step 5. The location extractor searches for anything that seems like a location in the text and translates that to Latitude and Longitude information.

Step 6. The loop simply cleans up the formatting of the meta-data.

Mashup Issues, Controversies, Problems

Educational data mashups are in their infancy and present serious ethical issues to both educa-

Figure 4. Search-Cube volcanoes

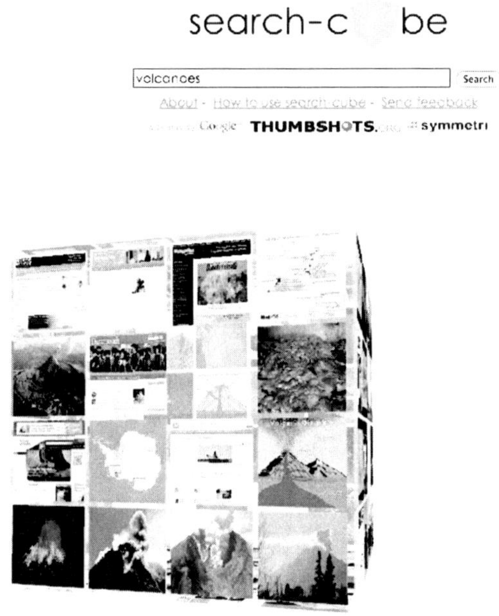

tor and student. As O'Reilly (2007) stated, "At present, these mashups are mostly innovative experiments, done by hackers" (p. 10). Despite the educational potential of data mashups, four main areas of concern must be considered. First, intellectual property rights, fair use, and copyright must be considered. Second, because mashups are comprised of data and logic from multiple sources on the Web, each one of those sources represents a potential point of failure if the resource is moved (Gartner, Inc., 2007). Third, any new technology should be carefully and critically assessed before

Table 2. Mashup Editors comparison

Mashup Editor	**Site**	**Strengths**	**Weaknesses**	**Notes**
Dapper	http://www.dapper.net/	Easy to use	More focused on web ads than other types of mashups	Reinvented as an on-the-fly ad generator
Microsoft's Popfly	http://www.popfly.com	Easy to use Simple interface	Less advanced customization features Still in alpha	Discontinued 8/24/09
Mozilla Ubiquity	https://ubiquity.mozilla.com/	Built-in set of commands to streamline and simplify mashup creation	Macintosh users must install an additional application before using Ubiquity	Still in beta
Yahoo! Pipes	http://pipes.yahoo.com/pipes	Customization and flexibility Hosting built-in	Steep learning curve for less experienced users	
Zembly	http://zembly.com	Easy to use Templates Hosting built-in	Less advanced customization features	Discontinued 12/30/09

Figure 5. Yahoo! pipes example

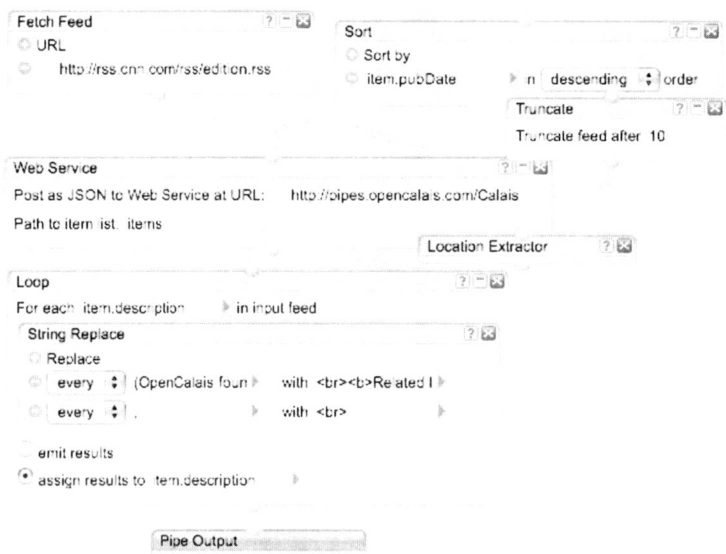

integrating into teaching and learning. Finally, not all web sites and services have made their underlying code available for inclusion in data mashups. However, mashup creators can find a way around open APIs and feeds through a process known as screen scraping. Lamb (2007) notes educators and policy-makers are already struggling with the challenges posed by readily accessible and reconfigurable digital technologies. The culture and ethical considerations of mashups pose a singular challenge.

Copyright, Intellectual Property Rights, and Fair Use

Given the ease with which Web services can be combined and mashed up to create a visually rich, content dense educational tool, making the determination of what constitutes an original work or derivative work is important. As Lethem (2007) stated, visual, sound, and text collage "might be called ***the*** art form of the twentieth century, never mind the twenty-first century" (p.1).

Knowing when a work is considered copyrighted is critical to the proper use of information found on the Internet. Since March 1, 1989, a work has been protected under copyright law from the moment it was created and produced in a tangible form so that it could be accessed with the aid of a machine or a device (United States Copyright Office, n.d.; Grossman, 1998) whether or not it bore a copyright notice (Stanford University, n.d.; Grossman; Hall, 1997).

The formal process of registering for a copyright ensures that the copyright owner is eligible for statutory damages and attorney's fees in successful litigation if the copyright is violated. The following sources may be freely used without citation:

- Works that lack originality like the phone book or unoriginal reprints of public domain works;
- Works in the public domain;
- Freeware;
- United States (U.S.) Government works;
- Facts, ideas, processes, methods, and systems described in copyrighted works.

Originally, copyrights lasted 14 years and provided protection for printing, reprinting, publishing, and vending. However, the Law had evolved to reflect changes in technology and society. The Sonny Bono Copyright Term Extension Act (CTEA) was passed October 27, 1998 for the purpose of extending copyrights an additional 20 years. Thus, works created after 1978, once covered for the life of the author plus 50 years, are now covered for the life of the author plus 70 years (Johnston, 1999). Works created and first published between 1950 and 1978 have a copyright lasting 75 years. Once the copyright on a work expires the work becomes public domain and is available for use and duplication. The copyright law has also been broadened to include dramatic works, motion pictures and other audiovisual works, sound recordings, sculpture, architecture, photographs, and computer programs. These changes in copyright law prompted the evolution of fair use. While copyright law will likely continue to evolve to deal with new technologies as they emerge, this information represents the current state of copyright law and fair use as they apply to digital technologies.

Fair use is explained and defined in Section 107 of the Copyright Act of 1976, in Title 17 of the U.S. Code. Section 107 contains a list of purposes for which duplication of a particular work may be considered "fair," such as criticism, comment, news reporting, teaching, scholarship, and research (United States Copyright Office, n.d.; University of Texas, n.d.; Effross, 1998; Nag, 1999; Walters, 1998). Section 107 (Appendix D) is seven pages in length, filled with legal and technical jargon, and difficult to comprehend. Many legal scholars, politicians, copyright owners, users, and their lawyers agree that fair use is so hard to understand that it fails to provide effective guidance for the use of others' works today (Cornell University, n.d.; Harper, 1998; Nag, 1999; Walters, 1998). Nevertheless, university faculty, staff, and students must develop a working understanding of copyright law and the fair use provisions to avoid infringement.

As no explicit legal specification exists to dictate when and how much information an individual can copy, the four-factor fair use guidelines exist to help make the determination:

1. What is the character of the use? If the copying will be used to illustrate or support a point in a lesson; will not be distributed for gain; will be intended for temporary use; or will be intended for nonprofit, educational, personal, criticism, commentary, news reporting, or parody, the copying would likely fall under fair use.
2. What is the nature of the work to be used? Articles from a newspaper would be treated differently than information from a workbook made for instruction. Graphics, audio, and video would be treated differently, on a case-by-case basis. Generally, if the work is fact-based or published it may fall under fair use.
3. How much of the work will be used? Copying an excerpt from a considerably longer work could fall under the fair use provision. "Be aware that in some cases, a small portion could capture the heart or essence of a work and be considered infringement," (Groton Public Schools, n.d.).
4. What effect would this use have on the market for the original or for permissions if the use were widespread? If copying information has an impact on the market it will likely be considered an infringement. However, the market test is not a litmus test for infringement because even works that do not have market impact can be considered an infringement (Cornell University, n.d.; Stanford University, n.d.; D'Amico, 1996a; Effross, 1998; Kaufman, 1999; Nag, 1999; Smith, 1999; Walters, 1998).

While all of these factors should be considered, the last factor is the most important in determining if a particular use qualifies as fair; even if copying part of a work falls under the fair use provision, the author or creator of the work should be credited. However, merely acknowledging the source of the copyrighted material does not substitute for obtaining permission if the use does not fall under the fair use umbrella. Regardless, the safest course of action is to get permission from the copyright owner before using copyrighted material.

The penalty for infringing upon a copyright owner's rights can be very costly (D' Amico, 1996b; Harper, 1998; Weiant, 1999). The court can award up to $100,000 for each act of intentional infringement (D'Amico, 1996b; Harper, 1998; Weiant, 1999). Intentional or willful infringement applies to a case where the individual knew a copyright infringement was being perpetrated and copied the material anyway (D'Amico, 1996a). Proof that the individual was ignorant of the law might reduce the ultimate monetary settlement but would not excuse the infringement. If the use of the copyrighted material should have reasonably been discovered by the institution or was sanctioned by the institution, they too would be held liable for infringement and be subject to the same penalties. Unfortunately, no set guidelines exist to obtain permission but there are recommended procedures that are likely to produce positive results (University of Texas, n.d.; Copyright Clearance Center, n.d.).

To update copyright law for digital technologies, the Digital Millennium Copyright Act of 1998 (DMCA), was signed by President Clinton October 28, 1998. The DMCA is considered by many legislators to be the most important copyright legislation since 1976 (Groton Public Schools, n.d.; Berman, 1998; Downing & Zelson, 1998; Leibowitz, 1998; Oman, 1999; Raul & Gomez, 1999; Schwartz & Metalitz, 1998; Sutin & Goldberg, 1998; Young, 1999). This legislation amended the U.S. Copyright Act to conform to two international copyright treaties from the World Intellectual Property Organization (WIPO) and the WIPO Performances and Phonograms Treaty of 1996 (Raysman & Brown, 1998; Raysman & Brown, 1999). The DMCA (1998) made the following provisions specifically pertaining to public and other nonprofit institutions of higher education:

- Limit liability of public and nonprofit institutions acting as Internet service providers;
- Require the U.S. Copyright Office to consult with copyright owners, nonprofit educational institutions, and nonprofit libraries and archives and submit to Congress recommendations on distance education exemptions to revise Section 110 of the Copyright Act for the digital age while maintaining an appropriate balance between the rights of copyright owners and the needs of users of copyrighted works;
- Update section 108, Limitations on exclusive rights: Reproduction by libraries and archives, of the Copyright Act to allow up to three copies of a work (including digital ones) to be made instead of one for preservation or replacement purposes.

The DMCA also included a provision that exempts online service providers and Internet access providers from copyright liability if customers infringe on copyrights (Berman, 1998; Downing & Zelson, 1998; Leibowitz, 1998; Oman, 1999; Raul & Gomez, 1999; Schwartz & Metalitz, 1998; Sutin & Goldberg, 1998; Young, 1999).

The Internet provides a means to seamlessly connect or link to other sites. Thus, understanding when linking constitutes copyright infringement is important (Harris, 1999; Mirchin, 1998). Though most organizations want to optimize exposure to their web sites, linking can pose problems when using deep linking (linking to a page other than the home page), IMG links (using trademarked logos or images), and when the link implies an endorsement or an affiliation that does not exist (Mirchin). Web site owners should follow two legal rules when linking:

- Linking without consent is presumed legal if the three conditions listed above have been taken into account.
- Consent to link should be obtained when a link would violate commercial fair play or owner has reasonable expectation of privacy.

Determining when material is copyrighted, when the four-factor analysis fair use test legalizes copying an excerpt from a copyrighted work, and when trademark use and linking are legal, is a tricky proposition. In order to successfully avoid infringing upon the copyrights of others on the web, keep the four-factor fair use analysis in mind and follow these pointers (Harris, 1999):

- Make sure information and materials used belong to the individual, belong to the web page creator, were in public domain, had been assigned or licensed to the Web page creator or the individual;
- Use written Web site agreements; negotiate all rights before use;
- Do not use unauthorized materials; never assume the defenses of fair use or implied license.

Mashup Logistics

Each component, API, feed, or web service of a data mashup is included from another site. At any time a web site could choose to change the assets or change the availability of assets being integrated into the mashup. As Gartner Research in David Berlind's Microsoft's Cloud Ecosystem Czar: 'When Mashups Fail, Whose Throat Do You Choke?' (2008) noted that "By 2010, Web mashups will be the dominant model (80 percent) for the creation of composite enterprise applications" (p. 1). Integration of this magnitude is truly a leap of faith that the resources used in these mashups will be stable.

A "mashup" is a lightweight tactical integration of multi-sourced applications or content into a single offering. Because mashups leverage data and services from public Web sites and Web applications, they're lightweight in implementation and built with a minimal amount of code. Their primary business benefit is that they can quickly meet tactical needs with reduced development costs and improved user satisfaction. Gartner warns that because they combine data and logic from multiple sources, they're vulnerable to failures in any one of those sources. (Gartner, Inc., 2007).

Berlind (2008) poses a number of questions about the wide spread use of composite enterprise applications developed through mashup technology. These well articulated questions include troublesome issues such as who do you call when your mashup application fails; how do you diagnose the cause of the failure; and "what happens when your cloud provider has multiple datacenters and has the ability to move your code around based on their need (read: not your need)?" (p. 2). These are the types of issues that arise out of a meteoric rise of a technology. The technology is advancing so quickly it is far outstripping the ability to regulate, set policy, or control. Add to the mix the remarkable number of players and the situation becomes even stickier.

Mashup Evaluation and the Digital Divide

What are the risks of encouraging and permitting teacher and learner created data mashups from an institutional perspective? Do we risk the same type of outcry encountered when students began to download music at an unprecedented rate from Napster? How do we address the needs of learners who may not have access to the technology necessary to participate in data mashup use or creation?

The National Center for Education Statistics (Lewis, Snow, Farris, Levin & Greene, 2000) recognized over a decade ago that students needed to have access to appropriate, and sometimes costly, technology with specific configurations. This need is even more compelling with the prospective use of educational mashups. Hardware requirements may include a particular processor speed, Internet connection speed, and sufficient memory for the use of the mashup editor. Software requirements may include a specific version of a particular browser and special plug-ins depending on the type of mashup editor, APIs, web services, and feeds needed for the mashup. For students without access to sophisticated computer technology, participating in this participatory learning experience may not be a choice in educational options. This phenomenon has been dubbed the "digital divide." The digital divide is often associated with a similar phenomenon, the "have and have-nots" in regard to technology access. However, other social factors also contribute to the digital divide. Participating technology dependent learning is complicated, if not impossible, for those with physical or learning disabilities. Gender equity and race issues also contribute to the digital divide.

Mashup Screen Scraping

Many sites, Google, Flickr, Yahoo, and others, have open content and APIs to facilitate automated machine consumption as used in data mashups. However, other sites were designed for human consumption not for machine consumption. Many of these sites have data that mashup developers may want to include in their creation. Screen scraping, the parsing and analyzing of content to extract semantic data structures that can be manipulated programmatically for sites designed for human, not automated machine consumption, allows mashup creators to use data that the site owner did not intend (Hoffman, 2009; Merrill, 2006). Intellectual property rights and copyright must be considered as educators and students create mashups creating a new resource by combining various resources created by someone else. The trade-off between protection of intellectual property and consumer privacy, fair use versus free flow of information, and the rights of unwitting content providers (data obtained through screen scraping) are a major concern. Creative Commons licensing provides a middle ground between restrictive copyright and the public domain and reuse with proper attribution.

SOLUTIONS AND RECOMMENDATIONS

Because data mashups fall under the umbrella of new and emerging technology, how we will deal with the complex issues discussed in the previous section is also emerging. Mashup integration will very likely require changes in practice, policy, and attitude. The Creative Commons allows users to license their work as either all rights reserved or some rights reserved. In other words, if the creator of a work wanted to share his or her work with others and allow them to make derivative works with attribution. "As technology becomes more sophisticated, developing the capacity to help us make moral and ethical choices as well as more pragmatic decisions, what we call 'human wisdom' will reach new levels" (Prensky, 2009, p. 2).

FUTURE RESEARCH DIRECTIONS

Leadership in the area of technology will become increasingly important as we strive to integrate interactive Web 2.0 technologies like data mashups into our teaching and learning strategies. Other new and emerging trends will also impact the ways in which data mashups are deployed and integrated. Because data mashups are still in their infancy, a dearth of solid, reliable, research is available. Data mashup research in all areas from policy to standardization to copyright to educational application needs to be conducted in order to fully understand the implications and potential of using data mashups from a user or creator of data mashups in an educational setting.

As educators and students begin to consider the integration of data mashups into the educational context, the following questions and concerns will need to be explored (adapted from Johnson et al., 2008):

- How do data mashups affect the learning process? Do they help students understand concepts?
- Do data mashups complement or enhance the understanding of information?
- Establish best practices in the development and use of data mashups through research.
- What visual formats are most effective in conveying concepts for learning?
- Is the data represented by the mashup valid?
- How are data mashups being used in learning? How effective are these strategies and practices?
- Do data mashups increase the personalization of learning?
- What standards should be developed for the use of data mashups?
- Do we need new or expanded copyright, intellectual property, and other laws and regulations for the use of data mashups?

CONCLUSION

The potential of mashups for education lies in the very serendipity they encourage. Even unorthodox mashups might be one creative instructor away from being compelling educational tools. With a nod to the future and knowing that intellectual property rights, copyright, cultural and ethical issues, and the stability of Web resources must be addressed, data mashups might just be the next big thing in teaching and learning.

REFERENCES

Alexander, B. (2006, March/April). Web 2.0: A new wave of innovation for teaching and learning? *EducauseReview*.

Barabasi, A. (2003). *Linked: How everything is connected to everything else and what it means for business, science, and everyday life*. New York: Penguin Press.

Batson, T. (2008). Using mashups to teach IT concepts at Bentley College. *Campus Technology*. Retrieved February 6, 2008 from http://campustechnology.com/Articles/2008/02/Using-Mashups-to-Teach-IT-Concepts-at-Bentley-College.aspx

Berlind, D. (2006). Mashup ecosystem poised to explode. *ZDNet*. Retrieved February 6, 2008, from http://blogs.zdnet.com/BTL/?p=2484

Berlind, D. (2008). *Microsoft's cloud ecosystem czar: 'When mashups fail, whose throat do you choke?'* Retrieved April 5, 2009 from http://www.informationweek.com/blog/main/archives/2008/11/micrososofts_cl.html

Berman, E. D. (1998). Preparing for the new millennium: Highlights of DMCA of 1998. *Multimedia & Web Strategist*, *5*(1), 1.

Bransford, J. D., Brown, A. L., & Cocking, R. R. (Eds.). (2000). How people learn: Brain, mind, experience, and school (Expanded Ed.). Washington, DC: National Academy Press.

Brown, J. S. (2005). *New Learning Environments for the 21st Century*. Retrieved from http://www.educause.edu/screencasts/JohnSeelyBrown@TWT_CU.pdf

Copyright clearance center. (1999). Retrieved March 24, 1999 from http://www.copyright.com

Cornell University. (n.d.). *Section 107. Limitations on exclusive rights: Fair use*. Retrieved March 24, 1999, from http://www4.law.cornell.edu/uscode/17/107.text.html

D'Amico, M. (1996a, May). Can I borrow a bit of digital? *NetGuide Magazine*.

D'Amico, M. (1996b, July). The web is not a legal quagmire. *Digital Media, 6*(2).

Davidson, C. N., & Goldberg, D. T. (2009). *The future of learning institutions in a digital age*. The John D., & Catherine T. MacArthur Foundation Reports on Digital Media Learning.

Downing, D. M., & Zelson, C. M. (1998). On intellectual property: The millennium arrives. *Intellectual Property, 7*(6).

Draves, W. A. (2002). *Teaching online*. River Falls, WI: LERN Books.

EDUCAUSE Learning Initiative. (2006). *7 things you should know about... Mapping mashups*. Retrieved February 24, 2008, from http://net.educause.edu/ir/library/pdf/ELI7016.pdf

Effross, W. A. (1998). Seamless seaminess? *Computer Law Strategist, 15*(8), 4.

Franklin, T., & van Harmelen, M. (2007, May). Web 2.0 for content for learning and teaching in higher education. *JISC*.

Gartner, Inc. (2007). *Mashups and the emerging technologies hype cycle*. Retrieved February 22, 2009, from http://www.webmashup.com/blog/2007/07/25/mashups-and-the-emerging-technoglogies-hype-cycle/

Grossman, M. (1998). Are you wrong about copyright? *Broward Daily Business Review*, December, B1.

Groton Public Schools. (n.d.). *Copyright implementation manual*. Retrieved March 24, 1999, from http://groton.k12.ct.us/mts/eg3.htm

Hall, B. (1997). *Web-based training cookbook*. New York: John Wiley & Sons, Inc.

Harper, G. (1998). *Fair use of copyrighted materials. Am I a crook on the Internet?*PBS Adult Learning Satellite Service.

Harris, R. D. (1999). Trademark and copyright law on the World Wide Web: A survey of the wild frontier. *Intellectual Property Today*, 44.

Hodgins, W. (2008). *The snowflake effect: The future of mashups and learning*. Retrieved January 8, 2009 from http://www.becta.org.uk

Hoffman, N. (2009). *Mashups using government data: A white paper*. Retrieved June 25, 2009 from http://www.mnhs.org/preserve/records/legislativerecords/docs_pdfs/DataMashups1.pdf

Johnson, L., Levine, A., & Smith, R. (2008). *The 2008 Horizon Report*. Austin, TX: The New Media Consortium.

Johnston, J. H. (1999, February). Putting Robert Frost on ice. *Legal Times*, 49.

Karch, M. (2009). *Mashup*. Retrieved April 2, 2009 from http://google.about.com/od/m/g/mashupdef.htm

Kaufman, J. (1999, March). The day the music web site died. *Legal Times,* 43.

Lamb, B. (2007, July/August). Dr. Mashup or why educations should learn to stop worrying and love the remix. *EDUCAUSE Review*, 13–24.

Leibowitz, W. (1998). The sound of one computer copy. *The National Law Journal*, A16.

Lethem, J. (2007). The ecstasy of influence. *Harper's Magazine*. Retrieved January 8, 2009 from http://www.harpers.org/archive/2007/02/0081387

Lewis, L., Snow, K., Farris, E., Levin, D., & Greene, B. (2000). Distance education at postsecondary education institutions: 1997-98. *National Center for Education Statistics*. Retrieved from http://nces.edu.gov/pubs2000/2000013.pdf

Mashup (Music). (2009). Retrieved June 2, 2009 from http://www.mashupshub.com/music/

McGee, P., & Diaz, V. (2007, September/October). Wikis and Podcasts and Blogs! Oh, My! What is a Faculty Member Supposed to Do? *EDUCAUSE Review*, 2007.

Merrill, D. (2006). *Mashups: The new breed of Web app*. Retrieved February 18, 2008 from http://www.ibm.com/developerworks/xml/library/x-mashups.html

Mirchin, D. M. (1998, October). Can you be held legally liable for hypertext linking? *Corporate Legal Times*, 22.

Nag, R. (1999, February). Parody or parasite? A copyright fair use analysis. *Intellectual Property Today*, 36.

Novak, J., & Voigt, B. (2008). *Mashing-up mashups: from collaborative mapping to community innovation toolkits*. Retrieved April 5, 2009 from http://www.ifi.uzh.ch/im/fileadmin/user_upload/personen_downloads/MCIS06.MashingUpMashups.Study.FullPaper.pdf

O'Reilly, T. (2007). Pipes and filters for the Internet. *O'Reilly Radar*. Retrieved February 6, 2008 from http://radar.oreilly.com/archives/2007/02/pipes-and-filte.html.

O'Reilly, T., & Battelle, J. (2009). *Web Squared: Web 2.0 five years on*.

Oman, R. (1999, January). US enacts new law on Internet copyright. *IP Worldwide*.

Palloff, R. M., & Pratt, K. (2003). *The virtual student: A profile and guide to working with online learners*. San Francisco: Jossey-Bass.

Prensky, M. (2001). *Digital natives, digital immigrants*. Retrieved February 19, 2004 from http://www.marcprensky.com

Prensky, M. (2005, September/October). Engage me or enrage me: What today's learners demand. *EDUCAUSE Review*, 2005.

Prensky, M. (2008a, November/December). The role of technology in teaching and the classroom. *Educational Technology*.

Prensky, M. (2008b, June). Young minds, fast times: The twenty-first century digital learner. *Edutopia*.

Prensky, M. (2009, February/March). H. Sapiens digital: From Digital Immigrants and Digital Natives to Digital Wisdom. *Innovate*.

Raul, A. C., & Gomez, M. A. (1999). Internet legislation in the 106th Congress, Several issues will vie for the limelight. *The Internet Newsletter: Legal & Business Aspects, 3*(10), 3.

Raysman, R., & Brown, P. (1998, December). The Digital Millennium Copyright Act. *New York Law Journal*.

Raysman, R., & Brown, P. (1999, March). Developments in trademark and domain-name disputes. *New York Law Journal*, 3–11.

Schmelzer, R. (2008). *Data mashups: Enabling ad hoc composite, headless, information services*. Retrieved June 26, 2009, from http://www.zapthink.com/report.html?id=ZAPFLASH-20081107

Schwartz, E. J., & Metalitz, S. J. (1998). The Digital Millennium Act: Why it is important. *The Intellectual Property Strategist, 5*(3).

Senge, P., Cambron-McCabe, N., Lucas, T., Smith, B., Dutton, J., & Kleiner, A. (2000). *Schools that learn: A fifth discipline fieldbook for educators, parents, and everyone who cares about education*. New York: Doubleday.

Slater, J. (2009). *42 things about Web 2.0 in 2008*. Retrieved June 26, 2009 from http://www.jasonslater.co.uk/2008/04/14/42-things-about-web-20-in-2008-part-1-of-3/

Smith, R. (n.d.). *Fair use: An online guide for educators*. Retrieved March 24, 1999 from http://www.fairuse.com

Stanford University. (n.d.). *Copyright law and fair use*. Retrieved March 24, 1999 from http://www.stanford.edu/group/CDL/copyright.html

Sutin, A. N., & Goldberg, E. (1998, December). High-tech agenda in Congress. *New York Law Journal*, S3.

United States Copyright Office. *Section 102*. (n.d.). Retrieved March 24, 1999 from http://lcweb.loc.gov/copyright/fls102/fl102.pdf

University of Texas. (n.d.). *Getting permission*. Retrieved February 3, 1999 from http://www.utsystem.edu/OGC/IntellectualProperty/permissn.htm

University of Texas. (n.d.). *Will we need fair use in the twenty-first century?* Retrieved February 3, 1999 from http://www.utsystem.edu/OGC/IntellectualProperty/fair_use.htm

Walters, M. D. (1998, October). Cyber-pirates beware. *Intellectual Property Magazine*.

Weiant, C. L. (1999, January). When computers cause mischief. *Legal Times*, S32.

Young, D. (1999). Congress modifies copyright protection for the digital age. *Legal Backgrounder, 14*(6).

ADDITIONAL READING

Cruger, R. (2003). *The mash-up revolution*. Retrieved April 1, 2009, from http://dir.salon.com/story/ent/music/feature/2003/08/09/mashups_cruger/index.html

Harvin, R. (2008). *Mash up your web site*. Retrieved March 28, 2009, from http://www.uschambermagazine.com/content/0802_tt.htm

Hof, R. (2005). Mix, match, and mutate. *Business Week*. Retrieved March 30, 2009, from http://www.businessweek.com/magazine/content/05_30/b3944108_mz063.htm

Kelley, M. (2008). Web 2.0 mashups and niche aggregators. Sebastopol, CA: O'Reilly Media, Inc.

Pattison, J. (2009). The sorry gap between shipping tech and customer expectations. *Ecommercetimes*. Retrieved March 30, 2009 from http://www.ecommercetimes.com/story/The-Sorry-Gap-Between-Shipping-Tech-and-Customer-Expectations-66527.html

Programmable Web. (n.d.). Retrieved January 3, 2009, from http://www.programmableweb.com/mashups

Schauland, D. (2009). What is a mashup? *Wise Geek*. Retrieved April 1, 2009, from http://www.wisegeek.com/what-is-a-mash-up.htm

Thompson, B. (2007). The mash-up future of the web. *BBC*. Retrieved March 28, 2009 from http://news.bbc.co.uk/1/hi/technology/6375525.stm

KEY TERMS AND DEFINITIONS

Mashup: Mashups include a wide variety of genres from music – primarily in the form of multiple sound tracks of multiple artists overlaying each other to create a new work; art - primarily in the form of collages of multiple artists' works to create a new work; data – primarily the leveraging of two or more application programming interfaces (APIs) and/or Web feeds to create a new work.

Data Mashup: Data mashups are a combination of multiple APIs and Web feeds from various sites to form a new work that was never intended or imagined by the original site creators.

Web 2.0: The use of second generation Web technology to encourage and enable human collaboration, sharing, communication, creativity, and innovation. Examples of Web 2.0 technologies include wikis, blogs, data mashups, social networking, and RSS or Atom feeds.

Copyright: Copyright provides legal protection to the creator of a work after it has been established in a fixed form (for instance a published work) whether the creator has marked the work with a copyright symbol or formally applied for copyright protection or not.

Intellectual Property: The legal intellectual property rights of an individual to maintain control over artistic and commercial innovations or creations of the person.

Remix: Reworking or adapting an existing work maintaining the essence of that original work.

Pedagogy: The art and science of being a teacher. The ability to weave interesting educational experiences into the fabric of the course content through instructional design and learning theory.

Engagement: As it is used in education, the degree to which a learning environment, strategy, process is able to immerse the student in the experience for deeper learning.

Section 6
Trends in Technology Education

Chapter 15
New Directions in the Research of Technology-Enhanced Education

Robert N. Ronau
University of Louisville, USA

Christopher R. Rakes
University of Louisville, USA

Margaret L. Niess
Oregon State University, USA

Lauren Wagener
University of Tennessee, USA

David Pugalee
University of North Carolina, USA

Christine Browning
Western Michigan University, USA

Shannon O. Driskell
University of Dayton, USA

Susann M. Mathews
Wright State University, USA

ABSTRACT

This chapter presents the results of a systematic review of literature in which the authors examined instructional technology integration in career and technical education, mathematics, language arts, social studies, and science. Three lenses were used to examine the literature: a research design framework, a teacher knowledge framework (CFTK), and a technology integration framework (TPACK). The research design framework revealed a low percentage of papers that were actually research studies (41.2%), favoring qualitative design (70% of the 41.2%). Consequently, educators may have difficulty

DOI: 10.4018/978-1-61520-899-9.ch015

sifting through high proportions of non-research to find the most informative, up-to-date instructional technology research. Three CFTK aspects of teacher knowledge were addressed less than others in the research studies: Individual Context (16%), Subject Matter (33%), and Discernment (29%). Pedagogical Knowledge was addressed the most (65%). The TPACK developmental framework revealed an emphasis on the lowest three levels of instructional technology integration (60%), indicating a gap in the research at the upper two levels. Mathematics studies accounted for almost half of all research addressing TPACK developmental stages (47%). From these findings, the authors conclude that pedagogical knowledge alone is not enough to ensure high levels of technology integration and offer recommendations for improving the disjointed nature of research on instructional technology.

INTRODUCTION

Teachers use instructional technology for online courses, video conferencing, electronic portfolios, and other exploratory projects. Literature reviews are important tools that teachers can use to evaluate instructional technology and develop strategies for its effective use. A systematic review of literature can make such evaluations far easier and more effective by synthesizing the results of the studies on a given topic using well-articulated methodological processes. The purpose of this chapter is to provide a systematic review of the impact of technology on teaching and learning and to propose a framework for looking at teacher knowledge from which gaps in the literature can be addressed. In this paper, the term "technology" refers to digital technology as opposed to other forms of instructional tools (e.g., overhead projectors, manipulatives).

Means, Wagner, Haertel, and Javitz (2003) identified two major issues regarding the use of technology for instruction: the pedagogical value of specific technology tools and the cumulative effects of technology exposure over time on student learning. In order to address these issues, educators need to assess specific sub-questions to gauge the effectiveness of technology as a teaching tool (e.g., What conditions foster learning with technology; what pedagogical strategies promote learning with technology; what teacher qualifications are related to content, technology, and implementation of pedagogical strategies; and to what internal and external classroom constraints must teachers attend when incorporating technology?). The complex nature of these questions requires multiple types of research and design.

Bell, Schrum, and Thompson (2009) suggested that the types of research needed to adequately address these issues include: (1) experimental or quasi-experimental studies, (2) large-scale studies, (3) studies with sufficient statistical information to be included in meta analysis and mixed-methodology studies, (4) studies with rich analysis of student content knowledge, and (5) studies that address the complexities of learners, classrooms, and schools. Recently, federal funding agencies such as the Institute of Education Sciences (IES; Whitehurst, 2003) have emphasized large scale experimental studies as the gold standard for scientific research. One such study, *Effectiveness of Reading and Mathematics Software Products: Findings from the First Student Cohort* (Dynarski et al., 2007), found that the technology programs used showed no significant improvement in student test scores in mathematics and reading. However, the results from a single study, even a large scale experimental study, are not conclusive in and of themselves. For example, Fitzer et al. (2007) challenged the generalizability of the Dynarski et al. (2007) study, noting that "this study oversimplifies the case by pushing aside these complicated relationships, and treating all the software programs as members of the same generic set of 'mathematics software' (or 'reading software')" (p. 3). Ronau et al. (2008) added that "The absence of teacher considerations along with a seemingly accepted view of a transmission model of learning with technology left the door open for better and richer technology research — research that addresses the complex situations occurring when various technologies are used in the mathematics classroom" (p. 19). From this example, we see that no one study or type of study can answer every pertinent question; small-scale empirical studies and qualitative studies fulfill an important role for research by answering focused questions in more detail than is feasible on a large scale. We suggest therefore that researchers seek a balance between various methodologies to better answer the multiple facets of key questions asked by stakeholders regarding the integration of technology in the classroom.

FRAMEWORKS FORTEACHER KNOWLEDGE

In addition to research design, this chapter is also interested in how previous studies have taken into account the impact of teacher knowledge on the effectiveness of the integration of technology in the classroom. Within the past few years, two new teacher knowledge frameworks have been proposed with the potential to support the research community in responding to questions on the impact of technology on learning. The Comprehensive Framework of Teacher Knowledge (CFTK) provides a three-dimensional model of teacher knowledge (Ronau et al., 2009). The Technology, Pedagogy, And Content Knowledge (TPACK) framework focuses on teachers' interconnected and interrelated knowledge of content, pedagogy, and technology (Mishra & Koehler, 2006; Niess, 2005a). Both structures emanate from the pedagogical content knowledge (PCK) framework proposed by Shulman (1986) as the specialized knowledge that teachers need for teaching.

Comprehensive Famework for Teacher Knowledge

CFTK organizes teacher knowledge into a three-dimensional model, each dimension comprised of two aspects: Field, comprised of the aspects Subject Matter Knowledge and Pedagogical Knowledge; Mode, consisting of the aspects Discernment and orientation; and Context, composed of the aspects Individual and Environment. This framework, depicted by the model in Figure 1, integrates multiple frameworks that address components of teacher knowledge to create an all-encompassing structure for studying and understanding the complex nature of knowledge required for the teaching profession (Ronau et al., 2009).

The first dimension of CFTK, Field, incorporates a broader scope and a more complex construct than simply the merging of pedagogy and subject matter as PCK (An, Kulm, & Wu, 2004; Davis & Simmt, 2003; Groth, 2007; Marks, 1990; Mishra & Koehler, 2006; Peressini, Borko, Romagnano, Knuth, & Willis, 2004; Wittmann, 1998; Zurita & Nussbaum, 2007). Instead, CFTK represents PCK as only one possible interaction within teacher knowledge. Subject matter and pedagogy also interact with teacher knowledge of Mode and Context to better capture the complexity of interplay between all three dimensions.

The second dimension of CFTK, Mode, describes the knowledge teachers rely on as they are engaged in their teaching profession; that is, knowledge about what to teach, how to teach, the ways students learn, and ways for a classroom to meet the needs of every student. The Orientation and Discernment aspects characterize knowledge of Mode. *Orientation* describes the knowledge of beliefs, dispositions, values, goals, and other personal qualities that embody and define an individual's views and actions toward learning and teaching. Teachers access this knowledge to understand and manage the way all affective issues impact a learning situation. *Discernment*,

Figure 1. CFTK framework of teacher knowledge as a three-dimensional structure

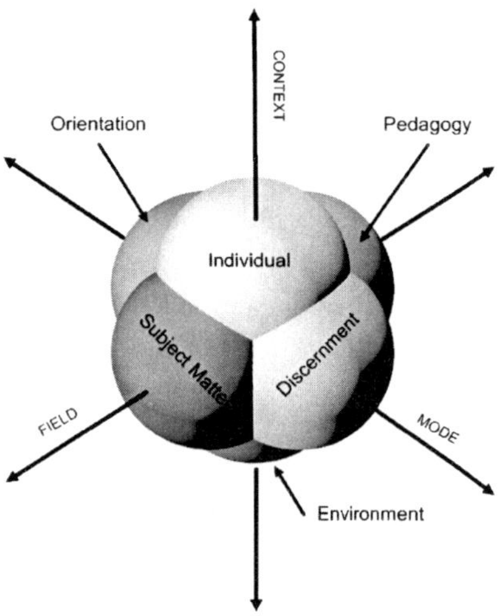

on the other hand, illustrates the knowledge lens through which teachers understand the impact of the cognitive domain (e.g., reflection in action, reflection on action, on-the-spot decision making). The interaction of these two aspects creates a dynamic knowledge base with which teachers can effectively manage multiple internal influences on student learning.

The third dimension of CFTK, Context, explains the knowledge teachers need of external factors that influence a learning situation. Two aspects of Context describe its sources: Individual and Environment. Contextual factors have a significant impact on the teaching and learning process, making knowledge of these factors essential to both teachers and researchers (for the importance of Context to teaching, see Bryk & Driscoll, 1998; Eraut, 1994; Felner et al., 1995, 2001; Scribner, 1999; for the importance of Context to research, see Cobb & Bowers, 1999; Datnow & Stringfield, 2000; diSessa & Cobb, 2004; Rossi & Stringfield, 1995a, 1995b; Stringfield, 1995; Teddlie & Stringfield, 1985; Wayman, Stringfield, & Yakimowski, 2004). *Individual* describes the knowledge of individual characteristics such as socioeconomic status (SES), gender, age, background, learning styles, and other contextual factors that impact an individual's approach to learning that teachers must understand and manage to be effective in a given learning situation. *Environment* describes knowledge on the impact of external factors on learning such as school climate, classroom climate, student teacher relationships, classroom organizational structures, school procedures, and other classroom, school, and community factors.

The understanding of learning contexts has evolved from simple considerations of individual characteristics and classroom environments to that of more all-encompassing, dynamic learning systems (Davis & Simmt, 2003; Davis & Sumara, 1997, 2001; Ding & Sherman, 2006). The interactions of the two aspects of Context with each other and with those of Field and Mode are able to more completely capture the complexity of learning under different demands and within a variety of situations.

Technology, Pedagogy, and Content Knowledge

TPACK provides a basic framework for more research attention to specifically address the role of technology in changing teacher behavior and in impacting student learning. TPACK is a response to the failure to actively integrate technologies in education during the 1980s and 1990s. During that period, many believed that increasing teacher awareness of the potential benefits of technology to learning would be enough to engender high levels of integration. Thus, teacher education programs were configured to provide teachers with opportunities to explore technology uses in the classroom. Yet, despite these educational supports, little active, meaningful, and continued integration of technology in learning environments occurred. With little evidence to suggest a reason for the lack of progress, multiple researchers began examining how teachers' understanding of technologies and PCK interact with one another to produce effective teaching with technology (Koehler & Mishra, 2008). Initially, the knowledge framework of Technological Pedagogical Content Knowledge (TPCK) was proposed as a complex interaction among three bodies of knowledge – technology, pedagogy, and subject matter content (Mishra & Koehler, 2006; Niess, 2005a). Late in 2007, TPCK was recast as TPACK, or the "total package" required for integrating technology, pedagogy, and content knowledge in the design of instruction for thinking and learning with technology; this recasting acknowledged the importance of the interactions between the individual constructs of the model technologies (Niess, 2007, 2008; Thompson & Mishra, 2007). Figure 2 shows the model used in visualizing this framework.

Figure 2. Venn diagram of TPACK as the intersection of content, pedagogy, and technology knowledge (adapted from Niess, 2008, p. 9)

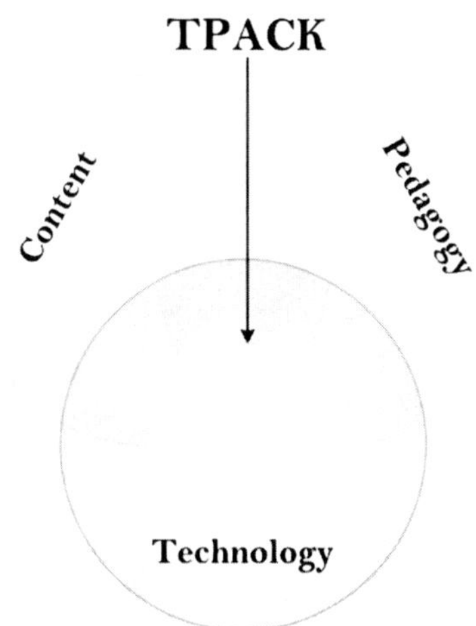

The TPACK framework provides a structure to guide research into the nature and development of teacher knowledge for teaching with technologies. Niess and colleagues (Niess, 2006; Niess, Lee, &Sadri, 2007; Niess et al., 2009) described teacher growth for technology integration in the classroom through five progressive stages:

1. **Recognizing (knowledge):** in which teachers are able to use the technology and recognize the alignment of the technology with subject matter content yet do not integrate the technology in the teaching and learning of subject matter.
2. **Accepting (persuasion):** in which teachers form a favorable or unfavorable attitude toward teaching and learning subject matter content with an appropriate technology.
3. **Adapting (decision):** in which teachers borrow from their prior experiences with the technology and implement the ideas in their classroom instruction, leading them to a choice to adopt or reject teaching and learning subject matter content with an appropriate technology.
4. **Exploring (implementation):** in which teachers actively integrate teaching and learning of subject matter content with an appropriate technology, designing their own ideas that allow more student-directed actions as they think about and plan their curriculum and instruction.
5. **Advancing (confirmation):** in which teachers make revisions in their curriculum as a result of the technology capabilities and evaluate the results of the decision to integrate teaching and learning subject matter content with an appropriate technology.

The Association Of Mathematics Teacher Educator's (AMTE) Technology Committee then created a visual description for thinking about these TPACK levels as they began the process of drafting a TPACK framework for mathematics teachers (Niess et al., 2009). Figure 3 portrays the levels that teachers engage in as they expand their knowledge and understandings in ways that merge multiple knowledge bases - technology, content, and pedagogy.

On the left side of the graphic, the figure highlights PCK as the intersection of pedagogy and content. As the knowledge of technology expands

Figure 3. Model of teacher thinking and understanding as their knowledge develops toward the intersection identified as important by TPACK (from Niess et al., 2009, p. 7)

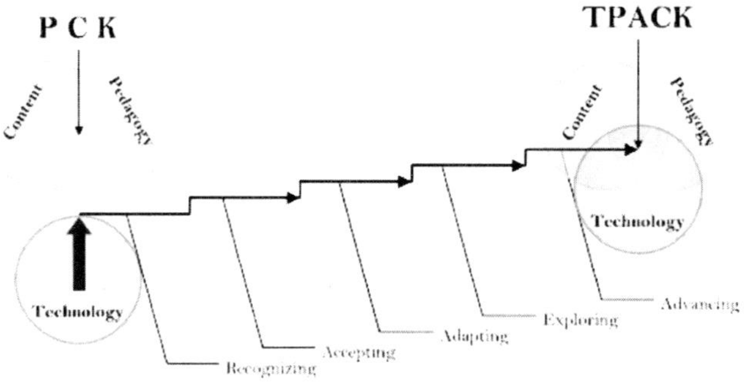

and begins to intersect with pedagogical and content knowledge, the teacher knowledge base described as TPACK emerges: This is a space in which teachers actively engage in guiding student learning of mathematics with appropriate technologies. The Committee's work in developing the framework considered the ideas provided by the National Educational Technology Standards for Teachers (NETS-T). These NETS-T standards were developed in 2002 and revised in 2008 by the International Society for Technology in Education (ISTE, 2008). The NETS-T standards were described for all teachers, regardless of content area. The Committee provided a content-specific view for mathematics teachers; Appendix A contains AMTE Board approved Mathematics TPACK framework.

Integrating the Frameworks

These two frameworks may seem to be competing images of the knowledge base teachers need for teaching with technology. However, a combination of the two frameworks may enhance our understanding of how technology integration and teacher knowledge interact in a learning environment. TPACK defines a framework that describes a series of levels for technology integration while CFTK provides insight into the teacher knowledge aspects and their interactions needed to implement the guidelines within that framework. For example, the first AMTE guideline for developing TPACK in the classroom, *Designing and developing digital-age learning environments and experiences - Teachers design and develop authentic learning environments and experiences incorporating appropriate digital-age tools and resources to maximize mathematical learning in Context* (Appendix A; Niess et al., 2009) requires more than just the knowledge of Subject Matter and Pedagogy, but also the knowledge of Orientation (for both teacher and student) and knowledge of individual and environmental contexts. In like fashion, the implementation of the second guideline (Teaching, Learning, and Curriculum) requires teacher knowledge best described by the knowledge of content and pedagogy (i.e., Field), student orientations and cognitive dynamics (i.e., Mode), and group dynamics (i.e., Context) integrated into a single construct. In a similar way, meeting the third AMTE guideline (Assessment and Evaluation) also requires the interaction of all six aspects of CFTK, particularly with the alignment of assessment tasks and procedures with that of classroom activities and expectations. Finally, the fourth guideline (Productivity and Professional Practice) incorporates the "Professional Identity" interaction described in the CFTK model (Ronau et al., 2009), originally defined by Peressini et al. (2004) and others.

In addition to these guidelines, the identification of the five developmental levels within TPACK for integrating technology into the classroom aligns easily with the interactions of the CFTK aspects, providing a way to gauge the degree or sophistication with which individuals incorporate technology into their teaching and learning. Treating technology as an interaction in CFTK expands the notion of TPACK from the one-dimensional foundation of PCK to a three-dimensional base that includes six aspects of teacher knowledge. For example, in moving from the Recognizing to the Accepting levels of TPACK, the teacher must not only merge Pedagogical knowledge with Subject Matter Knowledge but in the process, allow them to interact. They must also begin to tap into knowledge of Orientation.

To move from Accepting to Adapting, more sophisticated knowledge of subject matter is needed to facilitate the recognition of the fundamental differences of conceptual versus procedural knowledge. More development of pedagogical knowledge is also needed in order to construct new assessments and recognize the value of these new assessments over the old, procedural-based assessments. To progress from Adapting to Exploring, teachers develop their knowledge of student orientations and personal orientations further, recognizing the benefits of enhancing curriculum with technology-based instruction. Concurrently, the blending of subject matter and pedagogical knowledge continues through the Exploring stage. In order to begin exploring technology enhancements, teachers must also begin to tap into their knowledge of individual and environmental contexts. During the Exploring stage, teachers begin to mature in their understanding of the aspects of Field, and they begin to incorporate components of Mode and Context. As Exploring gives way to Advancing, the aspects of Mode and Context are further clarified and begin to interact. As teachers develop into higher levels of the Advancing TPACK stages, all six aspects of CFTK must be fully engaged and interacting.

The natural alignment between the TPACK and CFTK frameworks makes their integration uniquely capable of enabling researchers and practitioners to more fully understand the teacher knowledge required for the integration of technology into the classroom.

Methods

This study uses three frameworks (research design, CFTK, and TPACK) to interpret instructional technology research. We began by asking what types of research designs were used and how well the CFTK and TPACK models explained the teacher knowledge needed to integrate technology effectively in different content strands. To attend to these questions, we conducted a broad review of the research literature.

Study Inclusion Criteria

Three criteria were used to select the studies examined in this review: (1) Studies were found in scholarly, peer-reviewed journals, reports, dissertations, or conference proceedings, (2) Studies involved the use of technology in an educational setting, and (3) Studies focused on one of five specific fields (i.e., mathematics, science, career and technical education, language arts, or social studies).

Electronic Literature Search Strategy

In order to locate studies that met the criteria for this review, several electronic databases related to education and psychological sciences were searched. For mathematics, science, and career and technical education, these included the EBSCOhost databases: Academic Search Premier, Education Administration Abstracts, ERIC, Middle Search Plus, Psychology and Behavioral Sciences Collection, PsycINFO, Sociological Collection, and Teacher Reference Center; two H.W. Wilson databases: Education Full Text and the Social

Sciences Index; JSTOR; five ProQuest databases: Career and Technical Education, Dissertations & Theses, Ethnic NewsWatch, GenderWatch, and Research Library; the IEEE Electronic Library; and three ISI Web of Knowledge databases: the Science Citation Index Expanded, the Social Sciences Citation Index, and the Arts and Humanities Citation Index. Because some databases are specific to the language arts, extra H.W. Wilson databases were included when searching for literature in that field: Art Abstracts, Art Retrospective, Essay & General Lit, Humanities Index, and Short Story Index. Due to the overlapping nature of some social studies and language arts journal indexing, these extra databases were also used for searching social studies publications.

Keywords varied for each content area and database. Basic search terms were used to begin searching keywords and subject indices in each database (e.g., language arts, technology, education, social studies, history, geography, science, mathematics, career and technical education). Each database uses different keywords and search terms, so for each search, the basic search terms were altered to maximize the number of results and their relevance. For example, EBSCOhost databases used the subject term "Career and Technical Education," whereas ProQuest used the term "Vocational Education" (see Appendix C for full list of search terms).

Random Sample

The literature search identified a population of journal articles, reports, dissertations, and conference papers dating from 1967 to 2009. For the remainder of this paper, the term "study" refers to any one of these categories. To ensure equal representation, a stratified random sample of approximately 30 studies was extracted from the population of each content area using random number generator software from Minitab Version 15 (see Table 1).

Sample Coding

The coding instrument was developed by the team at the University of Louisville (Appendix B). The developers then tested and revised the instrument and eventually distributed it to the coding team. The coding protocol for this instrument captured information about the study itself (e.g., author, year the paper was published or the study was carried out), type of research design where applicable (e.g., qualitative, quantitative, theory development, or practitioner resource), the type of technology being examined or described, the type of knowledge being described/developed by the study, and TPACK level(s) supported by the study.

To code the sample studies, we began by screening titles and abstracts for eligibility based on the study inclusion criteria, as previously described. For studies that met inclusion criteria, we recorded all applicable information on the coding instrument.

Studies identified with a quantitative research design were also coded as being either randomized or quasi-experimental. We also recorded their outcome measures, reliability measures, and validity measures as well as their selection mechanisms and use of measures to control pre-existing differences. Studies identified as qualitative, were coded by their research design (e.g., narrative/historical, biography, design study, phenomenology, ethnography, grounded theory, or case study), the methodology employed (e.g., covert/overt observation, interview, or focus group), alignment of the study methodology with outcome(s) of interest, and evidence of trustworthiness. For studies with the purpose of theory development, we recorded as much applicable information as possible and marked the rest as "not applicable." In some fields, studies were intermingled with presentations of pedagogical strategies. These studies were not excluded if they were found in a peer-reviewed, scholarly journal. In these cases, the lack of research foundation was noted, and all other relevant information was coded.

Inter-rater reliability. In order to reduce the variation in coding decisions, we developed coding tables with closed response systems. Furthermore, coders began by examining exemplar studies with various research designs. Due to the expected variation across the five subject areas and the low degree of commonalities, we chose to rely on coordinated discussions with each coder to maintain uniformity of decisions. These discussions centered on difficulties deciding how a particular study's characteristics fit into the coding rubrics, mostly resulting from the emergent nature of the coding process (Patton, 2002). For example, every coder encountered a surprising number of papers that did not report research findings. We decided to add a non-research category to the coding results to fully report those findings. Another example of the evolving nature of this review surfaced as the types of qualitative inquiry from each content area were cross-checked. Specifically, the mathematics sample contained no narrative methodology studies, but the social studies and language arts fields did. Therefore, the mathematics sample was re-examined through that lens to ensure uniformity across the five content areas.

RESULTS

Summary of the Literature

Coders noted the distinctly low percentage of literature in scholarly, peer-reviewed journals actually dedicated to the presentation of research findings: 46% in career and technical education, 29% in social studies, 31% in science, 23% in language arts, 44% in mathematics, and 34% across all five subject matter areas (see Table 2). Of the non-research articles, 41% provided anecdotal descriptions of specific strategies used in classrooms for integrating technology. Only 20% of the non-empirical articles were dedicated to the development of theoretical models based on prior research. A few scholarly articles only offered opinions (9%). In Table 2 and in the descriptions that follow, studies may be counted more than once in the subcategories, so the totals in the subcategories may be greater than the number of studies in that category. For example, in the mathematics area, the 10 qualitative studies register as 12 subcategories.

Career and Technical Education (CTE). CTE research carried a distinctly international flavor. Studies included the use of email and discussion groups by rural farmers in Australia

Table 1. Stratified random sample of studies

Subject Matter	Number of Published Papers	Final Sample Size
Mathematics	309	30
Science	335	29
Career and Technical Education	497	28
Language Arts	179	30
Social Studies	465	28
Total	1785	145

Table 2. Breakdown of research designs

Research designs	Career & Technical Education	Social Studies	Science	Language Arts	Mathematics	Total[b]
Quantitative	2	0	4	0	5	11
Mixed Methods	0	1	2	1	0	4
Qualitative Overall[a]	10	7	3	5	10	35
Narrative/Historical	0	2	0	0	0	2
Case Study	2	3	1	1	9	14
Multi-Case Study	0	0	0	0	2	2
Ethnography	1	1	0	0	0	2
Action Research	0	0	1	0	1	2
Survey	3	1	0	1	0	5
Interview	1	0	2	4	0	7
Focus Groups	2	0	0	1	0	3
Observation	1	0	1	2	0	4
Non-Research	16	20	20	24	15	95
Theory Development	3	5	3	3	5	19
Instructional Strategy Description	2	7	6	3	6	24
Anecdotal Description	4	7	11	14	3	39
Book Review/Article Commentary	3	0	0	0	1	4
Opinion Papers	4	1	0	4	0	9
[a]Some studies used more than one method, so sub-scores may not add up to the overall number of studies using qualitative design. [b]$N = 145$.						

(Mulcahy, 1998), the introduction of Information and Communication Technology (ICT) into all of the schools in Estonia (Toots & Lanpere, 2004), the introduction of interactive whiteboards into African schools (Slay, Siebörger, & Hodgkinson-Williams, 2008), and the use of on-line discussion groups (De Smet, Van Keer, & Valcke, 2008; Steinkuehler & Duncan, 2008). These studies focused primarily on upper middle grades through adult education. Of the 28 studies in this sample, 57% were categorized as non-research, 36% qualitative, 7% were quantitative, and 0% were mixed methods (see Table 2). The non-research papers were mostly composed of anecdotal description (25%), opinion papers (25%), and theory development (19%).

Social Studies. The social studies sample also included an international scope. For example, in the United Kingdom (UK), studies have explored the impact and potential of web-based technologies (Fernandez-Cardenas, 2008; Richards & Wrigley, 1996; Selwyn, 2007); in Canada, researchers have viewed information technology as a vector for enhancing collaborative learning (Reed & Mitchell, 2001); in Japan, the use of geographic information systems has evolved far enough to be considered a distinct field (Sasaki, Oguchi, Okabe, & Sadahiro, 2008).

Approximately 33% of the sample literature of technology in social studies focused on the learning of history, 23.3% on bridging theory and practice, 20% on the learning of geography, 16.7% on the understanding of culture, and 6.7% on teacher education. These percentages indicated a potential gap in the area of teacher education and over-representation of practice related pieces.

These practice-related pieces often provided the description of one or two technology products and described how they could be applied in educational settings (e.g., Bodson, 2008; Lynch et al., 2008). These articles advocated for the versatility that was possible through technology for teaching geography, although the authors often failed to provide specific illustrative examples that would move the discussion about technology innovations forward. One promising work described the use of computer simulations as a tool for replicating real-life phenomenon through the exploration of visual interactions within artificial societies (Berson & Berson, 2007). Such models may hold the potential to assist students understanding of the complex dynamics that influence how societies evolve and adjust.

The paucity of research publications in social studies obscured potential trends in research design and methodology. The majority of this sample reported using qualitative methodologies (88%), primarily depending on interviews (e.g., Hess, 2007) and to a lesser extent, observations as the primary data collection tools. Ethnographic methods were also used to explore the communicative acts in the collaborative creation of web pages (e.g., Fernandez-Cardenal, 2008). Case studies using the class as the unit of analysis were also found (e.g., Reed & Mitchell, 2001), though some studies involved multiple sections of specific courses at different universities. Surveys were employed in several studies (e.g., Longhurst, 2003); however, the method of analysis varied widely, from the use of simple descriptive statistics to more sophisticated inferential techniques. Several studies offered ideas on a research agenda for the field (e.g., Defazio, 2006; Ely, 2008), lending support to the belief that current literature lacks the ability to link instructional theory to practice.

The 28 studies in the social studies sample were categorized as 71% non-research, 25% qualitative, 4% mixed methods, and 0% quantitative (see Table 2). The 20 non-research papers were mostly composed of instructional strategies (35%), anecdotal description (35%), theory development (19%), and opinion papers (5%).

Science. The science sample included studies from multiple fields of science education (e.g., middle school science, high school science, computer science education, and first-year engineering learning communities). These studies varied widely in focus. For example, Lawrence (2000) developed a framework for curriculum development in science education using apprenticeship activities with high school students. Bowman, Koirala, and Edmonds (2000), on the other hand, investigated how one teacher altered her pedagogy to include graphing calculators. Boulet, Boudreault, and Guerette (1997) compared the effects of distance education versus the traditional classroom in computer science education and found a slight advantage for distance over traditional education. Jenkins (2006) reported on the attitudes of students in England toward their secondary school science education. Min (2005) examined the effect of a hypermedia-enhanced problem-based learning environment in astronomy on sixth-graders' science knolwedge, attitudes toward learning science with technology, and motivation toward learning. The 29 studies in the science sample were categorized as 69% non-research, 14% quantitative, 10% qualitative, and 7% mixed methods (see Table 2). The 20 non-research papers included anecdotal description (55%), instructional strategies (30%), and theory development (15%).

Language arts. A review of the literature in language arts revealed that many of these studies also did not present research findings. These studies discussed the integration of technology through multiple tools and strategies (e.g., interactive whiteboards, computer-assisted instruction, computer-assisted discussions, computer-aided peer review, use of the internet, multimedia presentation of museum education, and digital technology to enhance literacy).

The six studies reporting research findings represented three distinct types of inquiry: (1) investigating teachers' perception of the use of case methodology for instruction in a graduate level course (Baker, 2005; Gray, 2001); (2) examining the nature of English language arts teachers' learning during technology professional development activities and the impact on their later technology-supported pedagogy (Hughes, 2005); and, (3) studying language arts teachers from the United States, Canada, and Australia and their use of literature-based collaborative Internet projects in their elementary classrooms (Karchmer-Klein & Layton, 2006; Malloy & Gambrell, 2006; Siegel, 2006).

The 30 studies in the language arts sample were categorized as 80% non-research, 17% qualitative, 3% mixed methods, and 0% quantitative (see Table 2). The non-research papers were mostly composed of anecdotal descriptions of experiences with technology use in the classroom (58%), followed by opinion pieces (16.7%), theory development (13%), and instructional strategies (13%).

Mathematics. The mathematics sample studies investigated and discussed a wide variety of technology (e.g., computers, computer software, online courses and course materials and grading, web-based learning environments, multimedia, and interactive whiteboards) with over half of the studies focusing on computers and the Internet. With the emergence of new web-based technologies and the rise of java- and flash-based applications (i.e., virtual manipulatives as in Cavanaugh et al., 2008; Suh & Moyer, 2007), this new emphasis caused little surprise or concern. However, we also expected that the large number of debates surrounding the effectiveness of calculators and graphing calculators (e.g., Ellington, 2003, 2006) would have resulted in another cluster of studies reporting such research. In this sample, none of the articles discussed the use of calculators in the classroom. Although the absence of such research in the sample does not translate into a complete absence of the topic from the greater population of studies, it does raise a concern about a potential weak point or gap in the mathematics research literature.

Finally, in three studies, approximately 10% of the sample, methodology was either not addressed or lacked sampling information such as sample sizes (Hayes & Mayerick, 2001; O'Connell & Phye, 2005; Zucker, Tinker, Staudt, Mansfield, & Metcalf, 2008). Other reviews have called for better reporting of standard information such as methodology, sample sizes, and standard deviations (e.g., McCoy, 1998; Mervielde, 1977; Nowak, 1969; Triandis, 1976). In light of these calls, we concluded that these studies may be indicative of a general weakness in the research literature. So, not only are there gaps in the existing literature, but the studies that have been completed in this area may be limited by their design and the information they provide. As a result, educators are left to evaluate the effectiveness of some types of instructional technology on their own without a dependable research foundation.

We identified50% of the 30 mathematics sample studies as non-research, 33% as qualitative, 17% as quantitative, and 0% as mixed methods (see Table 2). The non-research papers were mostly composed of instructional strategies (40%), followed by theory development (33%), anecdotal description (20%), and book reviews (7%).

RESEARCH DESIGNS

An examination of research designs revealed an imbalance across all five subject areas. Quantitative designs accounted for only 22% of all studies;

mixed methodology was only 8%, and qualitative designs accounted for the remaining 70% (see Table 2). These research methodologies represent fundamentally different beliefs. Quantitative methodology, seeks to capture the essence of reality, setting the researcher as a dispassionate, objective observer. In this methodology, controls are set in place to isolate causal factors in a system (Hewitt, 2006). Qualitative methodology, on the other hand, recognizes the need to understand the unquantifiable factors that influence the way people behave in different settings. Postmodernist, constructionist, and advocacy researchers tend to gravitate toward these methodologies (Cresswell, 2007; Patton, 2002). Rather than attempting to create generalizability or lay claim to causal inference, qualitative inquiry seeks to understand why something happens in a particular setting. In both cases, the research question should drive the methodology rather than the reverse (Tashakkori & Teddlie, 1998). Researchers need to be well-versed in both types of methodology so that the types of questions they can ask are not limited by methodological concerns.

Alternatively, pragmatists choose whatever methodologies fit the question, taking advantage of the power of both quantitative and qualitative methodology (Cresswell, 2007; Patton, 2002). Tashakkori and Teddlie (1998) and Datta (1994) described several practical reasons for using mixed methodology (historical use of both quantitative and qualitative methods, support of research community and funding agencies for both methods, the influence of both methods on educational policy, and the demonstrable effectiveness of both methods). Shadish (1995) also made a case for the complementary nature of quantitative and qualitative methods. With such important advantages to mixed methodology, its low representation in every subject matter reveals a significant weakness in educational technology research.

TEACHER KNOWLEDGE

We used the CFTK framework to identify aspects of teacher knowledge in technology studies across the five fields. Of the 145 studies, 48 addressed teacher knowledge in some manner (see Table 3). Only eight of the 48 addressed knowledge of Individual Context. In fact, the samples for language arts and science failed to address Individual Context at all. Surprisingly, only one third addressed knowledge of Subject Matter. Finally, less than one third included knowledge of Discernment.

Individual Context represents the aspect of knowledge related to understanding the way student characteristics affect a learning situation. Distinct from the internal factors of Orientation (e.g., beliefs, affect, efficacy), these Contextual factors (e.g., gender, culture) may influence the way students react to cooperative learning, mastery learning, and peer tutoring or to technology or the Subject Matter (Ronau et al., 2009). Because technology tools often rely heavily on each of these strategies, the lack of research to address the effect teacher knowledge of contextual differences limits the ability of that research to adequately address the needs of educators wishing to integrate technology effectively.

STAGES OF TECHNOLOGY INTEGRATION

Table 4 reveals a large imbalance in the number of studies across each subject matter area addressing the stages of TPACK favoring the mathematics field. Because TPACK has been more actively pursued in the mathematics field, it came as no surprise to see that this field demonstrated a more comprehensive examination of each stage of technology integration, accounting for a minimum of 60% of all studies addressing any particular aspect.

Although 65% of the sample studies addressed pedagogical knowledge, very few studies addressed TPACK stages of integrating technol-

Table 3. Aspects of teacher knowledge addressed

CFTK Aspects	Career & Technical Education	Social Studies	Science	Language Arts	Mathematics	Total
Subject Matter	2	5	1	1	7	16
Pedagogical Knowledge	3	6	5	4	13	31
Orientation	2	6	4	4	10	26
Discernment	3	4	1	3	3	14
Individual Context	1	2	0	0	5	8
Environmental Context	5	6	7	4	7	29
Total Number Relevant	11	8	9	5	15	48
Note. Some studies addressed more than one aspect, so aspect numbers may not add up to the overall number of relevant studies.						

Table 4. TPACK stages addressed

TPACK Stages	Career & Technical Education	Social Studies	Science	Language Arts	Mathematics	Total
Recognizing	4	7	3	3	21	38
Accepting	4	4	0	3	21	32
Adapting	4	2	5	3	21	35
Exploring	1	0	0	2	17	20
Advancing	0	0	1	3	18	22
Total Number of Studies	5	8	9	5	25	53
Note. Some studies addressed more than one stage of TPACK, so studies addressing a particular stage may not add up to the total number of studies addressing TPACK.						

ogy, explicitly or implicitly, in any area besides mathematics. By blending CFTK and TPACK developmental views, a new understanding of instructional technology emerges: Pedagogical knowledge alone will not ensure effective technology integration. Tankersley, Landrum, and Cook (2004) suggested that one reason teachers fail to make instructional changes may be a lack of support. In the case of instructional technology, support may simply mean providing access to technology tools. It may also include professional development that familiarizes teachers with the TPACK framework and methods of integrating technology into instruction.

DISCUSSION

This chapter endeavored to provide a systematic review of the literature about instructional technology. The authors hope that this information increases the ease with which teacher educators can synthesize research findings to integrate the most effective instructional technology tools into their courses. We also hope that the three frameworks presented here inform future instructional technology studies regarding the needs of the research community and educators. To summarize, we consider the limitations of this review along with the findings and the utility of our three research lenses: research design, teacher knowledge, and technology integration. We conclude with some final recommendations.

LIMITATIONS

The subjective nature of much of the coding constituted the greatest limitation to this study. Although great effort was made to coordinate responses through the use of coding tables and discussions for each ambiguous decision, some variability was unavoidable. However, we did attempt to ensure a systematic process through coordinating discussions to increase the possibility of replication and verification.

A second limitation arose from the use of a single random sample from each subject area. The randomization process is the most robust way to ensure representativeness and lack of sampling bias (Shadish, Cook, & Campbell, 2002), and each subject area had a large enough sample size to achieve sufficient power to realize that representativeness. However, multiple samples could have been used to cross-validate our findings.

The new design of using the CFTK and TPACK models together as a lens for examining research designs created a third limitation to this study. With the relatively new nature of each framework (TPACK from Niess, 2005a, 2008; CFTK from Ronau et al., 2009), a certain degree of misalignment between the vocabulary of the sample studies and the frameworks was inevitable.

FINDINGS

The use of the research design lens revealed a surprisingly low percentage (34%) of research studies. Of these research studies, qualitative research designs constituted a disproportionate amount of the methodology types (70%). Mixed methodology, on the other hand, was nearly nonexistent (8%). Finally, rather than an even 20% for each field, the breakdown of studies indicated an imbalance in the number of papers on instructional technology across the fields (mathematics, 17%; science, 19%; CTE, 28%; language arts, 10%; and social studies, 26%), highlighting a lack of focus on language arts technology education.

THE RESEARCH LENSES

As a byproduct of the review, we also considered the degree to which the lenses of research design, teacher knowledge, and technology integration interacted to contribute to understanding of the depth, scope, and balance of the available research in educational technology. The research design lens allowed us to compare published papers and study methodologies. The CFTK lens contributed an understanding of the types of teacher knowledge addressed by the sample literature. The TPACK lens offered insight into the way papers addressed technology integration in education. Taken together, these three frameworks revealed significant bias toward the use of certain designs, aspects of teacher knowledge, and only moderate levels of technology integration. Broad research interests and findings exist; however, the large percentages of anecdotal descriptions and opinion papers disguise the lower number of research reports and theoretical models. The continuation of such a trend only hinders the ease with which teacher educators and researchers can integrate existing theory into practice.

RECOMMENDATIONS

The results of this study indicated that 65% of the sample studies on educational technology did not actually report research, and 70% of the research studies employed qualitative designs. This finding does not address the relative value of qualitative or quantitative studies or of research versus non-research studies: All of these designs have the potential of being valuable for understanding the role and impact of technology in education. On the other hand, if the assumption is that all of these study types are of equivalent value, then a reasonable conclusion would be a call for a balance among these designs in order to provide a broader lens to increase the understanding of educational technology. Currently, the evidence suggests that an imbalance exists in our research data that is biased toward non-research papers and qualitative designs among the research studies. Furthermore, as Whitehurst (2002) suggested, all types of evidence are not equal; their value to compare, evaluate, and monitor progress of the target of study forms a hierarchy of evidence or of study designs that are ranked from 1 (high value) to 6 (low value): (1) randomized trial (true experiment), (2) comparison groups (quasi-experiment), (3) pre-post comparison, (4) correlational studies, (5) case studies, and (6) anecdotes. Using his hierarchy as a lens, we see from the present study that the trend in educational technology study designs is to emphasize these methodologies in reverse order. Therefore, we recommend that the educational community work toward a balance of evidence quality.

One way to address this imbalance is to use more mixed methodology designs. Tashakkori & Teddlie (1998) rejected the notion that qualitative and quantitative research designs are opposing sides of a long-standing argument; instead, they adopted a pragmatic viewpoint that uses each as a complementary tool to answer the complex educational questions that researchers are being challenged to answer today. They developed mixed methodology models that structurally employ both qualitative and quantitative designs at various stages of a research project. Only four papers out of the 145 papers analyzed in this chapter contained mixed methodology reports. As the research community strives toward balance in research design, mixed methodology should become a predominant design.

Further use of the CFTK and TPACK frameworks combined with a consideration for design and methodology may also help increase balance in educational technology research. TPACK offers a balance of developmental levels of technology integration by providing a structure for focus and scale, whereas CFTK contributes balances six different aspects of teacher knowledge. Taken together, educators have a robust tool for analyzing the effectiveness of instructional technology methods and bringing the best tools to the classroom.

REFERENCES

Aberg-Bengtsson, L. (2006). Then you can take half. almost--Elementary students learning bar graphs and pie charts in a computer-based Context. *The Journal of Mathematical Behavior, 25*, 116–135. doi:10.1016/j.jmathb.2006.02.007

Abramovich, S., & Norton, A. (2006). Equations with parameters: A locus approach. *Journal of Computers in Mathematics and Science Teaching, 25*, 5–28.

Adams, J. L., & Stephens, L. J. (1991). A comparison of computer-assisted instructional methods. *International Journal of Mathematical Education in Science and Technology, 22*, 889–893. doi:10.1080/0020739910220604

Agre, P. E. (2000). Infrastructure and institutional change in the networked university. *Information Communication and Society, 3*, 494–507. doi:10.1080/13691180010002323

Ainley, J., & Pratt, D. (1995). Supporting teachers' and children's mathematical thinking: A strategy for the effective use of information technology. *Technology, Pedagogy and Education, 4*, 81–92. doi:10.1080/0962029950040107

Alavi, M., Wheeler, B. C., & Valacich, J. S. (1995). Using IT to reengineer business education: An exploratory investigation of collaborative telelearning. *Management Information Systems Quarterly, 19*, 293–312. doi:10.2307/249597

An, S., Kulm, G., & Wu, Z. (2004). The pedagogical content knowledge of middle school, mathematics teachers in China and the U.S. *Journal of Mathematics Teacher Education, 7*, 145–172. doi:10.1023/B:JMTE.0000021943.35739.1c

Antonitsch, P. K., Kleinhagauer, R., & Micheuz, P. (2008). Incorporating history in secondary education informatics courses. *IEEE Annals of the History of Computing, 30*, 56–63. doi:10.1109/MAHC.2008.49

Baggott, L., Wishart, J., McFarlane, A., Brawn, R., & John, P. (2007). Teaching and learning with ICT within the subject culture of secondary school science. *Research in Science & Technological Education, 25*, 339–350. doi:10.1080/02635140701535158

Baker, E. A. (2005). Can preservice teacher education really help me grow as a literacy teacher? Examining preservice teachers' perceptions of multimedia case-based instruction. *Journal of Technology and Teacher Education, 13*, 415–431.

Barbas, M. P. (2006). Expanding knowledge: From the classroom into cyberspace. *Educational Media International, 43*, 65–73. doi:10.1080/09523980500490885

Bell, L., Schrum, L., & Thompson, E. A. (Eds.). (2009). *Framing the research on digital technologies and student learning in mathematics*. Charlotte, NC: Information Age Publishing.

Berson, I. R., & Berson, M. J. (2007). Exploring complex social phenomena with computer simulations. *Social Education, 71*, 136–139.

Bodzin, A. M. (2008). Integrating instructional technologies in a local watershed investigation with urban elementary learners. *The Journal of Environmental Education, 39*, 47–58. doi:10.3200/JOEE.39.2.47-58

Boechler, P. M., Foth, D., & Watchorn, R. (2007). Educational technology research with older adults: Adjustments in protocol, materials, and procedures. *Educational Gerontology, 33*, 221–235. doi:10.1080/03601270600894089

Boulet, M. M., Boudreault, S., & Guerette, L. (1997, November). *Distance education: Integrating technology into computer science education.* Paper presented at the 27th annual Frontiers in Education Conference, Pittsburg, PA.

Bowman, J. K., Koirala, H. P., & Edmonds, L. E. (2000). Graphing calculators: Critical tools for actively teaching math and science. *Computers in the Schools, 16*, 135–149. doi:10.1300/J025v16n03_03

Bricout, J. C. (2001). Making computer-mediated education responsive to the accommodation needs of students with disabilities. *Journal of Social Work Education, 37*, 267–281.

Bryk, A. S., & Driscoll, M. E. (1988). The high school as community: Contextual influences and consequences for students and teachers. Madison, WI: National Center on Effective Secondary Schools. (ERIC Document Reproduction Service No. ED302539)

Buxton, C. A. (2005). Creating a culture of academic success in an urban science and math magnet high school. *Science Education, 89*, 392–417. doi:10.1002/sce.20057

*Call for a national policy on science education. (1989). *Bioscience, 39,* 130-130.

Cavanaugh, C., Gillan, K. J., Bosnick, J., Hess, M., & Scott, H. (2008). Effectiveness of interactive online algebra learning tools. *Journal of Educational Computing Research, 38*, 67–95. doi:10.2190/EC.38.1.d

Chua, B. L., & Wu, Y. (2005). Designing technology-based mathematics lessons: A pedagogical framework. *Journal of Computers in Mathematics and Science Teaching, 24*, 387–402.

Cobb, P., & Bowers, J. (1999). Cognitive and situated learning perspectives in theory and practice. *Educational Researcher, 28*, 4–15. doi:10.2307/1177185

Cornford, J. (2000). The virtual university is... the university made concrete? *Information Communication and Society, 3*, 508–525. doi:10.1080/13691180010002314

Cowan, C., Hartleb, D., & Neves, D. (2007). Collaboration on technology projects results in cost sharing opportunities. *Community College Journal of Research and Practice, 31*, 503–504. doi:10.1080/10668920701359615

Creswell, J. W. (2007). *Qualitative inquiry and research design* (2nd ed.). Thousand Oaks, CA: Sage.

Dannelly, R. S., Michaud, P., Patterson-McNeill, H., & Steidley, C. W. (2002, October). *A multi-disciplinary student-centered laboratory.* Paper presented at the 32nd annual Frontiers in Education Conference, Boston, MA.

Datnow, A., & Stringfield, S. (2000). Working together for reliable school reform. [JESPAR]. *Journal of Education for Students Placed at Risk, 5*, 183–204. doi:10.1207/s15327671espr0501&2_11

Datta, L. (1994). Paradigm wars: A basis for peaceful coexistence and beyond. In Reichardt, C. S., & Rallis, S. F. (Eds.), *The qualitative-quantitative debate: New perspectives* (pp. 53–70). San Francisco: Jossey-Bass.

Davis, B., & Simmt, E. (2003). Understanding learning systems: Mathematics education and complexity science. *Journal for Research in Mathematics Education, 34*, 137–167. doi:10.2307/30034903

Davis, B., & Sumara, D. J. (1997). Cognition, complexity, and teacher education. *Harvard Educational Review, 67*, 105–125.

Davis, B., & Sumara, D. J. (2001). Learning communities: Understanding the workplace as a complex system. *New Directions for Adult and Continuing Education, 2001*, 85–95. doi:10.1002/ace.43

De Smet, M., Van Keer, H., & Valcke, M. (2008). Cross-age peer tutors in asynchronous discussion groups: studying the impact of tutors labelling their interventions. *Journal of Computer Assisted Learning, 24*, 462–473.

Deaney, R., Ruthven, K., & Hennessy, S. (2003). Pupil perspectives on the contribution of information and communication technology to teaching and learning in the secondary school. *Research Papers in Education, 18*, 141–165. doi:10.1080/0267152032000081913

Defazio, J. (2006). Theory into practice: A bridge too far? *AACE Journal, 14*, 221–233.

Ding, C., & Sherman, H. (2006). Teaching effectiveness and student achievement: Examining the relationship. *Educational Research Quarterly, 29*, 40–51.

diSessa, A. A., & Cobb, P. (2004). Ontological innovation and the role of theory in design experiments. *Journal of the Learning Sciences, 13*, 77–103. doi:10.1207/s15327809jls1301_4

Douglas, S. C. (2001, October). *The INFINITY project: Digital signal processing and digital music in high school engineering education.* Paper presented at the IEEE workshop on the Applications of Signal Processing to Audio and Acoustics, New Paltz, NY.

Dynarski, M., Agodini, R., Heaviside, S., Novak, T., Carey, N., Campuzano, L., et al. (2007). *Effectiveness of reading and mathematics software products: Findings from the first student cohort.* Washington, DC: National Center for Education Evaluation and Regional Assistance. Retrieved on February 12, 2009, from http://ies.ed.gov/ncee/pdf/20074005.pdf

Dyrud, M. A. (1997). Learning styles. *Business Communication Quarterly, 60*, 124–125. doi:10.1177/108056999706000211

Ellington, A. J. (2003). A meta-analysis of the effects of calculators on students' achievement and attitude levels in precollege mathematics classes. *Journal for Research in Mathematics Education, 34*, 433–463. doi:10.2307/30034795

Ellington, A. J. (2006). The effects of non-CAS graphing calculators on student achievement and attitude levels in mathematics: A meta-analysis. *International Journal of Instructional Media, 106*, 16–26.

Ellis, J. D. (1989). An evaluation of a project for preparing science teachers to use microcomputers. *Journal of Computers in Mathematics and Science Teaching, 8*, 51–65.

Ely, D. (2008). Frameworks of educational technology. *British Journal of Educational Technology, 39*, 244–250. doi:10.1111/j.1467-8535.2008.00810.x

Eraut, M. (1994). *Developing professional knowledge and competence.* London: Falmer Press.

Erbas, A. K., Ledford, S., Polly, D., & Orrill, C. H. (2004). Engaging students through technology. *Mathematics Teaching in the Middle School, 9*, 300–305.

Felner, R. D., Brand, S., Dubois, D. L., Adan, A. M., Mulhall, P. F., & Evans, E. G. (1995). Socioeconomic disadvantage, proximal environmental experiences, and socioemotional and academic adjustment in early adolescence: Investigation of a mediated effects model. *Child Development, 66*, 774–792. doi:10.2307/1131950

Felner, R. D., Favazza, A., Shim, M., Brand, S., Gu, K., & Noonan, N. (2001). Whole school improvement and restructuring as prevention and promotion, Lessons from step and the project on high performance learning communities. *Journal of School Psychology, 39*, 177–202. doi:10.1016/S0022-4405(01)00057-7

Fernandez-Cardenas, J. M. (2008). The situated aspect of creativity in communicative events: How do children design web pages together? *Thinking Skills and Creativity, 3*, 203–216. doi:10.1016/j.tsc.2008.09.007

Fisher, F. D. (1989). The electronic lumberyard and builders' rights. *Change, 21*, 13–21.

Fitzer, K. M., Freidhoff, J. R., Fritzen, A., Heintz, A., Koehler, M. J., & Mishra, P. (2007). Guest editorial: More questions than answers: Responding to the reading and mathematics software effectiveness study. *Contemporary Issues in Technology & Teacher Education, 7*, 1–6.

Fletcher, G. H. (2006). Power up, don't power down. *T.H.E. Journal, 33*, 24–26.

Gray, K. C. (2001). Teachers' perceptions of innovation adoption. *Action in Teacher Education, 23*, 30–35.

Groth, R. E. (2007). Toward a conceptualization of statistical knowledge for teaching. *Journal for Research in Mathematics Education, 38*, 427–437. doi:10.2307/30034960

Guri-Rosenblit, S. (2005). Distance education and e-learning: Not the same thing. *Higher Education, 49*, 467–493. doi:10.1007/s10734-004-0040-0

Hayes, M. H., & Mayercik, M. (2001). Distance learning across the Atlantic. *Education. IEEE Transactions on, 44*, 201–211.

Heath, R. D. (1987). The effect of calculators and computers on problem-solving ability and attitude toward mathematics. (Doctoral Dissertation, Northern Arizona University, 1987). *Dissertation Abstracts International-A, 48*(05), 1102.

Helling, H. E., & Solomon, E. M. (2003, September). *Bridging the gap between ocean science and education: Creating effective partnerships through informal educational institutions.* Paper presented at the annual meeting of the OCEANS 2003 Conference, San Diego, CA.

Hess, D. (2007). From Banished to Brother Outsider, Miss Navajo to An Inconvenient Truth: Documentary films as perspective-laden narratives. *Social Education, 71*, 194–199.

Hewitt, T. W. (2006). *Understanding curriculum: What we teach and why.* Thousand Oaks, CA: Sage Publications.

Hodges, C. B. (2006). Lessons learned from a first instructional design experience. *International Journal of Instructional Media, 33*, 397–403.

Holmes, A., Polhemus, L., & Jennings, S. (2005). CATIE: A blended approach to situated professional development. *Journal of Educational Computing Research, 32*, 381–394. doi:10.2190/F97W-QUJ4-G7YG-FPXC

Hughes, J. (2005). The role of teacher knowledge and learning experiences in forming technology-integrated pedagogy. *Journal of Technology and Teacher Education, 13*, 277–302.

International Society for Technology in Education. (2008). *National educational technology standards and performance indicators for teachers.* Eugene, OR: Author. Retrieved on February 1, 2009, from http://www.iste.org/Content/NavigationMenu/NETS/ForTeachers/2008Standards/NETS_T_Standards_Final.pdf

International Technology Education Association. (2005). Testimony pertaining to the science framework for the 2009 national assessment of education progress. *Technology Teacher, 65*, 36–37.

James, R. K., Lamb, C. E., Bailey, M. A., & Householder, D. L. (2000). Integrating science, mathematics, and technology in middle school technology-rich environments: A study of implementation and change. *International Journal of Instructional Media, 100*, 27–35.

Jenkins, E. W. (2006). Student opinion in England about science and technology. *Research in Science & Technological Education, 24*, 59–68. doi:10.1080/02635140500485365

John, P. (2005). The sacred and the profane: Subject sub–culture, pedagogical practice and teachers' perceptions of the classroom uses of ICT. *Educational Review, 57*, 471–490. doi:10.1080/00131910500279577

Jones, S. (2005). Fizz in the field: Toward a basis for an emergent internet studies. *The Information Society, 21*, 233–237. doi:10.1080/01972240591007544

Kalyuga, S., & Sweller, J. (2005). Rapid dynamic assessment of expertise to improve the efficiency of adaptive e-learning. *Educational Technology Research and Development, 53*, 83–93. doi:10.1007/BF02504800

Karchmer-Klein, R., & Layton, V. (2006). Literature-based collaborative internet projects in elementary classrooms. *Reading Research and Instruction*, *45*, 261–294.

Kaur, M. (2008). Cryptography as a pedagogical tool. *PRIMUS (Terre Haute, Ind.)*, *18*, 198–206. doi:10.1080/10511970701298833

Koehler, M. J., & Mishra, P. (2008). Introducing TPCK. In Colbert, J. A., Boyd, K. E., Clark, K. A., Guan, S., Harris, J. B., Kelly, M. A., & Thompson, A. D. (Eds.), *Handbook of Technological Pedagogical Content Knowledge (TPCK) for educators* (pp. 3–30). New York: Routledge.

Kordaki, M., Miatidis, M., & Kapsampelis, G. (2008). A computer environment for beginners' learning of sorting algorithms: design and pilot evaluation. *Computers & Education*, *51*, 708–723. doi:10.1016/j.compedu.2007.07.006

Lai, K. W., & Pratt, K. (2007). Positive to a degree: The effects of ICT use in New Zealand secondary schools. *Computers in the Schools*, *24*, 95–109. doi:10.1300/J025v24n03_07

Larkin, T., & Budny, D. (2005, July). *Learning styles in the classroom: Approaches to enhance student motivation and learning.* Paper presented at the 6th International Conference on Information Technology Based Higher Education and Training, Santo Domingo, Dominican Republic.

Lau, S. H., & Woods, P. C. (2009). Understanding the behavior changes in belief and attitude among experienced and inexperienced learning object users. *Computers & Education*, *52*, 333–342. doi:10.1016/j.compedu.2008.09.002

Lawrence, B. J. (2000). Procedural apprenticeship in school science: Constructivist enabling of connoisseurship. *Science Education*, *84*, 727–739. doi:10.1002/1098-237X(200011)84:6<727::AID-SCE3>3.0.CO;2-O

Longhurst, J. (2003). World history on the World Wide Web: A student satisfaction survey and a blinding flash of the obvious. *The History Teacher*, *36*, 343–356. doi:10.2307/1555691

Lowe, P. D., & Worboys, M. (1975). The teaching of social studies of science and technology in British polytechnics. *Social Studies of Science (Sage)*, *5*, 177–192. doi:10.1177/030631277500500204

Lynch, K., Bednarz, B., Boxall, J., Chalmers, L., France, D., & Kesby, J. (2008). E-learning for Geography's Teaching and Learning Spaces. *Journal of Geography in Higher Education*, *32*, 135–149. doi:10.1080/03098260701731694

Main, L. (1998). WOOing the millennium. *Journal of Education for Library and Information Science*, *39*, 339–342.

Malloy, J. A., & Gambrell, L. B. (2006). Approaching the unavoidable: Literacy instruction and the Internet. *The Reading Teacher*, *59*, 482–484. doi:10.1598/RT.59.5.8

Marks, R. (1990). Pedagogical content knowledge: From a mathematical case to a modified conception. *Journal of Teacher Education*, *41*, 3–11. doi:10.1177/002248719004100302

Martin, A. (1967). Industrial training: Current research and future needs. *Occupational Psychology*, *41*, 109–119.

Martin, H. E. (1996). Tracking weather satellites. *Science Teacher (Normal, Ill.)*, *63*, 30–32.

Massey, A. P., Ramesh, V., & Khatri, V. (2006). Design, development, and assessment of mobile applications: The case for problem-based learning. *IEEE Transactions on Education*, *49*, 183–192. doi:10.1109/TE.2006.875700

McCoy, N. L. (1998). Methodological problems in the study of sexuality and the menopause. *Maturitas*, *29*, 51–60. doi:10.1016/S0378-5122(98)00028-0

Means, B., Wagner, M., Haertel, G. D., & Javitz, H. S. (2003). Studying the cumulative impacts of educational technology. In Haertel, G. D., & Means, B. (Eds.), *Evaluating educational technology: Effective research designs for improving learning* (pp. 230–256). New York: Teachers College Press.

Mervielde, I. (1977). Methodological problems of research about attitude-behavior consistency. *Quality & Quantity*, *11*, 259–281. doi:10.1007/BF00138839

Miller, D., & Glover, D. (2007). Into the unknown: The professional development induction experience of secondary mathematics teachers using interactive whiteboard technology. *Learning, Media and Technology*, *32*, 319–331. doi:10.1080/17439880701511156

Min, L. (2005). The effect of a hypermedia learning environment on middle school students' motivation, attitude, and science knowledge. *Computers in the Schools*, *22*, 159–171.

Mishra, P., & Koehler, M. J. (2006). Technological pedagogical content knowledge: A framework for teacher knowledge. *Teachers College Record*, *108*, 1017–1054. doi:10.1111/j.1467-9620.2006.00684.x

Moursund, D. G. (1995). Site-based management: Saving our schools. *Association for Computing Machinery. Communications of the ACM*, *38*, 15–17. doi:10.1145/203241.203243

Mulcahy, M. D. (1998). Designing the user/using the design: The shifting relations of a curriculum technology change. *Social Studies of Science (Sage)*, *28*, 5–38. doi:10.1177/030631298028001001

Neal, J. G. (2006). The research and development imperative in the academic library: Path to the future. *Portal: Libraries & the Academy*, *6*, 1–3. doi:10.1353/pla.2006.0007

Niess, M., Ronau, R. N., Shafer, K. G., Driskell, S. O., Harper, S. R., & Johnston, C. (2009). Mathematics teacher TPACK standards and development model. *Contemporary Issues in Technology and Mathematics Teacher Education*, *9*, 4–24.

Niess, M. L. (2005a). Preparing teachers to teach science and mathematics with technology: Developing a Technology Pedagogical Content Knowledge. *Teaching and Teacher Education*, *21*, 509–523. doi:10.1016/j.tate.2005.03.006

Niess, M. L. (2005b). Scaffolding math learning with spreadsheets. Learning connections--mathematics. *Learning and Leading with Technology*, *32*, 24–25.

Niess, M. L. (2006). Preparing Teachers to Teach Mathematics With Technology. *Contemporary Issues in Technology and Mathematics Teacher Education*, *6*, 195–203.

Niess, M. L. (2007, June). *Mathematics teachers developing Technology, Pedagogy and Content Knowledge (TPCK)*. Paper presented at the Informatics, Mathematics, Information and Communication Technology (IMICT) conference, Boston, MA.

Niess, M. L. (2008). Knowledge needed for teaching with technologies — Call it TPACK. *AMTE Connections*, *17*, 9–10.

Niess, M. L., Lee, K., & Sadri, P. (2007). *Dynamic spreadsheets as learning technology tools: developing teachers' technology pedagogical content knowledge (TPCK)*. Paper presented at the annual meeting of the American Educational Research Association, Chicago, IL.

Niess, M. L., Lee, K., Sadri, P., & Suharwoto, G. (2006). *Guiding inservice mathematics teachers in developing a Technology Pedagogical Knowledge (TPCK)*. Paper presented at the annual meeting of the American Educational Research Association, San Francisco, CA.

No Child Left Behind Act of 2002, 20 U.S.C. § 6301 et seq. (West, 2002). Retrieved on February 1, 2009, from http://www.ed.gov/policy/elsec/leg/esea02/107-110.pdf

Nowak, S. (1969). Methodological dilemmas. *Studia Socjologiczne, 3*, 29–44.

O'Connell, J., & Phye, G. (2005). Creating strategies for improved teaching and learning. *T.H.E. Journal, 32*, 26–29.

O'Donnell, S. (2005). IT education and training for disadvantaged students: Lessons from Europe. *IEEE Technology and Society Magazine, 24*, 23–31. doi:10.1109/MTAS.2005.1507537

Parker, J., Cordes, D., Laurie, C., Hopenwasser, A., Izatt, J., & Nikles, D. (1995, November). *Curriculum integration in the freshman year at the University of Alabama-foundation coalition program.* Paper presented at the Frontiers in Education Conference, Atlanta, GA.

Patton, M. Q. (2002). *Qualitative research and evaluation methods* (3rd ed.). Thousand Oaks: Sage.

Peressini, D., Borko, H., Romagnano, L., Knuth, E., & Willis, C. (2004). A conceptual framework for learning to teach secondary mathematics: A situative perspective. *Educational Studies in Mathematics, 56*, 67–96. doi:10.1023/B:EDUC.0000028398.80108.87

Reed, M., & Mitchell, B. (2001). Using information technologies for collaborative learning in geography: A case study from Canada. *Journal of Geography in Higher Education, 25*, 321–339. doi:10.1080/03098260120067619

Reinthaler, J. (1990). Just teach them the basics and leave the applications to us. *Communications Magazine, IEEE, 28*, 56–57. doi:10.1109/35.61723

Rhoads, T. R. (2001, October). *Will you throw out the baby with the bathwater?* Paper presented at the 31st annual Frontiers in Education Conference, Reno, NV.

Rice, W. R., Beg, Y., Waters, C., Bokreta, M. K., & Santiago-Aviles, J. J. (1999, November). *New pedagogical approaches to computer science education: A case study in peer learning.* Paper presented at the 29th annual Frontiers in Education Conference, San Juan, Puerto Rico.

Richards, K., & Wrigley, N. (1996). Geography in the United Kingdom 1992-1996. *The Geographical Journal, 162*, 41–62. doi:10.2307/3060215

Riggs, H. (2006). Technology-supported mathematics learning environments: Sixty-seventh yearbook of the National Council of Teachers of Mathematics. *Teaching Children Mathematics, 12*, 333–333.

Roach, S. (2001, October). *The impact of technology on engineering and computer science education in the 21st century: Changing classroom instructional methods.* Paper presented at the 31st annual Frontiers in Education Conference, Reno, NV.

Rodgers, G., & Jones, G. (1997, November). *Science and technology in the workplace: A decade of experimentation with post-calculus H. S. Math.* Paper presented at the 27th annual Frontiers in Education Conference, Pittsburg, PA.

Rodriguez, C. M. (1998). Commentary on: 'Technology in the classroom: Teaching business marketing in the 21st century,' by Richard P. Vlosky and David T. Wilson. *Journal of Business-To-Business Marketing, 5*, 157–160. doi:10.1300/J033v05n01_15

Ronau, R. N., Niess, M. L., Browning, C. A., Pugalee, D., Driskell, S. O., & Harrington, R. (2008). Framing the research on digital technologies and student learning in mathematics. In Bell, L., Thompson, E. A., & Schrum, L. (Eds.), *Framing research on technology and student learning in the content areas* (pp. 13–31). Charlotte, NC: Information Age Publishing.

Ronau, R. N., Taylor, P. M., Dougherty, B. J., Pyper, J., Wagener, L. L., & Rakes, C. R. (2009). *A comprehensive framework for teacher knowledge: A lens for examining research.* Manuscript in preparation.

Roschelle, J., Tatar, D., Shechtman, N., & Knudsen, J. (2008). The role of scaling up research in designing for and evaluating robustness. *Educational Studies in Mathematics*, *68*, 149–170. doi:10.1007/s10649-008-9119-3

Rosenthal, L. (1974). A course in technology for artists. *Leonardo*, *7*, 27–29. doi:10.2307/1572733

Rossi, R. J., & Stringfield, S. C. (1995a). Education reform and students at risk. Volume I: Findings and recommendations. Studies of education reform. Baltimore, MD: John Hopkins University, Center for Research on the Education of Students Placed At Risk & American Institutes for Research in the Behavioral Sciences. (ERIC Document Reproduction Service No. ED397541)

Rossi, R. J., & Stringfield, S. C. (1995b). Education reform and students at risk. Volume II: Case study descriptions. Studies of education reform. Baltimore, MD: John Hopkins University, Center for Research on the Education of Students Placed At Risk & American Institutes for Research in the Behavioral Sciences. (ERIC Document Reproduction Service No. ED397542)

Rudd, E. (1986). The value of a Ph.D. in science or technology in Britain. *European Journal of Education*, *21*, 223–250. doi:10.2307/1503069

Sasaki, M., Oguchi, T., Okabe, A., & Sadahiro, Y. (2008). GIS education at geographical departments in Japanese universities in relation to the Japan standard GIS core curriculum. *International Research in Geographical and Environmental Education*, *17*, 298–306. doi:10.1080/10382040802401540

Scribner, J. P. (1999). Professional development: Untangling the influence of work Context on teacher learning. *Educational Administration Quarterly*, *35*, 238–266.

Segrave, R. (2004). Communication technologies and knowledge building in agriculture. *Australian Journal of Adult Learning*, *44*, 27–43.

Selwyn, N. (2007). Curriculum online? Exploring the political and commercial construction of the UK digital learning marketplace. *British Journal of Sociology of Education*, *28*, 223–240. doi:10.1080/01425690701192729

Shadish, W. R. (1995). The logic of generalization: Five principles common to experiments and ethnographies. *American Journal of Community Psychology*, *23*, 419–428. doi:10.1007/BF02506951

Shadish, W. R., Cook, T. D., & Campbell, D. T. (2002). *Experimental and quasi-experimental design*. Boston: Houghton Mifflin Company.

Sharp, B. D. (2007). Making the most of digital imagery. *Mathematics Teacher*, *100*, 590–593.

Shimony, R., Russo, J. W., Ciaccio, L., Sanders, J. W., Rimpici, R., & Takvorian, P. M. (2002). Medical laboratory technology: A New York state tech-prep model that improves academic skills. *The Journal of Educational Research*, *95*, 300–307. doi:10.1080/00220670209596603

Shulman, L. S. (1986). Those who understand: A conception of teacher knowledge. *American Educator*, *10*, 9–15.

Siegel, M. (2006). Rereading the signs: Multimodal transformations in the field of literacy education. *Language Arts*, *84*, 65–77.

Sinkinson, A. J. (2006). The impact of specialist school status: A case study of two contrasting mathematics and computing colleges. *Educational Studies*, *32*, 87–99. doi:10.1080/03055690500416041

Slator, B. M., Clark, J., Juell, P., McClean, P., Saini-Eidukat, B., Schwert, D. P., & White, A. R. (2001, August). *Research on role-based learning technologies.* Paper presented at the IEEE International Conference on Advanced Learning Technologies, Madison, WI.

Slay, H., Siebörger, I., & Hodgkinson-Williams, C. (2008). Interactive whiteboards: Real beauty or just lipstick? *Computers & Education*, *51*, 1321–1341. doi:10.1016/j.compedu.2007.12.006

Slough, S. W., & Chamblee, G. E. (2007). Technology as an innovation in science and mathematics teaching. *International Journal of Instructional Media*, *107*, 222–224.

Spector, B. S., & Burkett, R. S. (2003). MSTS inquiry for career-change teachers. *Bulletin of Science, Technology & Society*, *23*, 297–301. doi:10.1177/0270467603256080

Spellman, K. (2004). A national Sufi Order with trans-national dimensions: The Maktab Tarighat Oveyssi Shahmaghsoudi Sufi Order in London. *Journal of Ethnic and Migration Studies*, *30*, 945–960. doi:10.1080/1369183042000245633

Steinkuehler, C., & Duncan, S. (2008). Scientific habits of mind in virtual worlds. *Journal of Science Education and Technology*, *17*, 530–543. doi:10.1007/s10956-008-9120-8

Steve, W. (2005). Learning in school, home and community: ICT for early and elementary education. *Cambridge Journal of Education*, *35*, 282.

Stevens, K. K., & Schlossberg, S. (1997, November). *Connection technology.* Paper presented at the 27th annual Frontiers in Education Conference, Pittsburg, PA.

Stringfield, S. (1995). Attempting to enhance students' learning through innovative programs: The case for schools evolving into high reliability organizations. *School Effectiveness and School Improvement*, *6*, 67–96. doi:10.1080/0924345950060104

Suh, J., & Moyer, P. S. (2007). Developing students' representational fluency using virtual and physical algebra balances. *Journal of Computers in Mathematics and Science Teaching*, *26*, 155–173.

Suharwoto, G., & Lee, K. H. (2005, March). *Assembling the pieces together: What are the most influential components in mathematics preservice teachers' development of Technology Pedagogical Content Knowledge (TPCK)?* Paper presented at the annual meeting of the Society for Information Technology & Teacher Education (SITE), Phoenix, AZ.

Swan, B., & Dixon, J. (2006). The effects of mentor-supported technology professional development on middle school mathematics teachers' attitudes and practice. *Contemporary Issues in Technology & Teacher Education*, *6*, 67–86.

Tall, D. (2008). James J. Kaput (1942-2005), Imagineer and futurologist of mathematics education. *Educational Studies in Mathematics*, *68*, 185–193. doi:10.1007/s10649-008-9121-9

Tankersley, M., Landrum, T. J., & Cook, B. G. (2004). How research informs practice in the field of emotional and behavioral disorders. In Rutherford, R. B., Quinn, M. M., & Mathur, S. R. (Eds.), *Handbook of research in emotional and behavioral disorders* (pp. 98–116). New York: Guilford Press.

Tashakkori, A., & Teddlie, C. (1998). *Mixed methodology: Combining qualitative and quantitative approaches*. Thousand Oaks, CA: Sage Publications.

Teddlie, C., & Stringfield, S. (1985). A differential analysis of effectiveness in middle and low socioeconomic status schools. *Journal of Classroom Interaction, 20*, 38–44.

Thompson, A. D., & Mishra, P. (2007). Breaking news: TPCK becomes TPACK! *Journal of Computing in Teacher Education, 24*, 38, 64.

Thompson, M., Oakes, W., & Bodner, G. (2005, October). *A qualitative investigation of students in a first-year engineering learning community.* Paper presented at the 35th annual Frontiers in Education Conference, Indianapolis, IN.

Toots, A., & Lanpere, M. (2004). Tiger in focus -- A national survey of ICT in Estonian schools. *Educational Media International, 41*, 7–18. doi:10.1080/0952398032000105049

Triandis, H. C. (1976). Methodological problems of comparative research. *International Journal of Psychology, 11*, 155–159. doi:10.1080/00207597608247355

Vanderburg, W. H. (1992). Education for sustainability: A report card on engineering. *Technology and Society Magazine, IEEE, 11*, 26–31. doi:10.1109/44.141672

Wayman, J. C., Stringfield, S., & Yakimowski, M. (2004). Software enabling school improvement through analysis of student data (Rep. No. 67). Baltimore, MD: John Hopkins University, Center for Research on the Education of Students Placed at Risk (CRESPAR). (ERIC Document Reproduction Service No. EJ330697)

Webb, M. E. (2005). Affordances of ICT in science learning: Implications for an integrated pedagogy. *International Journal of Science Education, 27*, 705–735. doi:10.1080/09500690500038520

Whitehurst, G. J. (2002, October). *Evidence-based education.* Presentation given at the annual meeting of the School Accountability Conference, Orlando, FL. Retrieved on May 5, 2006 from http://www.ed.gov/offices/OERI/presentations/evidencebase.html

Whitehurst, G. J. (2003). *Identifying and implementing educational practices supported by rigorous evidence: A user-friendly guide.* Washington, D. C.: U. S. Department of Education, Institute of Education Sciences, National Center for Education Evaluation and Regional Assistance. Retrieved on June 1, 2009 from http://www.ed.gov/rschstat/research/pubs/rigorousevid/rigorousevid.pdf

Wittmann, E. C. (1998). Mathematics education as a 'design science. In Sierpinska, A., & Kilpatrick, J. (Eds.), *Mathematics education as a research domain: A search for identity*. Dordrecht: Kluwer Academic Publishers.

Wolf, M. A. (2008). High schools: An equation that works. *T.H.E. Journal, 35*, 24–26.

Woodgate, D., & Fraser, D. S. (2006, December). *EScience, science education and technology integration in the classroom: Some practical considerations.* Paper presented at the IEEE International Conference on e-Science and Grid Computing, Amsterdam, The Netherlands.

Woody, K. (2006). Designs for learning with new technologies. *Peer Review, 8*, 23–25.

Young-Suk, S. (2004). Virtual experiment environment's design for science education. *International Journal of Distance Education Technologies, 2*, 62–76.

Zia, L. L., & Mulder, M. C. (1996). NSF workshop on information technology and undergraduate science, mathematics, engineering, and technology education: Challenges and opportunities. *Education. IEEE Transactions on, 39*, 452–454.

Zucker, A. A., & Hug, S. (2008). Teaching and learning physics in a 1:1 laptop school. *Journal of Science Education and Technology, 17*, 586–594. doi:10.1007/s10956-008-9125-3

Zucker, A. A., Tinker, R., Staudt, C., Mansfield, A., & Metcalf, S. (2008). Learning science in grades 3-8 using probeware and computers: Findings from the TEEMSS II project. *Journal of Science Education and Technology, 17*, 42–48. doi:10.1007/s10956-007-9086-y

Zurita, G., & Nussbaum, M. (2007). A conceptual framework based on activity theory for mobile CSCL. *British Journal of Educational Technology, 38*, 211–235. doi:10.1111/j.1467-8535.2006.00580.x

APPENDIX A

American Mathematics Teacher Educators Association Guidelines for Implementing the TPACK Framework

(Adopted June 19, 2009)

I. Design and develop technology-enhanced mathematics learning environments and experiences. Educators use their knowledge of technology, pedagogy, and content to design and develop learning environments and experiences to maximize mathematics learning. They:

a. Establish and utilize mathematical environments, tasks, experiences and resources to integrate technology tools that support learners' individual and collaborative mathematical learning and creativity;

b. Design challenging and engaging mathematical learning experiences that utilize appropriate technologies to support the diverse needs of learners; and

c. Identify and utilize strategies and activities that promote equitable access to and facility with technology resources.

II. **Facilitate mathematics instruction with technology as an integrated tool.** Educators implement curricular plans that integrate appropriate technology to maximize mathematical learning and creativity. They:

a. Incorporate knowledge of learner characteristics, orientation, and thinking to foster learning of mathematics with technology;

b. Facilitate technology-enriched, mathematical experiences that foster creativity, develop conceptual understanding, and cultivate higher order thinking skills;

c. Promote mathematical discourse between and among instructors and learners in a technology-enriched learning community;

d. Use technology to support learner-centered strategies that address the diverse needs of all learners of mathematics; and

e. Encourage learners to become responsible for and reflect upon their own technology-enriched mathematics learning.

III. Assess and evaluate technology-enriched mathematics teaching and learning. Educators assess and evaluate mathematics teaching and learning using appropriate assessment tools and strategies. They:

a. Assess learning of mathematics applying technologies when appropriate, reflect upon the assessment results, and communicate those results using a variety of tools and techniques;

b. Assess learners' appropriate and ethical use of technology resources in learning and communicating mathematics;

c. Use formative assessment of technology-enriched lessons and activities to evaluate mathematics learning and adjust instructional strategies accordingly;

d. Align the technology expectations for assessment tasks and practices with that of mathematics instructional activities; and

e. Evaluate and reflect on the effective use of existing and emerging technologies to enhance the mathematical learning of all.

IV. Engage in ongoing professional development to enhance technological pedagogical content knowledge. Educators seek, identify, and use technology to enhance their knowledge, productivity, and professional practice. They:

a. Collaborate with others in ongoing professional activities to promote excellence in learning mathematics in technology-enriched environments;

b. Promote social justice for access to and facility with technology in learning mathematics;

c. Advocate, model, and promote safe, legal, and ethical use of technology for learning and exploring mathematics with learners, families and caregivers, and colleagues;

d. Communicate and collaborate with families and caregivers, colleagues, and the larger community using appropriate technologies in order to nurture mathematical learners; and

e. Exhibit leadership by demonstrating a research-based vision for integrating technology in teaching mathematics.

Appendix B

Coding Instrument

Report Characteristics	**Description**
Author(s)	
Year	
Title	
1. Journal	
2. Volume	
3. Pages	
4. Content Area	

Report Characteristics	Description
5. Content Topic	
6. Grade Level	
7. Description of Technology Tool:	
8. Description of the Outcome of Interest (Mark all that apply)	a) Student Achievement b) Teacher Knowledge c) Teacher Orientation d) Student Orientation e) Knowledge Transfer f) Other____________________ g) Can't Tell
9. Was the study population well described?	a) Yes b) No c) Can't Tell
10. Did the authors specify the sampling frame or universe of selection for the study population?	a) Yes b) No c) Can't Tell
11. Were the exposure variables valid measures of the intervention under study?	a) Yes b) No c) Can't Tell
12. Were the outcome and other independent (or predictor) variables reliable (consistent and reproducible) measures of the outcome of interest?	a) Yes b) No c) Can't Tell
13. Did the authors conduct appropriate analysis by conducting statistical testing (where appropriate)?	a) Yes b) No c) Can't Tell d) Not appropriate for this study e) Explain:__________________
14. Did at least 80% of enrolled participants complete the study?	a) Yes b) No c) Can't Tell
15. Did the authors correct for controllable variables or institute study procedures to limit bias appropriately?	a) Yes b) No c) Can't Tell
16. Describe all potential biases or unmeasured/contextual confounders described by the authors.	
17. Other important limitations of the study not identified elsewhere?	
18. CFTK Aspects Explicitly Addressed for teachers	a) Subject Matter b) Pedagogical Knowledge c) Orientation d) Discernment e) Individual Context f) Environmental Context g) Can't Tell
19. CFTK Aspects Explicitly addressed for students	a) Subject Matter b) Pedagogical Knowledge c) Orientation d) Discernment e) Individual Context f) Environmental Context g) Can't Tell

Report Characteristics	**Description**
20. TPACK Stages described (teachers only)	a) Recognizing b) Accepting c) Adapting d) Exploring e) Advancing f) Can't Tell
21. What type of research does this study conduct?	a) Quantitative b) Qualitative c) Theory Development/Literature Driven d) Other____________________
For Quantitative Studies	
22. Research design	a) Randomized experiment b) Non-equivalent control group c) Other _________________________ d) Can't tell
23. Group assignment mechanism	a) Random assignment b) Haphazard assignment c) Other nonrandom assignment d) Can't tell
24. Selection mechanism	a) Self-selected into groups b) Selected into groups by others on a basis related to outcome (e.g., good readers placed in the expectancy group) c) Selected into groups by others not known to be related to outcome (e.g., randomized experiment) d) Can't tell
25. Equating variables	a) None b) Prior achievement c) Other __________________ d) Can't tell
26. If equating was done, was it done using a statistical process (e.g., ANCOVA, weighting) or manually (e.g., hand matching)?	a) n/a, equating was not done b) Statistically c) Manual matching
27. Sample Sizes	
28. Achievement measure used in study	a) Researcher Designed Assessment b) Teacher Made Assessment c) Standardized Assessment d) Other ______________ e) Can't tell ______________
29. Score reliability for achievement measure (note: if a range is given, code the median value)	
30. Metric for score reliability	a) Internal consistency b) Split-half c) Test-retest d) Can't tell e) None given

Report Characteristics	Description
31. Source of score reliability estimate	a) Current sample b) Citation from another study c) Can't tell d) None given
32. Is the validity of the achievement measure mentioned?	a) No b) Yes
33. If yes, was a specific validity estimate given?	a) No b) Yes
34. If yes, what was the estimate?	
35. If a validity estimate was given in the report, what was the source of the estimate?	a) Current sample b) Citation from another study c) Can't tell d) n/a, validity was not mentioned in the report
36. What was the nature of the validity estimate?	a) Concurrent validity b) Convergent validity c) Predictive validity d) Other e) Can't tell (e.g., simply asserted that the measure is "valid") f) n/a, validity was not mentioned in the report
For Qualitative Studies	
37. Type of Study	a) Narrative/Historical b) Biography c) Design Study d) Phenomenology e) Ethnography f) Grounded theory g) Case Study
38. Describe the methodology. (Mark all that apply)	a) Covert Observation b) Overt Observation c) Interview d) Focus Group e) Other____________________ f) Can't Tell
39. Was there alignment between the nature of the data collected and the questions posed?	a) No Describe Issue: b) Yes Summarize: c) Can't Tell
40. Did the author proceed systematically (with the logic of decisions addressed)?	a) No b) Yes c) Can't tell

Report Characteristics	Description
41. Was trustworthiness addressed?	a) No b) Yes Describe: 1) Persistent observation 2) Use of triangulation techniques 3) Peer debriefing 4) Negative case analysis 5) Referential adequacy 6) Member checks 7) Thick description 8) Dependability audit 9) Confirmability audit 10) Reflexive journal c) Can't tell
42. Any gaps in the coherence of the methodology?	a) No b) Yes Describe: c) Can't Tell

Appendix C

Subject Terms Used in Literature Search

Databases	Career & Technical Education	Social Studies	Science	Language Arts	Mathematics
EBSCOhost	CTE or "Career and Technical Education" or "Career & Technical Education" or "Career Education" or "Technical Education" or "Workforce Education" or "Adult Education" or "Agriculture" or "Information Technology" or "Health Science" or "Human Services" or "Communications" or "Construction" or "Manufacturing" or "Public Services" or "Transportation" or "Business Education" or "Marketing Education" and "Educational Technology" or "High Technology & Education"	Technology, Education, and ("Social Studies" or "History" or "Geography" or "Political Science" or "Politics")	(Technology or "Educational Technology") and Education and (Science or "Science-Study & Teaching")	Technology And (Education or "Educational Technology) and ("Language Arts" or "Reading" or Writing")	(Technology or "Educational Technology") and Education and Math

Databases	Career & Technical Education	Social Studies	Science	Language Arts	Mathematics
ProQuest	(Vocational Education or Vocational Schools or Vocational Training or Work-force Planning or Information Technology or Agriculture or Agriculture Teachers) and (Technology or Technology Assessment or Technology Education or Technology Standards or Technology Transfer or Technology Acquisition or Technology Adoption or Educational Technology) and (Education or Education & Schools or Education and Schools or Education Discrimination or Education For All Handicapped Children Act 1975-Us or Education History or Education Philosophy)	(Social Studies or Social Studies Education or History or History Education or Geography or Political Science) and (Education or Education & Schools or Education and Schools or Education Discrimination or Education For All Handicapped Children Act 1975-Us or Education History or Education Philosophy) and (Technology or Technology Assessment or Technology Education or Technology Standards or Technology Transfer or Technology Acquisition or Technology Adoption or Educational Technology)	(Science or Science Activities or Science Centers or Science Education or Science Fairs) and (Science & Technology Policy or Science and Technology or Technology or Technology Assessment or Technology Education or Technology Standards or Technology Transfer or Technology Acquisition or Technology Adoption or Educational Technology) and (Education or Education & Schools or Education and Schools or Education Discrimination or Education For All Handicapped Children Act 1975-Us or Education History or Education Philosophy)	(Language Arts and (Education or Education & Schools or Education and Schools or Education Discrimination or Education For All Handicapped Children Act 1975-Us or Education History or Education Philosophy)) and (Technology or Technology Assessment or Technology Education or Technology Standards or Technology Transfer or Technology Acquisition or Technology Adoption or Educational Technology)	(Mathematics or Mathematical Ability or Mathematics Education or Mathematics Teachers or Mathematical Programming) and (Science & Technology Policy or Science and Technology or Technology or Technology Assessment or Technology Education or Technology Standards or Technology Transfer or Technology Acquisition or Technology Adoption or Educational Technology) and (Education or Education & Schools or Education and Schools or Education Discrimination or Education For All Handicapped Children Act 1975-Us or Education History or Education Philosophy)

Databases	Career & Technical Education	Social Studies	Science	Language Arts	Mathematics
JSTOR	(((Education and (Science) and (Technology))) and ("Educational Technology")	(((Education and ("Social Studies" or "History" or "Geography" or "Political Science")) and (Technology))) and ("Educational Technology")	Education and (Science) and (Technology)	(((Education and "Language Arts") and (Technology))) and ("Educational Technology")	(((Education and (Math) and (Technology)))
IEEE Explore	Education and Mathematics and (Technology or "Educational Technology")	("Education" and ("Social Studies" or "History" or "Geography" or "Political Science")) and (Technology or "Educational Technology")	("Education" and Science and (Technology or "Educational Technology")	("Language Arts" and "Education") and (Technology or "Educational Technology")	Education and Mathematics and (Technology or "Educational Technology")
H.W. Wilson	Education and (Technology or "Educational Technology") and "Educational Technology / Use" or "Educational Technology / Teacher Education" and Mathematics or "Mathematics Education"	(Technology or "Educational Technology") and ("Social Studies" or "History" or "Geography" or "Political Science")	Education and (Technology or "Educational Technology") and "Educational Technology / Use" or "Educational Technology / Teacher Education" and Science or "Science Education"	Education and Technology and "Language Arts"	Education and (Technology or "Educational Technology") and "Educational Technology / Use" or "Educational Technology / Teacher Education" and Mathematics or "Mathematics Education"

Chapter 16
Designing and Delivering Technology Integration to Engage Students

Kevin D. Biesinger
University of Nevada Las Vegas, USA

Kent J. Crippen
University of Nevada Las Vegas, USA

ABSTRACT

In order for educators to effectively build, select and integrate technology into the delivery of curriculum and pedagogy, an accepted set of critical program design and delivery elements is needed. The authors propose that research based components such as user validation functions, trace methods, and worked examples be among these accepted design elements of technology supported learning environments. As for the pedagogical methods employed to effectively integrate technology into K-12 curricula, an epistemological shift is needed by which more instructors view learning from a student-centered perspective. Systematic changes needed to foster this view include a migration away from the traditional computer lab scenario, on-going professional development as a continuous support system, and the expectation that technology integration is required as an indication of quality instruction as evidenced in teacher evaluations.

INTRODUCTION

Providing teachers with pedagogically sound methods for introducing technology into their instruction has become a newly needed skill in order to keep students of the 21st century engaged. Recent research has noted the importance of not only creating effective e-learning environments, but remaining cognizant of student behaviors within such systems through the use of trace methods (Winne & Hadwin, 1998). In addition, education's most recent paradigm shift has moved the goals of instruction from teacher-centered to student-centered, promoting motivational constructs such as goal orientation and engagement to center stage when conducting educational research. It is our contention that the importance of motivational constructs is even more pronounced within e-learning environments, with engagement and self-efficacy serving as key predictors of performance (Pajares, 2002).

DOI: 10.4018/978-1-61520-899-9.ch016

In addition to creating effective learning systems, the onset of technology supported learning environments has made it possible for both researchers as well as instructors to obtain more authentic indications of student behaviors while engaged in academic tasks. While recent advancements made in this area have made it possible to find out what learners actually do as opposed to what they claim to do (i.e. self-report), this additional data point should enhance, and not replace learner perceptions. Using the additional information to better triangulate learner behaviors, instructional designers can keep closely informed of effective instructional strategies and better yet, design dynamic systems that can change based on learner characteristics as well as the content to be learned.

This chapter will outline the theoretical foundations of self-regulated learning (SRL) within technology supported learning environments with an emphasis on critical motivational constructs such as goal orientation (Elliot, 1999). Specific pragmatic examples will be used to illustrate important considerations for building efficient technology supported learning environments such as cognitive load (Sweller, 1988), worked example usage (Crippen & Earl, 2007), and feedback (Bower, 2005). In addition, we will introduce the concept of technology *integration* rather than implementation as well as the critical elements necessary to put these instructional practices into place. Our intent is to provide the reader with a sampling of empirically sound studies in order to gain the knowledge needed to select or build effective and engaging technology supported learning environments as well as the ideal conditions to ensure a successful migration into this new arena.

BACKGROUND

Using technology supported learning environments to engage students is a critical antecedent to positive changes in self-efficacy, goal orientation, and achievement. Self-Regulated Learning (SRL) is the theoretical model which will be used to demonstrate the importance of engagement. Pintrich (1995) defined self-regulated learners as those who regulate their own learning by deliberately engaging cognitive, metacognitive and motivational efforts to attend to tasks with perseverance while incorporating prior knowledge efficiently. By taking responsibility for one's own learning (and not because of some external source such as a teacher or extrinsic reward), these learners are typically more successful in making recurring and accurate assessments of their progress towards a clear and predefined goal. A good metaphor which demonstrates the concept of SRL is that of a thermostat. When the temperature of a controlled environment reaches a certain "cut point", an efficient ventilation system will start or stop the flow of hot or cold air. In the same fashion, a learner who possesses good self-regulation skills will effectively gauge his or her learning environment, the critical details of the task to be completed, and monitor their progress through self-evaluation and feedback until the task is successfully completed. It is important to note that this process is quite complex in contrast to the thermostat metaphor and can vary significantly dependent upon the task, the environment, and the intrinsic characteristics of the learner. Indeed, more recent theoretical developments made within SRL theory reflect the influence of social cognitive theory (Bandura, 1997) and remain grounded in the triadic reciprocal causation model (Bandura, 1986), whereby the agency of a learner represents an interdependent relationship between behavior, personality factors (cognition, motivation and biology) and the learning environment. Events and dispositions from each of these three factors "operate as interacting determinants that influence one another bi-directionally" (Bandura, 1997). Although other sub-factors such as feedback (Winne & Hadwin, 1998; Zimmerman, 1990) and goal orientation (Pintrich, 2000a) have shed new light on the theory, most variation in recent models of self-regulated learning have involved changes to the structure of similar constructs from each of Bandura's three main social cognitive arenas and the relative influence or contribution attributed to each.

Figure 1 demonstrates the authors' model of effective technology integration. Specifically, the middle section or the "what" of technology integration consists of two major functions, the design and delivery of technology supported learning environments. While instructional technology designers work primarily with system design and educators work primarily with system delivery (indicated by the "who" at the bottom of the figure) the goals of both populations should be measured in terms of the learner, hence the overlap in the middle. In addition, while each population will utilize a unique set of techniques to develop the design and delivery of these systems (as indicated in the "how" at the top of the diagram), professional development is the key to ensuring that a bridge between these two functions is in place for two reasons; first, to ensure that implementation fidelity is upheld, and second, to keep designers in conversation with instructors to design systems which integrate effectively into the curriculum and provide accurate, targeted, and ongoing feedback.

FOUNDATIONS OF SELF-REGULATED LEARNING: A SET OF PHASES

Perhaps the best and most appropriate way to think of SRL is a set of phases that a learner progresses through when engaged in an academic task. Earlier research conducted with SRL (Zimmerman, 1990) emphasized three components; forethought (task analysis and motivation), performance (self-control and self-observation) and self-reflection (self-judgment and self-reaction). Self-regulation involves monitoring activities within each arena and making adjustments to work towards personal goal attainment. These adjustments are believed to be made continuously throughout the learning process as factors can change frequently. Furthermore, the theory is referred to as recursive since self-reflection is believed to influence

Figure 1. The design and delivery of technology

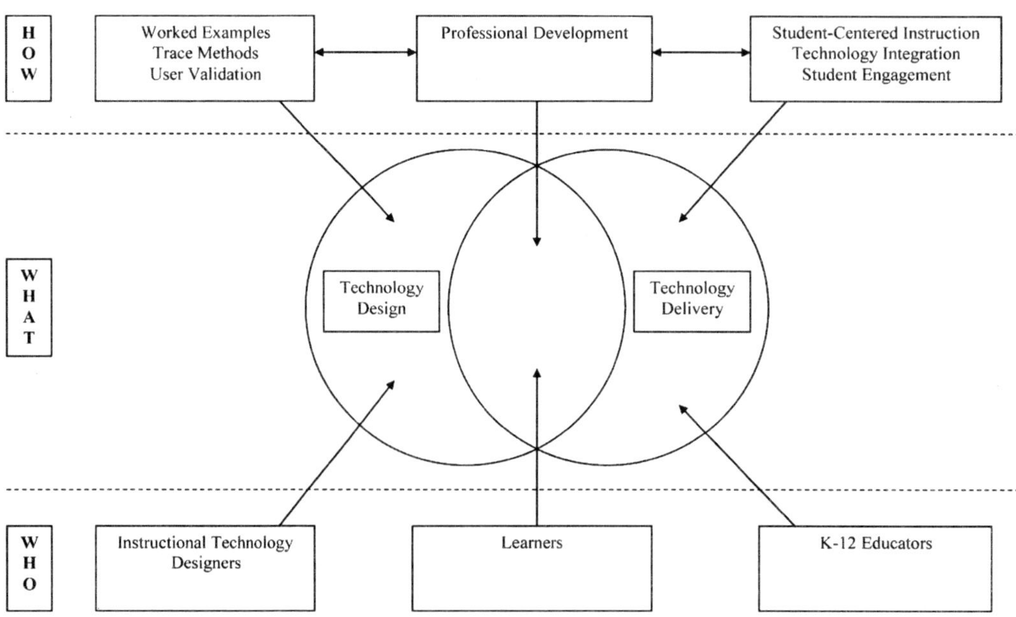

future processes of forethought. In the case of Zimmerman's model, the environment (referred to as context) and the amount of control exercised by the learner to manipulate it are held in high regard (i.e. volition). However, the results of a path analysis by Zimmerman and Bandura (1994) contributed more predictive power to this model only when a goal setting measure was introduced, thus substantiating a need for investigations with motivational constructs.

The groundwork in SRL discussed here was important in that it established a foundation for which SRL could be framed within the context of social cognitive theory. Additionally, the learner was emphasized as a deliberating agent in the educational process, selecting and adapting different strategies based on feedback and motivation in a recursive fashion. In summary, commensurate with other SRL theories under review and within the framework of social cognitive ideals, the learner is seen as an active participant in the process, constructing knowledge in conjunction with the environment. In addition, the theoretical influences of social cognitive theory place a significant focus on the potential for control. SRL activities are defined largely as attempts by the learner to monitor, control and adjust their cognition, metacognition, motivation and even certain aspects of the environment. This pertains to the current chapter as a key reason for the need for a shift to a student-centered learning environment. In addition, technology supported learning environments are often most effective when created from a student-centered point of view.

Goal Orientation

While these theoretical dispositions are somewhat distinct in their interpretations of social cognitive and information processing theories and the relative contributions and interactions of the pertinent constructs, all acknowledge the underlying importance and omnipresent influence of goal orientation dispositions of the learner. From early stages of engagement such as task definition and perceptions of instructor expectations to evaluative activities at task completion, it is goal orientation that sets the stage on which a learner's standards for success are built. This construct also shapes the perspective of the learner through which they will continually evaluate their progress against these standards, making cognitive, meta-cognitive and motivational adaptations due to fluctuations in the environment, the task and themselves.

The categories of goal orientation utilized in the current chapter are derivative of a two by two matrix (Table 1) which outlines two dimensions, perceived task definition and valance (Elliot & McGregor, 2001). This theoretical construct has evolved from the work of Dweck (1986), who suggested that individuals possess either a learning (i.e., mastery) goal orientation where the goal of learning is to master the material, or a performance goal orientation where individuals strive to obtain favorable evaluation from others. Individuals with a performance goal orientation typically prefer normative feedback and gauge their accomplishments based on ability and performance relative to others. These constructs have been assigned different labels across varying research environments such as task, mastery,

Table 1. Goal orientation definitions (Elliot & McGregor, 2001)

	Definition	
Valence	Absolute/intrapersonal (mastery)	Normative (performance)
Positive (approaching success)	Mastery approach goal	Performance approach goal
Negative (avoiding failure)	Mastery avoidance goal	Performance avoidance goal

or learning and performance, ability or ego goal orientations, but have fairly consistent operational definitions and have been accepted as equivalent for purposes of the current chapter.

Later research added another dimension to the theory by re-defining performance goal orientation as one with distinct characteristics at both ends of a continuum. The new dimension, valance, was conceptualized by approach versus avoidance. Approach behaviors are those that strive to achieve successful judgments from others or themselves and are thought of as having a positive valance. Conversely, avoidance behaviors refer to intrinsic motivations that stem from the evasion of failure and appearing incompetent in front of others. Avoidance orientations are regarded as containing a negative valance. Mastery avoidance has only recently been introduced as an addition to the original trichotomous framework to describe the learner who strives for perfection and avoidance of negative self-evaluations (Elliot & McGregor, 2001). Therefore, the four categories are (a) mastery approach (where a person is driven to achieve for the sake of learning how to successfully complete a task), (b) mastery avoidance (where a person strives to avoid misunderstanding or making an error), (c) performance approach (marks the goals of achievement to outperform others) and (d) performance avoidance (individuals who are most likely motivated for the sake of avoiding embarrassment compared to others on the same task).

Goal orientation is an important construct for the current chapter as it presents an opportunity for technology to serve as an effective vehicle to reach learners who may possess different goal orientations. Systems which give credence to the work of Elliot and McGregor and can be tailored to the needs and aspirations of individual students will most likely provide the most utility to K-12 instructors and can help teachers differentiate their instruction based on student needs.

Self-Efficacy

Self-efficacy (Bandura, 1977, 1997), under the implication of social cognitive theory, is defined by Bandura (1997) as "beliefs in one's capabilities to organize and execute the courses of action required to produce given attainments" (p. 3). While self-efficacy research cited here may not directly impact the design or delivery of technology-based instruction models, the authors feel that it is an important concept for K-12 instructors to be familiar with as it often serves as a desirable outcome of instructional technology research. The influence of perceived self-efficacy as a significant predictor of behavior is supported in the literature (Kennett & Keefer, 2006). Bandura's review of research also confirms the predictive validity of self-efficacy while accounting for other variables such as locus of control and ability. Similar to goal orientation, individuals with higher self-efficacy typically view successful task completion as highly dependent upon effort and persistence and will often choose more challenging tasks due to their perceived benefits (Dweck & Leggett, 1988; VandeWalle, Brown, Cron, & Slocum, 1999). Individuals with a lower self-efficacy may view increased effort as an indicator of lower ability and be drawn to the simplest of tasks as a coping mechanism to avoid failure (Dweck, 1999).

While a majority of research has demonstrated consistent empirical evidence of stronger relationships between a mastery approach goal orientation and intrinsic motivation, self-efficacy and deep processing cognitive strategies (Ames, 1992), its predictive power for self regulated learning has been restricted to self-reported measures (Pintrich, 2000b). The discussion of performance goal orientation as an antecedent of the same outcomes however, has received a mixture of results. While some research has focused on the maladaptive patterns that follow from a performance approach goal orientation (Dweck & Leggett, 1988), recent research has challenged this position when other factors such as context and motivation are considered. While VandeWalle et al (1999) found a positive relationship between performance goal orientation and sales commissions, Harackiewicz, Baron, Pintrich, Elliot and Thrash (2002) have also noted positive relationships with task value, academic concept, effort and performance. Furthermore, Pintrich (2000a) demonstrates some adaptive patterns for performance approach goals under a revised theory that allows for learners to progress through different goal orientations dependent upon the context and desired outcome. Elliot et al (1997, 2001) also identified performance approach goals as a significant predictor for graded performance with subjects high on performance approach goal orientation and low on mastery approach goal orientation receiving the highest grades. In fact, Harackiewicz et al (2002b) have gone so far as to claim that in a typical academic setting, mastery approach goals will only predict interest and enjoyment of a course, but performance goals will predict grades and subsequent grade point average.

Feedback

A key variable to be considered in the design and selection of educational technology programs is feedback. While a computer can consistently and tirelessly give feedback to learners, the type of feedback is a pivotal consideration. Typical protocols can be defined as the type of feedback that the learner receives; individualized (based on incremental benchmarks and the learner's own personal growth) or competitive (also referred to as normative, when the learner is informed of his or her progress in comparison to the performance of their peers). Historically, research into the effects of differing feedback protocols on achievement has been inconclusive (Johnson, Maruyama, Johnson, Nelson, & Skon, 1981) with the exception of some gender differences (Lewis & Cooney, 1987).

A more recent investigation into feedback effects by Bower (2005) made an interesting discovery. In his study, high school subjects used a computer-based math program to practice the quadratic equation. Each subject was randomly assigned to one of two feedback conditions; normative, where progress was compared to the performance of their peers or mastery, where progress was compared to their own prior performance. Results showed that learners did not necessarily perform better even when exposed to their preferred type of feedback. Denying learners of their feedback preference was negatively related to self-efficacy but unrelated to effort and showed differing (and indeed intriguing) effects on achievement. Specifically, learners with a preference for competitive feedback and who were assigned to this group made no significant gains in achievement. Learners with a mastery preference assigned to the normative feedback group did however realize significant gains in achievement (even though their assigned group did not match their preference). These findings are contrary to the matching concept proposed by Linnenbrink and Pintrich (2001) since assigning learners to their preferred method of feedback did not lead to increases in achievement.

Findings, such as the one just mentioned are important when considering the design and delivery of technology supported learning environments. As Bower's research indicates, allowing an end user complete freedom of choice in regard to the activities and type of feedback received might not always provide the most reliable course of action. Intelligent systems which are capable of interpreting the goals of a task as well as the personal characteristics of a learner in an effort to provide an efficient course of action with meaningful feedback aimed at keeping a learner engaged are more likely to be effective.

SUMMARY OF RELEVANT SELF-REGULATED LEARNING RESEARCH

Prior empirical work which demonstrates that goal orientation can differ depending upon the context (Mangos & Steele-Johnson, 2001; Pintrich, 2000a, 2000b), task (Mangos & Steele-Johnson, 2001) or learner characteristics (Patrick, Ryan, & Pintrich, 2000) supports the notion that SRL investigations can only be interpreted within context, bringing into question research that might attempt to globalize motivation or other constructs within SRL. Thus, the generalizability of research conducted with regard to these constructs is difficult to sustain and measurements collected at more rudimentary levels in domain specific environments will likely provide the most utility. This domain specific approach to measuring SRL characteristics has proven to be empirically fruitful when disaggregated at the course level (Wolters, Yu, & Pintrich, 1996) and along similar lines of data parsing such as task specificity (Winne & Perry, 2000), task demands (Steele-Johnson, Beauregard, Hoover, & Schmidt, 2000), or task complexity (Mangos & Steele-Johnson, 2001). In addition, self-reports are limited as these often can only give indications of learner behaviors at a broad level and are best interpreted in terms of a learner's propensity to include certain strategies in their repertoire of learning tactics.

It is important to note that like SRL theory, research which attempts to investigate the impact of different technology-based instruction models will most likely provide different results dependent upon the context, population, task, and most importantly the learning environment. Often times, those new to educational technology research are too concerned with what a technology-based instruction model does and turn a blind eye to its implementation and how it might be used by an instructor. This issue compounds when models are implemented across multiple classrooms or schools. Indeed, it is our opinion that implementation is more critical than the functions of a technology-based instruction model itself.

CURRENT ISSUES FACING TEACHER EDUCATION IN REGARD TO TECHNOLOGY IMPLEMENTATION

What Does Effective Technology Integration Look Like?

Both authors of the current chapter began their careers in education as high school instructors (math and science), and remain concerned with the lack of progress made in regard to effective technology integration in most typical K-12 settings. While the 1990s represented a time when millions of federal dollars were earmarked to get schools connected to the Web, the last decade attempted to focus (with limited success) on effectively using these connections in the classroom to enhance content delivery and knowledge acquisition. However, barriers caused by both infrastructure elements as well as limited training for teachers have resulted in an overall disjointed view of the role of technology in education.

Specifically, this disjointed view of technology implementation is characterized by a philosophy that students are only exposed to technology while in a computer lab. This flawed approach sends the wrong message to our teachers and students; specifically that technology use should be compartmentalized and that true learning of content only takes place in a traditional setting driven primarily by teacher centered activities. Indeed, what we propose more closely resembles technology *integration* than implementation. Namely, that technology becomes a support mechanism for the delivery of curriculum instead of an elective or enrichment activity.

There are three barriers which currently impede meaningful technology integration. First, current infrastructures in many K-12 schools were designed with the computer lab model. Indeed, moving from a building structure with a few rooms having 30 to 40 network drops to many rooms with 5 to 10 drops is no small chore. This would prove to be a costly and time consuming venture. However, the onset of wireless and mobile applications should allow educational leaders the additional flexibility to take at least some of the necessary steps needed. Second, training remains a paramount issue. Technology is often mistakenly seen as an end rather than a means to an end. True technology integration does not fit well into the teacher centered model where students remain quietly glued to a screen while an instructor gives directions from the front of a lab. Whereas technology can quickly build specific cognitive skills by providing targeted feedback and tireless repetition of tasks tailored to an individual student's needs, the true power of technology resides in a student-centered epistemology utilizing instructional techniques such as collaboration, project based learning, differentiated instruction, and authentic assessment. Failure to utilize technology as a route towards a more student-centered instructional model will detain educational technology to the tenants of Richard Clark (1983), where a computer simply represents another mode of transportation for academic content with little or no effect on its acquisition. This position, albeit one that is now dated by 25 years remains a challenge to the educational community to redefine the role of technology as it relates to curriculum integration. The third (and perhaps most ill-defined barrier) is teacher efficacy. School cultures are difficult to alter, and many teachers remain resilient to adapting their instructional approaches. Professional development can help in this regard, however many additional training opportunities are offered as optional activities attended primarily by instructors already amenable to change. In contrast, those truly in need of new and innovative approaches often settle for a handful of contractually obligated days devoted to staff development which continue to be consumed by peripheral administrative responsibilities. These one-shot training days typically lack the subsidence and continual supports necessary to definitively impact instruction.

While a teacher may have little influence over the technology infrastructure in place at a school, training and efficacy are within their realm of reach. Furthermore, as the demands for highly qualified teachers increases, particularly in low income neighborhoods, choice in work location may become more viable than before.

Motivation: The 800 Pound Gorilla that No One wants to Talk About

The previous sections of this chapter have used prior research to demonstrate the importance of a learner's volition and the importance of using technology not only to entice a learner to engage with content but as a window which can provide teachers and instructional designers with a glimpse of the needs and desires of the end user. What might be most disturbing is a lack of research published in this regard and even more so, the number of technology-based systems which fail to put what is known into place in regard to the design of these systems. Like the phases of self-regulation, system design and implementation should constitute an ongoing and emergent process rather than a design conducted in isolation.

The research base used to frame the current chapter is important in that it establishes the learner as an intelligent agent and relies heavily on newly accepted ideals that motivation can change over time and context. This research foundation also minimizes the emphasis on the role of ability since little can be done to change it. Motivation however, defined in large part by a learner's decision to engage or not engage with content will often serve as a viable predictor of academic success and represents an often untapped opportunity for instructors to impact their students.

Still, technology-based K-12 program research and product development is far too focused on distal outcomes and lacks the presence of engagement indicators that place a higher yield on motivational constructs. The stigma of "did it work?" was further amplified at the federal level when the age of accountability was born under the inception of No Child Left Behind in 2001 ("No Child Left Behind Act," 2001). The institutionalization of these performance benchmarks have distracted educators from more proximal programmatic impacts and forced attention towards bottom line indicators such as test scores and proficiency rates. While these are noble goals to pursue, a great deal of opportunity exists within the "black box" between implementation of an instructional technique and test day.

A great deal of this chapter has been devoted to motivational constructs and strategies as we believe that these topics receive far too little attention in K-12 technology program research and design. Teachers, as consumers of these products should look to programs that place value on student motivation and demonstrate evidence of engagement. Further, in addition to quantitative outcomes that K-12 and legislative leaders typically demand, it is important that instructors have clarity in regard to their role in technology integration. Innovative educational technology programs that fail to define the role of the instructor stand little chance of sustained success and those who see computer day as an opportunity to kick back and let the computer do the teaching are grossly misinformed about true technology integration.

RECOMMENTATIONS

As the current chapter has demonstrated, integration is a key predictor of technology's success in the classroom. Several critical elements should be evident both from teachers as well as K-12 leaders to best increase its likelihood of success. Namely, these are:

- A commitment from K-12 leaders to mandate technology integration
- Meaningful professional development with continuous systems of support
- Acknowledgement of student engagement as a critical outcome
- A willingness to move towards a student-centered instructional model
- Inclusion of research based engagement techniques in technology programs

A brief discussion of each of these critical elements follows.

A Commitment from K-12 Leaders to Mandate Technology Integration

Assuming that a general consensus exists within the educational community that technology has the potential to assist students and training is available to teachers to assist in the integration process, instructional leaders should look for evidence that technology integration is in fact occurring. Furthermore, educational leaders committed to technology integrated instruction should make this a priority by infusing requirements such as technology rich pedagogy into teacher evaluation criteria which include classroom observations and lesson plan reviews. Until this becomes part of the typical performance evaluation process, it is unlikely that teachers will see technology as anything more than an "optional" part of their assignment. Whether validated via observation, interview, or through a review of lesson plans, the message from each superintendent in America should be one that stresses the importance of using technology resources to enhance teaching and learning.

Meaningful Professional Development with Continuous Support Systems

From a survey sample of 1,027 mathematics and science teachers in the US, Garet et al (2001) identified six key components of professional development within two types of features that were reported as being effective at improving teacher practice:

Structure:

1. Organized as a reform (i.e. study group, teacher network, research study, etc.)
2. Duration
3. Collective Participation

Substance:

4. Active Learning
5. Coherence
6. Content Focus

It was also found that duration (both time span and contact hours) have a substantial positive influence on opportunities for active learning and coherence. Unfortunately, a national follow up study (Desimone, Porter, Garet, Yoon, & Birman, 2002) undertaken with 93% of US school districts nationwide found that only 23% of teachers from the sample of interest were engaged in reform types of professional development. Furthermore, the average time span of a professional development activity was less than one week. The results of these studies indicate that a majority of K-12 professional development conducted in the US lacks the duration necessary to spark significant changes in teacher practice.

One-time professional development workshops for teachers offer little in terms of truly impacting content knowledge or pedagogy. The lack of an appetite for many governmental agencies to appropriately fund school administrative teams and "extra" positions such as instructional coaches in the current economy make it difficult for site leaders to devote the time needed to make classroom observations and give appropriate feedback. In our experience, continual instructional support systems yield increases in teacher content knowledge, pedagogical practices, as well as student achievement (Crippen, Biesinger, & Ebert, 2009). Furthermore, action research projects have helped in this regard by training teachers to use a scientific approach of self-reflection to make instructional decisions based on empirical evidence.

Acknowledgement of Student Engagement as a Critical Outcome

Prior knowledge, that which a person currently knows about a topic, is the biggest predictor of new learning. Surprising to many, ability, as defined as an innate fixed quantity, plays a very small role. Though not as important as prior knowledge, the habits, strategies, and motivation of learners are malleable and can have strong effect on learning. A new paradigm for evaluating instructional strategies brings the focus away from summative indicators such as standardized tests and looks to more proximal outcomes to signify success. Our advocacy for this new model is that judging program efficacy based on only a few numbers complicates the potential reason for failures and often leaves educators wondering what specific component(s) of a program were (or were not) effective. For example, many programs fail due to a weak implementation and not because of an ill-conceived program (Reeves, 2008). Without formative data points throughout a program such as student engagement, it is difficult (if not impossible) to determine where and how programs or their implementation might be flawed. Second, student engagement is a valid and accepted predictor of achievement. How many times have we heard teachers tell us about the academic success possible if their students would only apply themselves? However, make no mistake, putting a child in front of a computer is not technology integration and the effort required for teachers to make this shift in pedagogy represents the most significant barrier.

Willingness to Move to a Student-Centered Instructional Model

How technology is used and integrated into teaching and learning is in large part determined by an instructor's epistemology (beliefs about the sources and acquisitions of knowledge). Still, too many instructional leaders view technology as the silver bullet rather than an opportunity to encourage a student-centered approach to learning. A major hurdle impeding this shift in thinking is caused by the structures currently in place at many public schools with separate computer labs mistakenly promoting technology as a mutually exclusive instructional activity and often one that is seen as ancillary. Additional hurdles in this area are outdated models of professional development which fail to acknowledge more innovative methods for integrating technology as well as a lack of initiative on the part of some instructors who were not exposed to this model as learners themselves. For many teachers, it is difficult to step outside of instructional techniques as teachers prior to experiencing them as learners, hence the heightened need for professional development that effectively models new and innovative educational technology methods.

Inclusion of Research Based Engagement Techniques in Technology Programs

The last 10 years or so have provided us with some notable advancements in educational technology components that teachers and K-12 leaders ought to verify before selecting programs, such as time out functions, trace method capability, and worked examples (where appropriate). Time out functions are a simple but almost necessary component for education technology programs. This simply means that a program should not remain idle for an extended period of time. Many educators and research analysts make the common mistake of anticipating positive correlations between time spent with a program and increased academic achievement. What actually matters is "what" learners do with a program and not necessarily the "how long" (quality not quantity). Without some type of time out mechanism, measurements of this nature for research purposes will be greatly flawed and the goals of engagement will be adversely impacted.

A second worthy addition to technology programs is trace methods. The onset of Web 2.0 offers educators a rich opportunity to use technology for discussion boards, blogs, and communication (either synchronous or asynchronous) while providing students with additional opportunities to communicate their thoughts in writing. In addition, mobile technology presents good opportunities for students to participate frequently and at any time desired. Furthermore, trace methods give instructors and researchers a great opportunity to gain insight into the needs, behaviors, and dispositions of their students. Indeed, the authors were pleasantly reminded of this when recently assisting a school district with the design and implementation of an innovative technology program to assist high school students in preparing for a state exit exam required for graduation (Biesinger & Crippen, 2008). Teachers were critical of the program due to its inability to give them detailed information about which students were logging in and how they were interacting with the program. Even functions such as a simple item analysis can be helpful in this regard.

Additionally, this line of data sheds a new light on what is known about the instructional strategies most likely to impact student engagement and highlights the fact that what students claim to do is not always the same as what they actually do. Additionally, self reports alone do not provide a comprehensive depiction of SRL and should be used in conjunction with distinct data points obtained through other methods such as trace to best triangulate a more complete scenario of self-regulated learning behaviors (Winne & Hadwin, 1998). The CoNoteS2 system has served as the primary data collection vehicle for Winne's more recent work with self-regulation (Hadwin & Winne, 2001) and should be considered an effective model for technology integration. The system is a multimedia user interface where learners interact with text (chapters). Each chapter contains a set of learning objectives, indexes, a glossary and links to other information. A series of organizer tools allow the user to highlight, categorize and prioritize text encountered in the reading assignment. One can also use the system to expound on salient details within the text, raise questions and build themes within the content. Learner behaviors are tracked and later compared to assessment results to indicate the effectiveness of the cognitive and metacognitive study strategies employed. Winne and colleagues have more recently pointed out some additional advantages of what is now referred to as "gStudy" (Perry & Winne, 2006). These include tracking capabilities over multiple academic episodes, complex task designs that address multiple goals and large-scale projects (individual or cooperative learning settings) and variation in the amount of feedback received from the system that is regulated by the learner.

Another instructional technology based strategy worthy of consideration is worked examples. Worked examples are an effective learning strategy for decreasing extraneous cognitive load (Paas & Van Merrienboer, 1994; Sweller, 1988; Van Merrienboer, Kirschnet, & Kester, 2003) and represent an exemplary self-regulation strategy. In recent years, self-regulation strategies to aid in the reduction of cognitive load have seen a resurgence for instructional design considerations (Pawley, Ayres, Cooper, & Sweller, 2005; Van Merrienboer, et al., 2003) particularly within the context of multimedia learning applications (Mayer & Moreno, 2003). Worked examples present a specific fundamental opportunity for technology to keep learners motivated by providing scaffolded instruction which can easily be adjusted to remain within a learner's zone of proximal development. The zone of proximal development was a concept originally conceived by Vygotsky (1978) and refers to instruction which is not deemed too easy nor too difficult in order to keep a learner engaged in an academic task. Worked examples could also serve as an excellent aide for instructors to differentiate instruction.

DIRECTIONS FOR FUTURE RESEARCH

The research and ideals discussed in this chapter offer two main directions for future research within the realm of educational technology research and development. First, we advocate for a student-centered position for both technology design as well as its integration into the classroom. As Linnenbrink (2005) argues, "[F]uture research should examine the stable effects of personal goals, perhaps based on motives or views of intelligence, as well as the changing nature of personal goal orientations based on the classroom environment. With this research, researchers may be better served by moving away from subjective perceptions of the goal context to more objective measures such as observations or experimental designs...Finally, a developmental perspective assessing personal goals and underlying dispositions and using objective measures of the goal context would allow one to more carefully trace the unique effects of these predictors to learning-related outcomes and the potential of a given classroom goal context to alter personal goal orientations over time (p.209)."

Second, teacher training and professional development programs should be traced to their outcomes on student engagement and achievement. The days of a simple Likert survey administered to teachers on their way out the door from a long day of "sit and get" do not fit the current and more desirable model of technology integration. Sadly, a majority of research conducted in regard to the effectiveness of professional development does not even investigate potential relationships to student achievement, much less engagement (Shymansky, Yore, Annetta, & Everett, 2008).

CONCLUSION

This chapter has drawn from current educational technology research and the authors' experience to provide the reader with critical elements to consider when building or selecting K-12 programs and their effective integration. Effective programs are those that utilize validation techniques such as time out functions, trace methods, and worked examples to ensure that a learner remains engaged with a program and provide additional information about what learners actually do while interacting with a program. While previous lines of data collection were often limited to self-reports, trace methods offer a critical additional data point since differences often emerge between what learners claim to do and actually do when engaged in a technology supported learning environment. When appropriate, worked examples serve as an effective tool to encourage learners to engage with a program and provide them a more enhanced experience compared to drill/practice exercises typically associated with more traditional technology supported learning environments.

In addition to program design concerns, perhaps even more important is the integration of technology programs. A primary concern of the authors is the philosophy of many educators who merely see technology as a supplementary activity which takes place occasionally in a remote lab as opposed to a continual support mechanism to enhance the delivery of content. Our hope is that more innovative professional development programs with continual support mechanisms will be able to effectively encourage a shift in epistemology focused on student-centered instructional techniques. In addition, K-12 leaders should place a higher premium on the expectation that instructors utilize technology effectively, which may encourage more teachers to make technology a part of their daily pedagogy.

REFERENCES

Ames, C. (1992). Classrooms: Goals, structures, and student motivation. *Journal of Educational Psychology*, *84*(3), 261–271. doi:10.1037/0022-0663.84.3.261

Bandura, A. (1977). Self-efficacy: Toward a unifying theory of behaviorial change. *Psychological Review*, *84*(2), 191–215. doi:10.1037/0033-295X.84.2.191

Bandura, A. (1986). *Social Foundations of Thought and Action: A Social Cognitive Theory*. Englewood Cliffs, N.J.: Prentice-Hall.

Bandura, A. (1997). *Self-Efficacy: The Exercise of Control*. New York: W.H. Freeman.

Biesinger, K., & Crippen, K. J. (2008). The impact of an online remediation site on performance related to high school mathematics proficiency. *Journal of Computers in Mathematics and Science Teaching*, *27*(1), 5–17.

Bower, M. (2005). Online assessment feedback: Competitive, individualistic, or preferred form! *Journal of Computers in Mathematics and Science Teaching*, *24*(2), 121–147.

Clark, R. E. (1983). Reconsidering research on learning from media. *Review of Educational Research*, *53*(4), 445–459.

Crippen, K. J., Biesinger, K. D., & Ebert, E. E. (in press). Using professional development to achieve classroom reform and science proficiency: An urban success story from southern Nevada USA. *Professional Development in Education.*

Crippen, K. J., & Earl, B. L. (2007). The impact of Web-based worked examples and self-explanation on performance, problem solving, and self-efficacy. *Computers & Education, 49*(3), 809–821. doi:10.1016/j.compedu.2005.11.018

Desimone, L. M., Porter, A. C., Garet, M. S., Yoon, K. S., & Birman, B. F. (2002). Effects of professional development on teachers' instruction: Results from a three-year longitudinal study. *Educational Evaluation and Policy Analysis, 24*(2), 81–112. doi:10.3102/01623737024002081

Dweck, C. S. (1986). Motivational processes affecting learning. *The American Psychologist, 41*(10), 1040–1048. doi:10.1037/0003-066X.41.10.1040

Dweck, C. S. (1999). *Self Theories: Their Role in Motivation, Personality, and Development.* Philadelphia, PA: Psychology Press.

Dweck, C. S., & Leggett, E. L. (1988). A social-cognitive approach to motivation and personality. *Psychological Review, 95*(2), 256–273. doi:10.1037/0033-295X.95.2.256

Elliot, A. J. (1999). Approach and avoidance motivation and achievement goals. *Educational Psychologist, 34*(3), 169–189. doi:10.1207/s15326985ep3403_3

Elliot, A. J., & McGregor, H. A. (2001). A 2 X 2 achievement goal framework. *Journal of Personality and Social Psychology, 80*(3), 501–519. doi:10.1037/0022-3514.80.3.501

Garet, M. S., Porter, A. C., Desimone, L., Birman, B. F., & Yoon, K. S. (2001). What makes professional development effective? Results from a national sample of teachers. *American Educational Research Journal, 38*(4), 915–945. doi:10.3102/00028312038004915

Hadwin, A. F., & Winne, P. H. (2001). CoNoteS2: A software tool for promoting self-regulation. *Educational Research and Evaluation, 7*(2-3), 313–334. doi:10.1076/edre.7.2.313.3868

Harackiewicz, J. M., Barron, K. E., Pintrich, P. R., Elliot, A. J., & Thrash, T. M. (2002). Revision of achievement goal theory: Necessary and illuminating. *Journal of Educational Psychology, 94*(3), 638–645. doi:10.1037/0022-0663.94.3.638

Johnson, D. W., Maruyama, G., Johnson, R., Nelson, D., & Skon, L. (1981). Effects of cooperative, competitive, and individualistic goal structures on achievement: A meta-analysis. *Psychological Bulletin, 89*(1), 47–62. doi:10.1037/0033-2909.89.1.47

Kennett, D. J., & Keefer, K. (2006). Impact of learned resourcefulness and theories of intelligence on academic achievement of university students: An integrated approach. *Educational Psychology, 26*(3), 441–457. doi:10.1080/01443410500342062

Lewis, M. A., & Cooney, J. B. (1987). Attributional and performance effects of competitive and individualistic feedback in computer assisted mathematics instruction. *Computers in Human Behavior, 3*(1), 1–13. doi:10.1016/0747-5632(87)90005-7

Linnenbrink, E. A. (2005). The dilemma of performance-approach goals: The use of multiple goal contexts to promopte students' motivation and learning. *Journal of Educational Psychology, 97*(2), 197–213. doi:10.1037/0022-0663.97.2.197

Linnenbrink, E. A., & Pintrich, P. R. (2001). Multiple goals, multiple contexts: The dynamic interplay between personal goals and contextual goal stresses. In Volet, S., & Jarvela, S. (Eds.), *Motivation in learning contexts: Theoretical and methodological implications* (pp. 251–269). Amsterdam: Pergamon Press.

Mangos, P. M., & Steele-Johnson, D. (2001). The role of subjective task complexity in goal orientation, self-efficacy, and performance relations. *Human Performance, 14*(2), 169–186. doi:10.1207/S15327043HUP1402_03

Mayer, R. E., & Moreno, R. (2003). Nine ways to reduce cognitive load in multimedia learning. *Educational Psychologist, 38*(1), 43–52. doi:10.1207/S15326985EP3801_6

No Child Left Behind Act. (2001). Retrieved November 15, 2006, from http://www.ed.gov/nclb

Paas, F. G. W. C., & Van Merrienboer, J. J. G. (1994). Variability of worked examples and transfer of geometrical problem solving skills: A cognitive load approach. *Journal of Educational Psychology, 86*(1), 122–133. doi:10.1037/0022-0663.86.1.122

Pajares (2002). Overview of social cognitive theory and of self-efficacy. Retreived 3/3/2010, from http://www.emory.edu/EDUCATION/mfp/eff.html

Patrick, H., Ryan, A. M., & Pintrich, P. R. (2000). The differential impact of extrinsic and mastery goal orientations on males' and females' self-regulated learning. *Learning and Individual Differences, 11*(2), 153–171. doi:10.1016/S1041-6080(00)80003-5

Pawley, D., Ayres, P., Cooper, M., & Sweller, J. (2005). Translating words into equations: A cognitive load theory approach. *Educational Psychology, 25*(1), 75–97. doi:10.1080/0144341042000294903

Perry, N. E., & Winne, P. H. (2006). Learning from learning kits: gStudy traces of students' self-regulated engagements with computerized content. *Educational Psychology Review, 18*(3), 211–228. doi:10.1007/s10648-006-9014-3

Pintrich, P. R. (1995). Understanding self-regulated learning. In P. R. Pintrich (Ed.), New Directions for Teaching and Learning: Vol. 63. Understanding Self-regulated Learning. San Fransisco: Jossey-Bass.

Pintrich, P. R. (2000a). Multiple goals, multiple pathways: The role of goal orientation in learning and achievement. *Journal of Educational Psychology, 92*(3), 544–555. doi:10.1037/0022-0663.92.3.544

Pintrich, P. R. (2000b). The Role of Goal Orientation in Self-Regulated Learning. In Pintrich, P. R., & Zeidner, M. (Eds.), *Handbook of Self Regulation.* San Diego, CA: Academic Press. doi:10.1016/B978-012109890-2/50043-3

Reeves, D. B. (2008). *Reframing Teacher Leadership to Improve Your School.* Alexandria, VA: ASCD.

Shymansky, J. A., Yore, L. D., Annetta, L. A., & Everett, S. A. (2008). Missouri-Iowa science cooperative (science co-op): Rural schools-rrban rniversities collaborative project. *Rural Educator, 29*(2), 1–3.

Steele-Johnson, D., Beauregard, R. S., Hoover, P. B., & Schmidt, A. M. (2000). Goal orientation and task cemand effects on motivation, affect, and performance. *The Journal of Applied Psychology, 85*(5), 724–738. doi:10.1037/0021-9010.85.5.724

Sweller, J. (1988). Cognitive load during problem solving: Effects on learning. *Cognitive Science, 12*(2), 257–285.

Van de Walle, D., Brown, S. P., Cron, W. L., & Slocum, J. W. (1999). The Influence of goal orientation and self-regulation tactics on sales performance: A longitudinal field test. *The Journal of Applied Psychology*, *84*(2), 249–259. doi:10.1037/0021-9010.84.2.249

Van Merrienboer, J. J. G., Kirschnet, P. A., & Kester, L. (2003). Taking the load off a learner's mind: Instructional design for complex learning. *Educational Psychologist*, *38*(1), 5–13. doi:10.1207/S15326985EP3801_2

Vygotsky, l. (1978). *Mind in Society: The Development of Higher Psychological Processes.* Cambridge, MA: MIT Press.

Winne, P. H., & Hadwin, A. F. (1998). Studying as self-regulated learning. In Hacker, D. J., Dunlosky, J., & Graesser, A. C. (Eds.), *Metacognition in educational theory and practice* (pp. 277–304). Manwah, NJ: Erlbaum.

Winne, P. H., & Perry, N. E. (2000). Measuring self-regulated learning. In Pintrich, P. R., & Zeidner, M. (Eds.), *Handbook of self-regulation* (pp. 531–566). San Diego, CA, US: Academic Press. doi:10.1016/B978-012109890-2/50045-7

Compilation of References

Aberg-Bengtsson, L. (2006). Then you can take half. almost--Elementary students learning bar graphs and pie charts in a computer-based Context. *The Journal of Mathematical Behavior*, *25*, 116–135. doi:10.1016/j.jmathb.2006.02.007

Abramovich, S., & Norton, A. (2006). Equations with parameters: A locus approach. *Journal of Computers in Mathematics and Science Teaching*, *25*, 5–28.

ACDE. (2001). New Learning: A Charter of Australian education. ACDE: RMIT University. Bigum, C. (1995). Schools and the internet: re-inventing the 1980s? Paper delivered at IARTV seminar, Melbourne 24 May 1995.

Adams, J. L., & Stephens, L. J. (1991). A comparison of computer-assisted instructional methods. *International Journal of Mathematical Education in Science and Technology*, *22*, 889–893. doi:10.1080/0020739910220604

Adobe Systems, Inc. (2001-2009). *Adobe Acrobat Connect Pro.* San Jose, CA: Adobe Systems, Inc.

Agre, P. E. (2000). Infrastructure and institutional change in the networked university. *Information Communication and Society*, *3*, 494–507. doi:10.1080/13691180010002323

Ainley, J., & Pratt, D. (1995). Supporting teachers' and children's mathematical thinking: A strategy for the effective use of information technology. *Technology, Pedagogy and Education*, *4*, 81–92. doi:10.1080/0962029950040107

Alavi, M., Wheeler, B. C., & Valacich, J. S. (1995). Using IT to reengineer business education: An exploratory investigation of collaborative telelearning. *Management Information Systems Quarterly*, *19*, 293–312. doi:10.2307/249597

Alexander, B. (2006, March/April). Web 2.0: A new innovation for teaching and learning? *Educause review.* Retrieved on January 20, 2008, from http://www.educause.edu/ir/library/pdf/ERM0621.pdf

Alexander, B. (2006, March/April). Web 2.0: A new wave of innovation for teaching and learning? *Educause Review.*

Allen, I. E., & Seaman, J. (2006). *Making the grade: Online education in the United States, 2006.* Retrieved April 2, 2009, from http://www.sloan-c.org/publications/survey/pdf/making_the_grade.pdf

Allen, I. E., & Seaman, J. (2008). *Staying the course: Online education in the United States, 2008.* Retrieved April 2, 2009, from http://www.sloan-c.org/publications/survey/pdf/staying_the_course.pdf

Alley, P., Blocher, M., & Markel, S. (2008 March). *The road to electronic assessment: An examination of one college's systematic process for evaluating and recommending electronic portfolio software.* Paper presented at Society for Information Technology & Teacher Education, Las Vegas, Nevada.

American Association for the Advancement of Science. (2005). *High school biology Textbooks: A benchmark-based evaluation.* Retrieved from the AAAS Project 2061 Textbook Evaluations Web site: http://www.project2061.org/publications/textbook/hsbio/report/default.htm

Ames, C. (1992). Classrooms: Goals, structures, and student motivation. *Journal of Educational Psychology*, *84*(3), 261–271. doi:10.1037/0022-0663.84.3.261

An, H., & Wilder, H. (2010, April). Preparing elementary preservice teachers from a non-traditional student population to teach with technology. In submission Paper session presented at The *Annual Meeting of the American Educational Research Association*, Denver, Colorado.

An, S., Kulm, G., & Wu, Z. (2004). The pedagogical content knowledge of middle school, mathematics teachers in China and the U.S. *Journal of Mathematics Teacher Education, 7*, 145–172. doi:10.1023/B:JMTE.0000021943.35739.1c

Anagnostopoulos, D., Basmadjian, K. G., & McCrory, R. S. (2005). The decentered teacher and the construction of social space in the virtual classroom. *Teachers College Record, 107*(8), 1699–1729. doi:10.1111/j.1467-9620.2005.00539.x

Anderson, L., & Krathwohl, D. (Eds.). (2001). *A Taxonomy for Learning, Teaching, and Assessing: A Revision of Blooms Taxonomy of Educational Objectives*. New York: Addison Wesley Longman, Inc.

Anonymous,. (2009). The 2.0 tech I can't live without. *Knowledge Quest, 37*(4), 34–36.

Antonitsch, P. K., Kleinhagauer, R., & Micheuz, P. (2008). Incorporating history in secondary education informatics courses. *IEEE Annals of the History of Computing, 30*, 56–63. doi:10.1109/MAHC.2008.49

Arbaugh, J. B., & Benbunan-Fich, R. (2006). An investigation of epistemological and social dimensions of teaching in online learning environments. *Academy of Management Learning & Education, 5*, 435–447.

Arnold, J., & Miller, H. (2001). Academic masters, mistresses, and apprentices: Gender and power in the real world of the web. *Mots Pluriels, 19*. Retrieved March 10, 2009, from http://www.arts.uwa.edu.au/MotsPluriels/MP1901jahm.html

Ashwin, A. (2006). GCSE business studies: The essentials. *Teaching Business & Economics, 10*(2), 42–44.

Ashworth, P. (2003). The origins of qualitative psychology. In Smith, J. (Ed.), *Qualitative psychology: A practical guide to research methods*. Thousand Oaks, CA: Sage.

Astin, A. (1985). *Achieving educational excellence: A critical assessment of priorities and practices in higher education*. San Francisco: Jossey-Bass.

Astin, A. W., Vogelsang, L. J., Ikeda, E. K., & Yee, J. A. (2000). *How service learning affects students*. Los Angeles: University of California, Higher Education Research Institute.

Aycock, A. (1995). Technologies of the self: Foucault and internet discourse. *Journal of Computer Mediated Communication, 1*(2). Retrieved November 10, 2006, from http://jcmc.indiana.edu/vol1/issue2/aycock.html

Baggott, L., Wishart, J., McFarlane, A., Brawn, R., & John, P. (2007). Teaching and learning with ICT within the subject culture of secondary school science. *Research in Science & Technological Education, 25*, 339–350. doi:10.1080/02635140701535158

Baines, L. (2006). Deconstructing Teacher Certification. *Phi Delta Kappan, 88*(4), 326–329.

Bakeman, R., & Gottman, J. (1997). *Observing Interaction: An introduction to sequential analysis*. Cambridge, UK: Cambridge University Press. doi:10.1017/CBO9780511527685

Baker, E. A. (2005). Can preservice teacher education really help me grow as a literacy teacher? Examining preservice teachers' perceptions of multimedia case-based instruction. *Journal of Technology and Teacher Education, 13*, 415–431.

Baker, J. D. (2001). The effects of instructor immediacy and student cohesiveness on affective and cognitive learning in the online classroom. (Doctoral dissertation, Regent University, 2001). *Dissertation Abstracts International, 62*, 06. 2081 UMI No. 3018333.

Ball, D. L., & Cohen, D. K. (1999). Developing practices, developing practitioners. In Darling-Hammond, L., & Sykes, G. (Eds.), *Teaching as the learning profession: Handbook of policy and practice* (pp. 3–32). San Francisco: Jossey-Bass.

Ball, D. L., Bass, H., & Hill, H. C. (2004). Knowing and using mathematical knowledge in teaching: Learning what matters. In A. Buffler & R. C. Laugksch (Eds.), *Proceedings of the 12th Annual Conference of the Southern African Association for Research in Mathematics, Science and Technology Education.* Durban: SAARMSTE.

Bandura, A. (1977). Self-efficacy: Toward a unifying theory of behavioral change. *Psychological Review, 84*(2), 191–215. doi:10.1037/0033-295X.84.2.191

Bandura, A. (1986). *Social Foundations of Thought and Action: A Social Cognitive Theory.* Englewood Cliffs, N.J.: Prentice-Hall.

Bandura, A. (1997). *Self-Efficacy: The Exercise of Control.* New York: W.H. Freeman.

Barabasi, A. (2003). *Linked: How everything is connected to everything else and what it means for business, science, and everyday life.* New York: Penguin Press.

Barbas, M. P. (2006). Expanding knowledge: From the classroom into cyberspace. *Educational Media International, 43*, 65–73. doi:10.1080/09523980500490885

Barnes, C. J. (2006). Preparing preservice teachers to teach in a culturally responsive way. *Negro Educational Review, 57*(1/2), 85–100.

Baron, N. S. (2004). See you online: Gender issues in American college student use of instant messaging. *Journal of Language and Social Psychology, 23*(4), 397–423. doi:10.1177/0261927X04269585

Barrett, H. (2000). Create your own electronic portfolio using off-the-shelf software to showcase your own or student work. *Learning & Leading with Technology.* Retrieved June 5, 2005, from http://electronicportfolios.com/portfolios/iste2k.html

Barrett, H. (2006). *Digital Stories in e-Portfolios: Multiple Purposes and Tools.* Retrieved June 2009, from http://electronicportfolios.org/digistory/purposesmac.html

Barrett, H. (2006). Using electronic portfolios for formative/classroom based assessment: The reflect initiative. *Connected Newsletter,* June 2006.

Barrett, H. (2007). Researching electronic portfolios and learner engagement: The Reflect Initiative. *Journal of Adolescent & Adult Literacy, 50*(6), 436–449. doi:10.1598/JAAL.50.6.2

Barrett, H., & Wilkerson, J. (2004). *Conflicting paradigms in electronic portfolio approaches.* Retrieved March 20, 2009, from http://electronicportfolios.org/systems/paradigms.html

Bartlett, A. (2002). Preparing preservice teachers to implement performance assessment and technology through electronic portfolios. *Action in Teacher Education, 24*(1), 90–97.

Batchelder, T., & Root, S. (1994). Effects of an undergraduate program to integrate academic learning and service: cognitive, prosocial cognitive and identity outcomes. *Journal of Adolescence, 17*, 341–356. doi:10.1006/jado.1994.1031

Batson, T. (2008). Using mashups to teach IT concepts at Bentley College. *Campus Technology.* Retrieved February 6, 2008 from http://campustechnology.com/Articles/2008/02/Using-Mashups-to-Teach-IT-Concepts-at-Bentley-College.aspx

Bauer, J., & Anderson, R. (2000). Evaluating students' written performance in the online classroom. *New Directions for Teaching and Learning, 84*(4), 65–71. doi:10.1002/tl.849

Baumeister, R. F., & Leary, M. R. (1995). The need to belong: Desire for interpersonal attachments as a fundamental human motivation. *Psychological Bulletin, 117*(3), 497–529. doi:10.1037/0033-2909.117.3.497

Beatty, A. (1997). *Learning from TIMSS: Results of the Third International Mathematics and Science Study, Summary of a Symposium.* Committee on Science Education K-12, National Research Council. Washington, DC: The National Academies Press. Retrieved from http://www.nap.edu/catalog.php?record_id=5937

Beck, R. J., King, A., & Marshall, S. K. (2002). Effects of videocase construction on pre-service teachers' observation of teaching. *Journal of Experimental Education, 70*(4), 345–361. doi:10.1080/00220970209599512

Beck, R., Livine, N., & Bear, S. (2005). Teachers' self assessment of the effects of formative and summative electronic portfolios on professional development. *European Journal of Teacher Education*, *28*(3), 221–244. doi:10.1080/02619760500268733

Becker, H. (2000). *Findings from the teaching, learning, and computing survey: Is Larry Cuban right?* Paper presented for the Council of Chief State School Officers' Annual Technology Leadership Conference, Washington, DC.

Beishuizen, J., Van Boxel, P., Banyard, P., Twiner, A., Vermeij, H., & Underwood, J. (2006). The introduction of portfolios in higher education: a comparative study in the UK and the Netherlands. *European Journal of Education*, *41*(3), 491–508. doi:10.1111/j.1465-3435.2006.00278.x

Beldarrain, Y. (2006). Distance Education Trends: Integrating new technologies to foster student interaction and collaboration. *Distance Education, 27*(2), 139-154. Retrieved from Proquest databases on September 2008.

Bell, L., Schrum, L., & Thompson, E. A. (Eds.). (2009). *Framing the research on digital technologies and student learning in mathematics*. Charlotte, NC: Information Age Publishing.

Bergman, T. (2004). *Feasible electronic portfolios: Global networking for the self-directed learner in the digital age*. Retrieved June 5, 2008, from, http://www.mehs.educ.state.ak.us/portfolios/why _digital _portfolios.html.

Berlind, D. (2006). Mashup ecosystem poised to explode. *ZDNet*. Retrieved February 6, 2008, from http://blogs.zdnet.com/BTL/?p=2484

Berlind, D. (2008). *Microsoft's cloud ecosystem czar: 'When mashups fail, whose throat do you choke?'* Retrieved April 5, 2009 from http://www.informationweek.com/blog/main/archives/2008/11/micrososofts_cl.html

Berman, E. D. (1998). Preparing for the new millennium: Highlights of DMCA of 1998. *Multimedia & Web Strategist*, *5*(1), 1.

Berson, I. R., & Berson, M. J. (2007). Exploring complex social phenomena with computer simulations. *Social Education*, *71*, 136–139.

Biesinger, K., & Crippen, K. J. (2008). The impact of an online remediation site on performance related to high school mathematics proficiency. *Journal of Computers in Mathematics and Science Teaching*, *27*(1), 5–17.

Black, S., & Smith, E. (2001). The integrity of the council accreditation process. *Journal of Family and Consumer Sciences*, *93*(3), 52–62.

Blackboard, Inc. (1997-2009). *Blackboard Learning System*. Washington, DC: Blackboard, Inc.

Bloom, B. S. (Ed.). Engelhart, M.D. Furst, E.J., Hill, W.H., & Krathwohl, D.R. (1956). Taxonomy of Educational Objectives: Handbook 1: Cognitive Domain. New York: David McKay.

Bodzin, A. M. (2008). Integrating instructional technologies in a local watershed investigation with urban elementary learners. *The Journal of Environmental Education*, *39*, 47–58. doi:10.3200/JOEE.39.2.47-58

Boechler, P. M., Foth, D., & Watchorn, R. (2007). Educational technology research with older adults: Adjustments in protocol, materials, and procedures. *Educational Gerontology*, *33*, 221–235. doi:10.1080/03601270600894089

Boler, M. (1999). *Feeling power: Emotions and education*. New York: Routledge.

Bonwell, C., & Eison, J. (1991, September 1). Active learning: Creating excitement in the classroom. *ERIC Digest*. (ERIC Document Reproduction Service No. ED340272) Retrieved August 18, 2009, from ERIC database.

Borsheim, C., Merrit, K., & Reed, D. (2008). Beyond technology for technology's take: Advancing multiliteracies in the twenty-first century. *Clearing House (Menasha, Wis.)*, *82*(2), 87–91. doi:10.3200/TCHS.82.2.87-90

Boulet, M. M., Boudreault, S., & Guerette, L. (1997, November). *Distance education: Integrating technology into computer science education.* Paper presented at the 27th annual Frontiers in Education Conference, Pittsburg, PA.

Bower, M. (2005). Online assessment feedback: Competitive, individualistic, or preferred form! *Journal of Computers in Mathematics and Science Teaching, 24*(2), 121–147.

Bowman, J. K., Koirala, H. P., & Edmonds, L. E. (2000). Graphing calculators: Critical tools for actively teaching math and science. *Computers in the Schools, 16*, 135–149. doi:10.1300/J025v16n03_03

Boyd, D., & Ellison, N. (2007). Social network sites: definition, history, and scholarship. *Journal of Computer-Mediated Communication, 13*(1), 210-230. Retrieved April 2009, from http://plcmcl2-things.blogspot.com/

Brand, B. R., & Wilkins, J. L. M. (2007). Using self-efficacy as a construct for evaluating science and mathematics methods courses. *Journal of Science Teacher Education, 18*(2), 297–317. doi:10.1007/s10972-007-9038-7

Brandes, G., & Boskic, N. (2008). E portfolios: From description to analysis. *International Review of Research in Open and Distance Learning, 9*(2), 1–17.

Bransford, J., Brown, A., & Cocking, R. (1999). *How People Learn: Brain, Mind, Experience and School.* National Research Council.

Bricout, J. C. (2001). Making computer-mediated education responsive to the accommodation needs of students with disabilities. *Journal of Social Work Education, 37*, 267–281.

Brown, D., & Warschauer, M. (2006). From the university to the elementary classroom: Students' experiences in learning to integrate technology in instruction. *Journal of Technology and Teacher Education, 14*(3), 599–62.

Brown, J. (2002). *Growing Up Digital: How the Web Changes Work, Education, and the Ways People Learn.* United States Distance Learning Association. Retrieved on March 10, 2009, from http://www.usdla.org/html/journal/FEB02_Issue/article01.html

Brown, J. S. (2005). *New Learning Environments for the 21st Century.* Retrieved from http://www.educause.edu/screencasts/JohnSeelyBrown@TWT_CU.pdf

Brown, J., & Adler, R. (2008). Minds on fire: Open education, the long tail, and learning 2.0. *EDUCAUSE Review, 43*(1), 16–32.

Brush, T., Igoe, A., Brinkerhoff, J., Glazewski, K., Ku, H., & Smith, T. C. (2001). Lessons from the field: Integrating technology into preservice teacher education. *Journal of Computing in Teacher Education, 17*(4), 16–20.

Bryk, A. S., & Driscoll, M. E. (1988). The high school as community: Contextual influences and consequences for students and teachers. Madison, WI: National Center on Effective Secondary Schools. (ERIC Document Reproduction Service No. ED302539)

BSCS. (2006). *The BSCS 5E instructional model: origins and effectiveness: a report prepared for the Office of Science Education, National Institutes of Health.* Retrieved from http://www.bscs.org/library/BSCS_5E_Model_Full_Report2006.pdf

Bull, G., Park, J., Searson, M., Thompson, A., Mishra, P., Koehler, M. J., & Knezek, G. (2007). Editorial: Developing technology policies for effective classroom practice. *Contemporary Issues in Technology & Teacher Education, 7*(3). Retrieved from http://www.citejournal.org/vol7/iss3/editorial/article1.cfm.

Bullock, D. (2004). Moving from theory to practice: An examination of the factors that preservice teachers encounter as the attempt to gain experience teaching with technology during field placement experiences. *Journal of Technology and Teacher Education, 12*(2), 211–237.

Burns, A. (1999). *Collaborative Action Research.* Cambridge, UK: Cambridge University Press.

Buxton, C. A. (2005). Creating a culture of academic success in an urban science and math magnet high school. *Science Education, 89*, 392–417. doi:10.1002/sce.20057

Bybee, R. (1993). An instructional model for science education. In Developing biological literacy. Colorado Springs, CO: Biological Science Curriculum Study.

Cambridge, D. (2008). Universities as responsive learning organizations through competency-based assessment with electronic portfolios. *JGE: The Journal of General Education, 57*(1), 51–64. doi:10.1353/jge.0.0007

Campbell, D., Cignetti, P., Melenyzer, B., Nettles, D., & Wyman, R. (2001). *How to develop a professional portfolio: A manual for teachers*. Boston, MA: Allyn & Bacon.

Capraro, M. (2003). *Electronic teaching portfolios: technology skills + portfolio development = powerful pre-service teachers*. ERIC Number ED476367. Retrieved from ERIC database on April 1, 2009.

Carlson, S. (2005). The net generation goes to college. *The Chronicle of Higher Education, 52*(7), A34. Retrieved from http://chronicle.com/free/v52/i07/07a03401.htm.

Carneval, D. (2005, June 28). Online Courses Continue to Grow Dramatically. *Chronicle of Higher Education*,14-26. Retrieved September 2, 2008 from http://chronicle.com/prm/daily/2005/06/2005062802t.htm

Carstens, A., & Beck, J. (2005). Get ready for the gamer generation. *TechTrends, 49*, 22–25. doi:10.1007/BF02763643

Casey, B., & Howson, P. (1993). Educating preservice students based on a problem-centered approach to teaching. *Journal of Teacher Education, 44*(5), 361–369. doi:10.1177/0022487193044005006

Cavanaugh, C., Gillan, K. J., Bosnick, J., Hess, M., & Scott, H. (2008). Effectiveness of interactive online algebra learning tools. *Journal of Educational Computing Research, 38*, 67–95. doi:10.2190/EC.38.1.d

Caywood, K., & Duckett, J. (2003). Online vs. on-campus learning in teacher education. *Teacher Education and Special Education, 26*(2), 98–105. doi:10.1177/088840640302600203

Cennamo, K. S., Abell, S. K., George, E. J., & Chung, M. L. (1996). The development of integrated media cases for use in elementary science teacher education. *Journal of Technology and Teacher Education, 4*(1), 19–36.

Center for Science, Mathematics, and Engineering Education. (1996). *National Science Education Standards*. Washington, DC: The National Academies Press. Retrieved from http://books.nap.edu/openbook.php?record_id=4962&page=1

Chambers, S., & Wickersham, L. (2007). The electronic portfolio journal: A year later. *Education, 127*(3), 351–360.

Chitpin, S., Simon, M., & Galipeau, J. (2008). Pre-service teachers' use of the Objective Knowledge Framework for Reflection during practicum. *Teaching and Teacher Education: An International Journal of Research and Studies, 24*(8), 2049–2058. doi:10.1016/j.tate.2008.04.001

Christensen, C. M. (1997). *The innovator's dilemma: When new technologies can cause great firms to fail*. Boston: Harvard Business School Press.

Chua, B. L., & Wu, Y. (2005). Designing technology-based mathematics lessons: A pedagogical framework. *Journal of Computers in Mathematics and Science Teaching, 24*, 387–402.

Chuang, H. (2007). Making connections: n international student's perspective. In Thompson, A.,

Chuang, H., & Sahin, I. (Eds.), *Faculty mentoring: The power of students in developing technology expertise* (pp. 59–69). Charlotte, NC: Information Age Publishing.

Chung Lee, J. (n.d.). Low-cost multi-point interactive whiteboards using the WiiMote. *WiiMote Project*. Retrieved on February 2, 2009, from http://www.cs.cmu.edu/~johnny/projects/wii/

Chyung, S. Y. (2001). Systematic and systemic approaches to reducing attrition rates in online higher education. *American Journal of Distance Education, 15*(3), 36–50. doi:10.1080/08923640109527092

Cibulka, J. (2008). Quality teaching: Moving forward to strengthen NCATE accreditation. *The Newsletter of the National Council for Accreditation of Teacher Education, 18*(1), 1–6.

Clark, D. A., Piper, S. C., Keeling, C. D., & Clark, D. B. (2003). Tropical rain forest tree growth and atmospheric carbon dynamics linked to interannual temperature variation during 1984-2000. *Proceedings of the National Academy of Sciences of the United States of America, 100*(10), 5852–5857. doi:10.1073/pnas.0935903100

Clark, R. E. (1983). Reconsidering research on learning from media. *Review of Educational Research, 53*(4), 445–459.

Clark, R. W., Foster, A., & Mantle-Bromley, C. (2005). *Hybrid educators and the simultaneous renewal of schools and the education of educators.* Seattle, WA: Institution for Educational Inquiry.

Clarke, O. (2005). Engaging the digital natives in learning. *Primary & Middle Years Educator, 3*(3), 20–25.

Cobb, P., & Bowers, J. (1999). Cognitive and situated learning perspectives in theory and practice. *Educational Researcher, 28*, 4–15. doi:10.2307/1177185

College LiveText Educational Solutions. (2009). Retrieved from http://www.livetext.com

Commission on Colleges of the Southern Association of Colleges and Schools. (2004). *Principles of Accreditation: Foundations for Quality Enhancement.* Retrieved April 1, 2009, from http://www.sacscoc.org/pdf/PrinciplesOfAccreditation.PDF

Conrad, D. (2008). Building knowledge through portfolio learning in prior learning assessment and recognition. *Quarterly Review of Distance Education, 9*(2), 139–150.

Conrad, D. (2008). Reflecting on strategies for a new learning culture: Can we do it? *Journal of Distance Education, 2*(3), 157–162.

Copyright clearance center. (1999). Retrieved March 24, 1999 from http://www.copyright.com

Cornell University. (n.d.). *Section 107. Limitations on exclusive rights: Fair use.* Retrieved March 24, 1999, from http://www4.law.cornell.edu/uscode/17/107.text.html

Cornford, J. (2000). The virtual university is... the university made concrete? *Information Communication and Society, 3*, 508–525. doi:10.1080/13691180010002314

Council for the Advancement of Standards in Higher Education. (2006). *CAS professional standards for higher education* (6th ed.). Washington, DC: Author.

Council of Chief State School Officers. (2005). State indicators of science and mathematics education 2005, Washington, DC.

Cowan, C., Hartleb, D., & Neves, D. (2007). Collaboration on technology projects results in cost sharing opportunities. *Community College Journal of Research and Practice, 31*, 503–504. doi:10.1080/10668920701359615

Cress, C. M., Collier, P. J., & Reitenauer, V. L. (2005). *Learning through serving: A student guidebook for service-learning across the disciplines.* Sterling, VA: Stylus Publishing.

Creswell, J. W. (2007). *Qualitative inquiry and research design* (2nd ed.). Thousand Oaks, CA: Sage.

Crippen, K. J., & Earl, B. L. (2007). The impact of Web-based worked examples and self-explanation on performance, problem solving, and self-efficacy. *Computers & Education, 49*(3), 809–821. doi:10.1016/j.compedu.2005.11.018

Crippen, K. J., Biesinger, K. D., & Ebert, E. E. (in press). Using professional development to achieve classroom reform and science proficiency: An urban success story from southern Nevada USA. *Professional Development in Education.*

Crook, C., & Harrison, C. (2008). *Web 2.0 technologies for learning at key stages 3 and 4: Summary report.* Retrieved April 2009, from http://schools.becta.org.uk/upload-dir/downloads/page_documents/research/web2_ks34_summary.pdf

Cross, T. L. (2006). Digital immigrants, natives, and "tweeners": A glimpse into the future for our students with gifts and talents. *Gifted Child Today, 29*(3), 52–53.

Cuban, L. (2001). *Oversold and Underused, Computers in the Classroom.* Boston, MA: Harvard University Press.

D'Amico, M. (1996a, May). Can I borrow a bit of digital? *NetGuide Magazine.*

D'Amico, M. (1996b, July). The web is not a legal quagmire. *Digital Media, 6*(2).

Danielson, C. (1996). *Enhancing professional practice: A framework for teaching.* Alexandria, VA: ASCD.

Dannelly, R. S., Michaud, P., Patterson-McNeill, H., & Steidley, C. W. (2002, October). *A multidisciplinary student-centered laboratory.* Paper presented at the 32nd annual Frontiers in Education Conference, Boston, MA.

Darlaston-Jones, D. (2007). Making connections: The relationship between epistemology and research methods. *The Australian Community Psychologist, 19*(1), 19–27.

Darling-Hammond, L., Wei, R. C., Andree, A., Richardson, N., & Orphanos, S. (2009). *Professional learning in the learning profession: A status report on teacher development in the United States and abroad.* Dallas, TX: National Staff Development Council.

Datnow, A., & Stringfield, S. (2000). Working together for reliable school reform. [JESPAR]. *Journal of Education for Students Placed at Risk, 5*, 183–204. doi:10.1207/s15327671espr0501&2_11

Datta, L. (1994). Paradigm wars: A basis for peaceful coexistence and beyond. In Reichardt, C. S., & Rallis, S. F. (Eds.), *The qualitative-quantitative debate: New perspectives* (pp. 53–70). San Francisco: Jossey-Bass.

Davidson, C. N., & Goldberg, D. T. (2009). *The future of learning institutions in a digital age.* The John D., & Catherine T. MacArthur Foundation Reports on Digital Media Learning.

Davis, B., & Simmt, E. (2003). Understanding learning systems: Mathematics education and complexity science. *Journal for Research in Mathematics Education, 34*, 137–167. doi:10.2307/30034903

Davis, B., & Sumara, D. J. (1997). Cognition, complexity, and teacher education. *Harvard Educational Review, 67*, 105–125.

Davis, B., & Sumara, D. J. (2001). Learning communities: Understanding the workplace as a complex system. *New Directions for Adult and Continuing Education, 2001*, 85–95. doi:10.1002/ace.43

De Smet, M., Van Keer, H., & Valcke, M. (2008). Cross-age peer tutors in asynchronous discussion groups: studying the impact of tutors labelling their interventions. *Journal of Computer Assisted Learning, 24*, 462–473.

Deaney, R., Ruthven, K., & Hennessy, S. (2003). Pupil perspectives on the contribution of information and communication technology to teaching and learning in the secondary school. *Research Papers in Education, 18*, 141–165. doi:10.1080/0267152032000081913

DeBell, M., & Chapman, C. (2006). *Computer and Internet Use by Students in 2003 (NCES 2006–065).* U.S. Department of Education. Washington, DC: National Center for Education Statistics. Retrieved from http://nces.ed.gov/pubsearch/pubsinfo.asp?pubid=2006065

DeBourgh, G. (2003). Predictors of student satisfaction in distance delivered graduate nursing courses: What matters most. *Journal of Professional Nursing, 19*, 149–163. doi:10.1016/S8755-7223(03)00072-3

Defazio, J. (2006). Theory into practice: A bridge too far? *AACE Journal, 14*, 221–233.

DeHaan, R. (2005). The impending revolution in undergraduate science education. *Journal of Science Education and Technology, 14*(2), 253–269. doi:10.1007/s10956-005-4425-3

Delmont, G. (2003). Using electronic portfolios to document learning. *Athletic Therapy Today, 8*(4), 22–23.

DeSalle, R., & Heithaus, M. (2008). *Biology.* New York: Holt, Rinehart and Winston.

Desimone, L. M., Porter, A. C., Garet, M. S., Yoon, K. S., & Birman, B. F. (2002). Effects of professional development on teachers' instruction: Results from a three-year longitudinal study. *Educational Evaluation and Policy Analysis, 24*(2), 81–112. doi:10.3102/01623737024002081

Dewey, J. (1933). *How we think: A restatement of the relation of reflective thinking to the educative process.* Boston: Heath and Company.

Dewey, J. (1966). *Democracy and Education.* New York: Free Press. Educational Encyclopedia. (2009). *Accreditation in the United States: Higher Education.* Retrieved June 17, 2009, from http://education.stateuniversity.com

Dexter, S., & Riedel, E. (2003). Why improving preservice teacher educational technology preparation must go beyond the college's walls. *Journal of Teacher Education*, *54*(4), 334–346. doi:10.1177/0022487103255319

Dickey, M. H., Wasko, M. M., Chudoba, K. M., & Thatcher, J. B. (2006). Do you know what I know?: A shared understandings perspective on text-based communication. *Journal of Computer-Mediated Communication, 12*(1). Retrieved March 16, 2009, from http://jcmc.indiana.edu/vol12/issue1/dickey.html

Ding, C., & Sherman, H. (2006). Teaching effectiveness and student achievement: Examining the relationship. *Educational Research Quarterly, 29*, 40–51.

diSessa, A. A., & Cobb, P. (2004). Ontological innovation and the role of theory in design experiments. *Journal of the Learning Sciences, 13*, 77–103. doi:10.1207/s15327809jls1301_4

Donath, J., Karahalios, K., & Viegas, F. (1999). Visualizing conversation. *Journal of Computer-Mediated Communication, 4*(4). Retrieved March 3, 2009, from http://jcmc.indiana.edu/vol4/issue4/donath.html

Donovan, M. S., Bransford, J. D., & Pellegrino, J. W. (Eds.). (1999). *How people learn: Bridging research and practice*. Washington, DC: National Academy Press.

Donovan, M., & Bransford, J. (2005). *How Students Learn: Science in the Classroom*. Washington, DC: The National Academies of Science Press. Retrieved from http://books.nap.edu/openbook.php?record_id=11102&page=1

Doolittle, P., & Hicks, D. (2003). Constructivism as a theoretical foundation for the use of technology in Social Studies. *Theory and Research in Social Education, 31*(1), 72–104.

Dornan, T., Carroll, C., & Parboosingh, J. (2002). An electronic learning portfolio for reflective continuing professional development. *Medical Education, 36*(1), 767–769. doi:10.1046/j.1365-2923.2002.01278.x

Dotterer, R. E., & Pasley, J. D. (2000). *New Frontiers in Physiology/ Physiology Insights and Final Evaluation Report*. Chapel Hill, NC: Horizon Research Inc.

Douglas, S. C. (2001, October). *The INFINITY project: Digital signal processing and digital music in high school engineering education*. Paper presented at the IEEE workshop on the Applications of Signal Processing to Audio and Acoustics, New Paltz, NY.

Downing, D. M., & Zelson, C. M. (1998). On intellectual property: The millennium arrives. *Intellectual Property, 7*(6).

Draves, W. A. (2002). *Teaching online*. River Falls, WI: LERN Books.

Duffy, F. M. (2003). I think, therefore I am resistant to change: What we know - or think we know - is our biggest roadblock to learning. *Journal of Staff Development, 24*(1).

Duffy, P., & Bruns, A. (2006). The use of blogs, wikis and RSS in education: a conversation of possibilities. In *Proceedings Online Learning and Teaching Conference 2006*, Brisbane (pp. 31–38). Retrieved September 2008, from http://www.scu.edu.au/twt/wiki01.html

Duschl, R., Schweingruber, H., & Shouse, A. (2007). *Taking Science to School: Learning and Teaching Science in Grades K-8*. Washington, DC: The National Academies of Science Press. Retrieved from http://books.nap.edu/openbook.php?record_id=11625&page=R1

Dweck, C. S. (1986). Motivational processes affecting learning. *The American Psychologist, 41*(10), 1040–1048. doi:10.1037/0003-066X.41.10.1040

Dweck, C. S. (1999). *Self Theories: Their Role in Motivation, Personality, and Development*. Philadelphia, PA: Psychology Press.

Dweck, C. S., & Leggett, E. L. (1988). A social-cognitive approach to motivation and personality. *Psychological Review, 95*(2), 256–273. doi:10.1037/0033-295X.95.2.256

Dykman, C. A., & Davis, C. K. (2008). Online education forum—part three: A quality online educational experience. *Journal of Information Systems Education, 19*(3), 281–289.

Dymond, S. K., & Bentz, J. L. (2006). Using digital videos to enhance teacher preparation. *Teacher*

Education and Special Education, *29*(2), 98–112. doi:10.1177/088840640602900202

Dynarski, M., Agodini, R., Heaviside, S., Novak, T., Carey, N., Campuzano, L., et al. (2007). *Effectiveness of reading and mathematics software products: Findings from the first student cohort.* Washington, DC: National Center for Education Evaluation and Regional Assistance. Retrieved on February 12, 2009, from http://ies.ed.gov/ncee/pdf/20074005.pdf

Dyrud, M. A. (1997). Learning styles. *Business Communication Quarterly*, *60*, 124–125. doi:10.1177/108056999706000211

Eastment, D. (2008). Social networking. *ELT Journal*, *62*(2), 217–221. doi:10.1093/elt/ccn007

EDUCAUSE Learning Initiative. (2006). *7 things you should know about... Mapping mashups.* Retrieved February 24, 2008, from http://net.educause.edu/ir/library/pdf/ELI7016.pdf

Effross, W. A. (1998). Seamless seaminess? *Computer Law Strategist*, *15*(8), 4.

Ellington, A. J. (2003). A meta-analysis of the effects of calculators on students' achievement and attitude levels in precollege mathematics classes. *Journal for Research in Mathematics Education*, *34*, 433–463. doi:10.2307/30034795

Ellington, A. J. (2006). The effects of non-CAS graphing calculators on student achievement and attitude levels in mathematics: A meta-analysis. *International Journal of Instructional Media*, *106*, 16–26.

Elliot, A. J. (1999). Approach and avoidance motivation and achievement goals. *Educational Psychologist*, *34*(3), 169–189. doi:10.1207/s15326985ep3403_3

Elliot, A. J., & McGregor, H. A. (2001). A 2 X 2 achievement goal framework. *Journal of Personality and Social Psychology*, *80*(3), 501–519. doi:10.1037/0022-3514.80.3.501

Ellis, J. D. (1989). An evaluation of a project for preparing science teachers to use microcomputers. *Journal of Computers in Mathematics and Science Teaching*, *8*, 51–65.

Ely, D. (2008). Frameworks of educational technology. *British Journal of Educational Technology*, *39*, 244–250. doi:10.1111/j.1467-8535.2008.00810.x

Eraut, M. (1994). *Developing professional knowledge and competence*. London: Falmer Press.

Erbas, A. K., Ledford, S., Polly, D., & Orrill, C. H. (2004). Engaging students through technology. *Mathematics Teaching in the Middle School*, *9*, 300–305.

eSchool News. (2008). *On the way: Nation's first tech-literacy exam.* Retrieved March 8, 2009, from http://www.eschoolnews.com/news/top-news/?i=55483

Ewing, J. M., Dowling, J. D., & Courts, N. (1998). Learning using the World Wide Web: A collaborative learning event. *Journal of Educational Multimedia and Hypermedia*, *8*, 3–22.

Eyler, J., & Giles, D. E. (1999). *Where's the learning in service learning?* San Francisco: Jossey-Bass.

Fagerberg, J. (2004). Innovation: A Guide to the Literature. In Fagerberg, J., Mowery, D., & Nelson, R. (Eds.), *The Oxford Handbook of Innovations* (pp. 1–26). Oxford, UK: Oxford University Press.

Fahy, P. (2002). Epistolary and Expository Interaction Patterns in a Computer Conference Transcript. *Journal of Distance Education*, *17*(1), 20–35.

Fahy, P. (2003). Indicators of support in online interaction. *International Review of Research in Open and Distance Learning*, *4*(1), 1-16. Retrieved April 28, 2008, from http://www.irrodl.org/index.php/irrodl/article/view/129

Fahy, P. J. (2005). Two methods for assessing critical thinking in computer-mediated communications (CMC) transcripts. *International Journal of Instructional Technology and Distance Learning*, *2*(3). Retrieved June 5, 2008, from http://www.itdl.org/Journal/Mar_05/article02.htm

Fahy, P., Crawford, G., & Ally, M. (2001). Patterns of interaction in a computer conference transcript. *The International Review of Research in Open and Distance Learning*, *2*(1). Retrieved September 30, 2008, from http://www.irrodl.org/index.php/irrodl/article/view/36

Felner, R. D., Brand, S., Dubois, D. L., Adan, A. M., Mulhall, P. F., & Evans, E. G. (1995). Socioeconomic disadvantage, proximal environmental experiences, and socioemotional and academic adjustment in early adolescence: Investigation of a mediated effects model. *Child Development*, *66*, 774–792. doi:10.2307/1131950

Felner, R. D., Favazza, A., Shim, M., Brand, S., Gu, K., & Noonan, N. (2001). Whole school improvement and restructuring as prevention and promotion, Lessons from step and the project on high performance learning communities. *Journal of School Psychology*, *39*, 177–202. doi:10.1016/S0022-4405(01)00057-7

Fernandez-Cardenas, J. M. (2008). The situated aspect of creativity in communicative events: How do children design web pages together? *Thinking Skills and Creativity*, *3*, 203–216. doi:10.1016/j.tsc.2008.09.007

Ferris, A., Roberts, N., & Skolnikoff, W. (1997). Technology and preservice education: Models that work, models that don't. *Educational Technology Review*, *7*, 13–19.

Ferry, B., Kervin, L., Cambourne, B., Turbill, J., Puglisi, S., Jonassen, D., & Hedberg, J. (2004). Online classroom simulation: The 'next wave' for pre-service teacher education? In R. Atkinson, C. McBeath, D. Jonas-Dwyer & R. Phillips (Eds.), *Beyond the comfort zone: Proceedings of the 21st ASCILITE Conference* (pp. 294-302). Retrieved from http://www.ascilite.org.au/conferences/perth04/procs/ferry.html

Fiedler, R., & Baumbach, D. (2008 March). *Portfolio as a Comprehensive Exam: Instigating Change*. Paper presented at Society for Information Technology & Teacher Education, Las Vegas, Nevada.

Fisher, F. D. (1989). The electronic lumberyard and builders' rights. *Change*, *21*, 13–21.

Fitzer, K. M., Freidhoff, J. R., Fritzen, A., Heintz, A., Koehler, M. J., & Mishra, P. (2007). Guest editorial: More questions than answers: Responding to the reading and mathematics software effectiveness study. *Contemporary Issues in Technology & Teacher Education*, *7*, 1–6.

Fletcher, G. H. (2006). Power up, don't power down. *T.H.E. Journal*, *33*, 24–26.

Flick, L., & Bell, R. (2000). Preparing tomorrow's science teachers to use technology: Guidelines for Science educators. *Contemporary Issues in Technology & Teacher Education*, *1*(1). Retrieved from http://www.citejournal.org/vol1/iss1/currentissues/science/article1.htm.

Foote, C. (2008). See me, hear Me: Skype in the classroom. *School Library Journal*, *1*(1), 4–8.

Foote, C. J. (2001). Teaching Portfolio 101: Implementing the Teaching Portfolio in Introductory Courses. *Journal of Instructional Psychology*, *28*(1).

Fox, S., & Livingston, G. (2007). Hispanics with lower levels of education and English proficiency remain largely disconnected from the internet. *Pew Internet & American Life Project: Latinos Online*. Retrieved March 8, 2009, from http://www.pewinternet.org/PPF/r/204/report_display.asp

Franklin, T., & van Harmelen, M. (2007, May). Web 2.0 for content for learning and teaching in higher education. *JISC*.

Freedom of Information Act. (1967). Retrieved July 23, 2009, from http://www.answers.com/topic/freedom-of-information-act

Gabriele, A. J., & Joram, E. (2007). Teachers' reflections on their reform-based teaching in mathematics: Implications for the development of teacher self-efficacy. *Action in Teacher Education*, *29*(3), 60–74.

Galan, J. (2004). Design of Educational Web Pages. *European Journal of Teacher Education*, *27*(1), 99–104. doi:10.1080/0261976042000211793

Garet, M. S., Porter, A. C., Desimone, L., Birman, B. F., & Yoon, K. S. (2001). What makes professional development effective? Results from a national sample of teachers. *American Educational Research Journal*, *38*(4), 915–945. doi:10.3102/00028312038004915

Gartner, Inc. (2007). *Mashups and the emerging technologies hype cycle*. Retrieved February 22, 2009, from http://www.webmashup.com/blog/2007/07/25/mashups-and-the-emerging-technoglogies-hype-cycle/

Gay, G. (2000). *Culturally responsive teaching: Theory, research, and practice*. New York: Teachers College Press.

Gaytan, J. (2005). Effective Assessment Techniques for Online Instruction. *Information Technology. Learning and Performance Journal*, *23*(1), 25–36.

Gergen, K. (1999). *An invitation to social construction*. London: Sage.

Gibson, D., & Barrett, H. (2003). Directions in electronic portfolio development. *Contemporary Issues in Technology & Teacher Education*, *2*(4), 559–576.

Gibson, S. E. (2002). Using a problem based multimedia enhanced approach in learning in the social studies classroom. *Australian Journal of Educational Technology*, *18*(3), 394–409.

Giroux, H. (1994). *Disturbing pleasures: Learning popular culture*. New York: Routledge.

Goldsborough, R. (2008). Web Design: Balancing Form and Function. [from Academic Search Premier database.]. *Tech Directions*, *67*(10), 11. Retrieved April 7, 2009.

Goldsmith, D. (2007). Enhancing learning and assessment through e-portfolios: A collaborative effort in Connecticut. *New Directions for Student Services*, *119*(1), 31–42. doi:10.1002/ss.247

Gomm, S. (2003). Computer Literacy Defined and Implemented as University Graduation Requirement. In C. Crawford et al. (Eds.), *Proceedings of Society for Information Technology and Teacher Education International Conference 2003* (pp. 941-944). Chesapeake, VA: AACE.

Goodlad, J. (1994). *Educational renewal: Better teachers, better schools*. San Francisco: Jossey-Bass.

Gray, K. C. (2001). Teachers' perceptions of innovation adoption. *Action in Teacher Education*, *23*, 30–35.

Graybill, S. W. (1997). Questions of race and culture: How they relate to the classroom for African American students. *Clearing House (Menasha, Wis.)*, *70*, 311–319.

Greenberg, E., Vojir, C., & Whitney, F. (2000). *Listening to MAPP online voices: Learning and teaching over the Internet*. Aurora, CO: University of Colorado Health Sciences Center.

Greene, M. (1973). *Teacher as stranger: Educational philosophy for the modern age*. Belmont, CA: Wadsworth.

Grossman, M. (1998). Are you wrong about copyright? *Broward Daily Business Review*, December, B1.

Groth, R. E. (2007). Toward a conceptualization of statistical knowledge for teaching. *Journal for Research in Mathematics Education*, *38*, 427–437. doi:10.2307/30034960

Groton Public Schools. (n.d.). *Copyright implementation manual*. Retrieved March 24, 1999, from http://groton.k12.ct.us/mts/eg3.htm

Guernsey, L. (1998). Distance education for the notso-distant. *The Chronicle of Higher Education*, *44*, A29–A30.

Guri-Rosenblit, S. (2005). Distance education and e-learning: Not the same thing. *Higher Education*, *49*, 467–493. doi:10.1007/s10734-004-0040-0

Hadwin, A. F., & Winne, P. H. (2001). CoNoteS2: A software tool for promoting self-regulation. *Educational Research and Evaluation*, *7*(2-3), 313–334. doi:10.1076/edre.7.2.313.3868

Hall, B. (1997). *Web-based training cookbook*. New York: John Wiley & Sons, Inc.

Hall, R. H., Watkins, S. E., & Ercal, F. (2000, April). *The horse and the cart in web-based instruction: Prevalence and efficacy*. Paper presented at the Annual Meeting of the American Educational Research Association, New Orleans, LA.

Hamilton, W. (2009). *Electronic evidence PowerPoint V6*. Retrieved June 17, 2009, from http://www.slideshare.net/williamfhamilton/electronic-evidence-powerpoint-v6final.

Hancock, J. T. (2004). Verbal irony use in face-to-face and computer-mediated communication. *Journal of Language and Social Psychology*, *23*(4), 447–463. doi:10.1177/0261927X04269587

Hanks, R. F. (2002). Environmental and personal factors effecting K-12 teacher utilization of technology. Paper presented at the *National Educational Computing Conference*, San Antonio, Texas (ERIC Reproduction Service No. ED475934). Retrieved April 3, 2009, from http://www.eric.ed.gov

Harackiewicz, J. M., Barron, K. E., Pintrich, P. R., Elliot, A. J., & Thrash, T. M. (2002). Revision of achievement goal theory: Necessary and illuminating. *Journal of Educational Psychology, 94*(3), 638–645. doi:10.1037/0022-0663.94.3.638

Harford, J., & MacRuairc, G. (2008). Engaging student teaches in meaningful reflective practice. *Teaching and Teacher Education: An International Journal of Research and Studies, 24*(7), 1884–1892. doi:10.1016/j.tate.2008.02.010

Harper, G. (1998). *Fair use of copyrighted materials. Am I a crook on the Internet?*PBS Adult Learning Satellite Service.

Harris, R. D. (1999). Trademark and copyright law on the World Wide Web: A survey of the wild frontier. *Intellectual Property Today*, 44.

Hawkins, C., & Black, S. (2004). Developing electronic portfolios across the state of Utah: Breaks, Breakdowns, and Breakthroughs. *Computers in Schools, 21*(1-2), 95-113. Hastie, P., & Sinelnikov, O. (2007). The use of web-based portfolios in college physical education activity courses. *Physical Educator, 64*(1), 21–28.

Hayes, M. H., & Mayercik, M. (2001). Distance learning across the Atlantic. *Education. IEEE Transactions on, 44*, 201–211.

Heath, M. (2002). Electronic portfolios for reflective self-assessment. *Teacher Librarian, 30*(1), 19–24.

Heath, R. D. (1987). The effect of calculators and computers on problem-solving ability and attitude toward mathematics. (Doctoral Dissertation, Northern Arizona University, 1987). *Dissertation Abstracts International-A, 48*(05), 1102.

Heffernan, K. (2001). *Fundamentals of service learning course construction*. Providence, RI: Campus Compact.

Helling, H. E., & Solomon, E. M. (2003, September). *Bridging the gap between ocean science and education: Creating effective partnerships through informal educational institutions*. Paper presented at the annual meeting of the OCEANS 2003 Conference, San Diego, CA.

Herring, S. C. (1993). Gender and democracy in computer-mediated communication. *EJC/REC, 3*(20). Retrieved May 18, 2008, from http://www.internetstudies.pe.kr/txt/Herring.txt

Herring, S. C. (1994). Politeness in computer culture: Why women thank and men flame. In M. Bucholtz, A. Liang, & L. Sutton (Eds.), *Cultural Performances: Proceedings of the Third Berkeley Women and Language Conference* (pp. 278-94). Berkeley, CA: Berkeley Women and Language Group.

Herring, S. C. (1996a). Two variants of an electronic message schema. In Herring, S. C. (Ed.), *Computer-mediated communication: Linguistic, social, and cross-cultural perspectives* (pp. 81–106). Philadelphia, PA: John Benjamins.

Herring, S. C. (1996b). Posting in a different voice: Gender and ethics in computer-mediated communication. In Ess, C. (Ed.), *Philosophical Perspectives on Computer-Mediated Communication* (pp. 115–145). Albany, NY: SUNY Press.

Herring, S. C. (2000). Gender Differences in CMC: Findings and Implications. *CPSR Newsletter, 18*(1). Retrieved May 30, 2008, from http://www.cpsr.org/issues/womenintech/herring

Herring, S. C. (2001). Computer-mediated discourse. In Schiffrin, D., Tannen, D., & Hamilton, H. E. (Eds.), *The Handbook of Discourse Analysis* (pp. 612–634). Malden, MA: Blackwell Publishers.

Herring, S. C. (2003). Gender and power in online communication. In Holmes, J., & Meyerhoff, M. (Eds.), *The Handbook of Language and Gender* (pp. 202–228). Oxford: Blackwell Publishers. doi:10.1002/9780470756942.ch9

Herring, S. C., & Paolillo, J. C. (2006). Gender and genre variation in weblogs. *Journal of Sociolinguistics, 10*(4), 439–459. doi:10.1111/j.1467-9841.2006.00287.x

Hess, D. (2007). From Banished to Brother Outsider, Miss Navajo to An Inconvenient Truth: Documentary films as perspective-laden narratives. *Social Education, 71*, 194–199.

Hewitt, T. W. (2006). *Understanding curriculum: What we teach and why*. Thousand Oaks, CA: Sage Publications.

Higdon, J., & Topaz, C. (2009). Blogs and wikis as Instructional tools: A Social software adaptation of just-in-time teaching. *College Teaching, 57*(2), 105-110. Retrieved May 2009, from http://web.mac.com/chad.topaz/ChadTopaz/Blogging_files/ht2009.pdf

Hiltz, R., & Wu, D. (2003). *Online Discussions and Perceived Learning*. Retrieved May 2009, from http://www.alnresearch.org/Data_Files/articles/full_text/wu_Hiltz(2003).pdf

Hodges, C. B. (2006). Lessons learned from a first instructional design experience. *International Journal of Instructional Media, 33*, 397–403.

Hodgins, W. (2008). *The snowflake effect: The future of mashups and learning*. Retrieved January 8, 2009 from http://www.becta.org.uk

Hoffman, N. (2009). *Mashups using government data: A white paper*. Retrieved June 25, 2009 from http://www.mnhs.org/preserve/records/legislativerecords/docs_pdfs/DataMashups1.pdf

Hofmeyr, B. (2006). The power not to be (what we are), the politics and ethics of self-creation in Foucault. *Journal of Moral Philosophy, 3*(2), 215–230. doi:10.1177/1740468106065493

Holmberg, S. (1997). Is accreditation worth the trouble? *Education Weekly, 16*, 32. Institutional Report Continuing Accreditation. (2008). *College of education professional education unit*. Jonesboro, AR: Arkansas State University.

Holmes, A., Polhemus, L., & Jennings, S. (2005). CATIE: A blended approach to situated professional development. *Journal of Educational Computing Research, 32*, 381–394. doi:10.2190/F97W-QUJ4-G7YG-FPXC

Honawar, V. (2008, December 14). NCATE commits to streamlining accrediting process. *Education Week, 28*(14), 6.

Howard, J. (Ed.). (2001, Summer). Service-learning course design workbook. Ann Arbor, MI: OCSL Press.

Howard, J. P. F. (Eds.), *Academic Service Learning: A Pedagogy of Action and Reflection* (pp. 24–29). San Francisco: Jossey-Bass.

Hricko, M. (2003). Understanding section 508 and its implications for distance learning. In Design and Implementation of Web-enabled Teaching Tools (pp. 25-45). Retrieved October 26, 2007, from InfoSci-Online database.

Huang, D., & Behara, R. (2007). Outcome-driven experiential learning with Web 2.0. *Journal of Information Systems Education, 18*(3), 329–337.

Hudson, P. (2006). Examining Preservice Teachers' Involvement in Online Science Education. *Journal of Interactive Learning Research, 17*(4), 367–385.

Huffaker, D. A., & Calvert, S. L. (2005). Gender, identity, and language use in teenage blogs. *Journal of Computer-Mediated Communication, 10*(2). Retrieved May 3, 2008, from http://jcmc.indiana.edu/vol10/issue2/huffaker.html

Hughes, J. (2005). The role of teacher knowledge and learning experiences in forming technology-integrated pedagogy. *Journal of Technology and Teacher Education, 13*, 277–302.

Hunt, B. (2008). *Writing for the Web*. Retrieved October 1, 2008, from http://www.webdesignfromscratch.com/writing_for_the_web.cfm

IESD Research Report. (2008). *Safe schools in a web 2.0 world initiative: National online survey of district technology directors exploring district use of Web 2.0 technologies*. Retrieved from http://www.prweb.com/releases/Web20/schools/prweb2300494.htm

Illustrator, A. (2007). *CS3 classroom in a book*. Berkeley, CA: Adobe Press.

International Society for Technology in Education. (1999). *Will new teachers be prepared to teach in a digital age? A national survey on information technology in teacher education.* Santa Monica, CA: Milken Exchange on Education Technology. Retrieved October 29, 2006 from http://www.milkenexchange.org/research/iste_results.html

International Society for Technology in Education. (2008). *National educational technology standards and performance indicators for teachers.* Eugene, OR: Author. Retrieved on February 1, 2009, from http://www.iste.org/Content/NavigationMenu/NETS/ForTeachers/2008Standards/NETS_T_Standards_Final.pdf

International Society for Technology in Education. (2008). *NETS for teachers 2008*. Retrieved March 13, 2009, from http://www.iste.org/Content/NavigationMenu/NETS/ForTeachers/2008Standards/NETS_for_Teachers_2008.htm

International Society for Technology in Education. (2009). *The ISTE National Educational Technology Standards and Performance Indicators for Teachers.* Retrieved February 11, 2009, from http://www.iste.org

International Technology Education Association. (2005). Testimony pertaining to the science framework for the 2009 national assessment of education progress. *Technology Teacher, 65*, 36–37.

Irvine, J. (2003). *Educating teachers for diversity: Seeing with a cultural eye.* New York: Teachers College Press.

Ivy, D. K., & Backlund, P. (1994). *Exploring GenderSpeak: Personal effectiveness in gender communication.* New York: McGraw-Hill.

Jacobs, V. R., Franke, M. L., Carpenter, T. P., Levi, L., & Battey, D. (2007). Professional development focused on children's algebraic reasoning in elementary school. *Journal for Research in Mathematics Education, 38*(3), 258–288.

Jaffe, J. M., Lee, Y., Huang, L., & Oshagan, H. (1995). *Gender, Pseudonyms, and CMC: Masking Identities and Baring Souls.* Presented at the 45th Annual Conference of the International Communication Association (ICA), Albuquerque, New Mexico, USA.

James, R. K., Lamb, C. E., Bailey, M. A., & Householder, D. L. (2000). Integrating science, mathematics, and technology in middle school technology-rich environments: A study of implementation and change. *International Journal of Instructional Media, 100*, 27–35.

Jenkins, E. W. (2006). Student opinion in England about science and technology. *Research in Science & Technological Education, 24*, 59–68. doi:10.1080/02635140500485365

Jenkins, H., Purushotma, R., Clinton, K., Weigel, M., & Robison, A. J. (2006). *Confronting the challenges of participatory culture: Media Education for the 21st Century.* Chicago, IL: John D. & Catherine T. MacArthur Foundation.

Jeong, A. (2003). *Gender interactions in online debates: Look who's arguing with whom.* Paper presented at the Annual Meeting of the American Educational Research Association, Chicago, Ill, April. Retrieved January, 2009, from http://mailer.fsu.edu/~ajeong/GenderInteraction2.doc

Jeong, A., & Davidson-Shivers, G. V. (2006). The effects of gender interaction patterns on student participation in computer-supported collaboration argumentation. *ETR&D, 54*(1), 543–569. doi:10.1007/s11423-006-0636-4

Jeong, A., & Joung, S. (2007). Scaffolding collaborative argumentation in asynchronous discussions with message constraints and message labels. *Computers & Education, 48*, 427–445. doi:10.1016/j.compedu.2005.02.002

Jiang, M., Parent, S., & Eastman, D. (2006). Effectiveness of web-based learning opportunities in a competency-based program. *International Journal on E-Learning, 5*, 353–360.

Jin, S. H. (2005). Analyzing student-student and student-instructor interaction through multiple communication tools in web-based learning. *International Journal of Instructional Media*, *32*(1), 59–67.

John, P. (2005). The sacred and the profane: Subject sub–culture, pedagogical practice and teachers' perceptions of the classroom uses of ICT. *Educational Review*, *57*, 471–490. doi:10.1080/00131910500279577

Johnson, D. W., Maruyama, G., Johnson, R., Nelson, D., & Skon, L. (1981). Effects of cooperative, competitive, and individualistic goal structures on achievement: A meta-analysis. *Psychological Bulletin*, *89*(1), 47–62. doi:10.1037/0033-2909.89.1.47

Johnson, L., Levine, A., & Smith, R. (2008). *The 2008 Horizon Report*. Austin, TX: The New Media Consortium.

Johnson-Leslie, N. (in press). Comparing the efficacy of an engineered-based system (College LiveText) with an off-the-shelf general tool (Hyperstudio) for developing electronic portfolios in teacher education. *Journal of Educational Technology Systems*, *37*(4), 385-404.

Johnston, J. (2008). *Piloting NCATE's streamlined system: positive Results*. Retrieved January 1, 2009 from http://www.NCATE. org/documents/news/Johnston_Streamlined.pdf

Johnston, J. H. (1999, February). Putting Robert Frost on ice. *Legal Times*, 49.

Jolly, G. (2007). *An overview of some of the social network web sites*. Retrieved May 15, 2009, from http://www.associatedcontent.com/article/465599/an_overview_of_some_of_the_social_network.html?cat=35

Jones, M. (2009). *What is social networking?* Retrieved June 2009 from http://tech.blorge.com/Structure:%20/2009/05/30/what-is-social-networking/

Jones, S. (2005). Fizz in the field: Toward a basis for an emergent internet studies. *The Information Society*, *21*, 233–237. doi:10.1080/01972240591007544

Juler, P. (1990). Promoting Interaction, Maintaining Independence: Swallowing the mixture. *Open Learning*, *5*(2), 24–33. doi:10.1080/0268051900050205

Kaiser Family Foundation. (2005). Generation M: media in the lives of 8-18 year-olds. *Kaiser Family Foundation Web Site*. Retrieved from http://www.kff.org/entmedia/entmedia030905pkg.cfm

Kalman, Y. M., & Rafaeli, S. (2005). Email chronemics: Unobtrusive profiling on response time. In *Proceedings of HICSS-38: Hawaii International Conference on System Sciences* (pp. 108b). Los Alamitos, CA: IEEE Computer Society Press.

Kalyuga, S., & Sweller, J. (2005). Rapid dynamic assessment of expertise to improve the efficiency of adaptive e-learning. *Educational Technology Research and Development*, *53*, 83–93. doi:10.1007/BF02504800

Karch, M. (2009). *Mashup*. Retrieved April 2, 2009 from http://google.about.com/od/m/g/mashupdef.htm

Karchmer-Klein, R., & Layton, V. (2006). Literature-based collaborative internet projects in elementary classrooms. *Reading Research and Instruction*, *45*, 261–294.

Kaufman, J. (1999, March). The day the music web site died. *Legal Times*, 43.

Kaur, M. (2008). Cryptography as a pedagogical tool. *PRIMUS (Terre Haute, Ind.)*, *18*, 198–206. doi:10.1080/10511970701298833

Kay, R. (2006). Evaluating strategies used to incorporate technology into preservice education: A review of the literature. *Journal of Research on Technology in Education*, *38*(4), 383–408.

Kemmis, S., & McTaggart, R. (1990). *The Action-research planner*. Geelong, Victoria: Deakin University.

Kennelly, P. (2009). An online social networking approach to reinforce learning of rocks and minerals. *Journal of Geo-science Education*, *57*(1), 33–35.

Kennett, D. J., & Keefer, K. (2006). Impact of learned resourcefulness and theories of intelligence on academic achievement of university students: An integrated approach. *Educational Psychology*, *26*(3), 441–457. doi:10.1080/01443410500342062

Khare, A., & Lam, H. (2008). Assessing Student Achievement and Progress with Online Examinations: Some Pedagogical and Technical Issues. *International Journal on E-Learning, 7*(3), 383–403.

Kirkland, A. (2007). Becoming librarian 2.0. partnership. *Canadian Journal of Library and Information Practice and Research, 2*(1), 25–31.

Knezek, D. (2008). *Providing leadership and service to improve teaching and learning by advancing the effective use of technology in education.* Retrieved November 12, 2008, from http://www.iste.org/AM/Template.cfm?Section=About_ISTE*LiveText Solutions, Inc.* (2004). Retrieved from http://www.livetext.com U. S. Department of Education. (2003). *No Child Left Behind.* Retrieved October 9, 2008, from http://www.ed.gov/news/pressreleases/2003/12/12092003.html

Koehler, M. J., & Mishra, P. (2008). Introducing TPCK. In Colbert, J. A., Boyd, K. E., Clark, K. A., Guan, S., Harris, J. B., Kelly, M. A., & Thompson, A. D. (Eds.), *Handbook of Technological Pedagogical Content Knowledge (TPCK) for educators* (pp. 3–30). New York: Routledge.

Kordaki, M., Miatidis, M., & Kapsampelis, G. (2008). A computer environment for beginners' learning of sorting algorithms: design and pilot evaluation. *Computers & Education, 51*, 708–723. doi:10.1016/j.compedu.2007.07.006

Kraft, N. (2001*). Standards in teacher education: a critical analysis of NCATE, INTASC, and NBPTS.* Retrieved September 4, 2008, from EBSCOhost database.

Kramarae, C. (1995). A backstage critique of virtual reality. In Jones, S. (Ed.), *Cybersociety: Computer-mediated communication and community* (pp. 35–56). Thousand Oaks, CA: Sage.

Kyong, J. K., & Bonk, C. J. (2006). The Future of Online Teaching and Learning in Higher Education. *EduCause Quarterly, 29*(4). Retrieved October 23, 2008 from http://net.eduause.edu/ir/library/pdf/eqm0644.pdf

Laff, M. (2007). Serious Gaming: The trainer's new best friend. *T + D, 61*, 52-57.

Lai, K. W., & Pratt, K. (2007). Positive to a degree: The effects of ICT use in New Zealand secondary schools. *Computers in the Schools, 24*, 95–109. doi:10.1300/J025v24n03_07

Lamb, B. (2007, July/August). Dr. Mashup or why educations should learn to stop worrying and love the remix. *EDUCAUSE Review*, 13–24.

Lambert, J., Yi, G., & Cuper, P. (2008). Technology, transfer, and teaching: The impact of a single technology course on pre-service teachers' computer attitudes and ability. *Journal of Technology and Teacher Education, 16*(4), 385–411.

Lao, T., & Gonzales, C. (2005). Understanding online learning through a qualitative description of professors and students' experiences. *Journal of Technology and Teacher Education, 13*, 459–474.

LaPointe, L., & Reisetter, M. (2008). Belonging Online: Students' Perceptions of the Value and Efficacy of an Online Learning Community. *International Journal on E-Learning, 7*(4), 641–666.

Larkin, T., & Budny, D. (2005, July). *Learning styles in the classroom: Approaches to enhance student motivation and learning.* Paper presented at the 6th International Conference on Information Technology Based Higher Education and Training, Santo Domingo, Dominican Republic.

Larrivee, B. (2008). Meeting the challenge of preparing reflective practitioners. *New Educator, 4*(2), 87–106. doi:10.1080/15476880802014132

Larson, A., & Clift, R. (1996). Technology education in teacher preparation: Perspectives from a year-long elementary education program. *Educational Foundations, 10*(4), 33–50.

Latham, G. (2007). *New Learning: Building surprise through the virtual.* Melbourne RMIT University.

Latham, G. Blaise, M., Dole, S., Faulkner, J., Lang, J., Malone, K. (2006). Learning to teach: New times, new practices. Melbourne, Australia: Oxford University Press.

Lau, S. H., & Woods, P. C. (2009). Understanding the behavior changes in belief and attitude among experienced and inexperienced learning object users. *Computers & Education, 52*, 333–342. doi:10.1016/j.compedu.2008.09.002

Laurel, B. (1991). *Computers as theatre*. Reading, MA: Addison-Wesley Publishing Company. Oblinger, D. (2003). Boomers, gen-Xers and millennial: Understanding the new students. *EDUCAUSE Review, 38*(4), 37–47.

Law, S. (n.d.). Retrieved July 23, 2009, from http://www.answers.com/topic/sunshine-laws

Lawrence, B. J. (2000). Procedural apprenticeship in school science: Constructivist enabling of connoisseurship. *Science Education, 84*, 727–739. doi:10.1002/1098-237X(200011)84:6<727::AID-SCE3>3.0.CO;2-O

Lee, G. B. (1996). Addressing anonymous messages in cyberspace. *Journal of Computer-Mediated Communication, 2*(1), Retrieved May 6, 2008, from http://jcmc.indiana.edu/vol2/issue1/anon.html

Lefor, P. J., Benke, M., & Ting, E. (2003). Information technology and adult learners at Empire State College. *New Directions for Student Services, 102*, 35–42. doi:10.1002/ss.87

Leibowitz, W. (1998). The sound of one computer copy. *The National Law Journal*, A16.

Lennex, L. (2003). *College of Education NCATE online exhibit room*. Retrieved May 10, 2004, from http://edu-tech.net/msucoe/

Lennex, L. (2007). The faculty Web page: contrivance or continuation? *TechTrends, 51*(5), 32–37. doi:10.1007/s11528-007-0067-z

Lennex, L., & Flynn, H. (2009). Wisely using cyberspace: needs analysis of P-12 teacher Web pages. In C. Crawford et al. (Eds.), *Proceedings of Society for Information Technology and Teacher Education International Conference 2009* (pp. 3473-3480). Chesapeake, VA: AACE.

Lennex, L., & Reynolds, A. (2008). Whose web page is this? Why faculty create web pages. In C. Crawford et al. (Eds.), *Proceedings of Society for Information Technology and Teacher Education International Conference 2008* (pp. 3840-3842). Chesapeake, VA: AACE.

Lennex, L., Swetnam, B., & Flynn, H. (2009). *Survey of NCATE constituents on Web features*. Unpublished manuscript, Morehead State University.

Lethem, J. (2007). The ecstasy of influence. *Harper's Magazine*. Retrieved January 8, 2009 from http://www.harpers.org/archive/2007/02/0081387

Levin, D., Arafeh, S., Lenhart, A., & Rainie, L. (2002). The digital disconnect: The widening gap between internet-savvy students and their Schools. *Pew Internet & American Life Project*. Retrieved April 2009 from http://epsl.asu.edu/epru/articles/EPRU-0208-36-OWI.pdf

Lewis, L., Snow, K., Farris, E., Levin, D., & Greene, B. (2000). Distance education at postsecondary education institutions: 1997-98. *National Center for Education Statistics*. Retrieved from http://nces.edu.gov/pubs2000/2000013.pdf

Lewis, M. A., & Cooney, J. B. (1987). Attributional and performance effects of competitive and individualistic feedback in computer assisted mathematics instruction. *Computers in Human Behavior, 3*(1), 1–13. doi:10.1016/0747-5632(87)90005-7

Linch & E. G. Stutevant (Ed.). *Growing Literacy* (pp. 173-187). Pittsburgh: PA. College Reading Association. Schlechty, P. C. (2005). *Creating the capacity to support innovations*. Occasional Paper No. 2. Louisville, KY: Schlechty Centre.

Linnenbrink, E. A. (2005). The dilemma of performance-approach goals: The use of multiple goal contexts to promopte students' motivation and learning. *Journal of Educational Psychology, 97*(2), 197–213. doi:10.1037/0022-0663.97.2.197

Linnenbrink, E. A., & Pintrich, P. R. (2001). Multiple goals, multiple contexts: The dynamic interplay between personal goals and contextual goal stresses. In Volet, S., & Jarvela, S. (Eds.), *Motivation in learning contexts: Theoretical and methodological implications* (pp. 251–269). Amsterdam: Pergamon Press.

Little, J. W. (2002). Locating learning in teachers' communities of practice: Opening up problems of analysis in records of everyday practice. *Teaching and Teacher Education, 18*, 917–946. doi:10.1016/S0742-051X(02)00052-5

Littlefield, J. (2008). Top 5 Distance Learning Myths. *About.com*. Retrieved October 30, 2008, from http://distancelearn.about.com/od/distancelearning101/a/5Myths.htm

Lock, J. V. (2006). A new image: Online communities to facilitate teacher professional development. *Journal of Technology and Teacher Education, 14*(4), 663–678.

Longhurst, J. (2003). World history on the World Wide Web: A student satisfaction survey and a blinding flash of the obvious. *The History Teacher, 36*, 343–356. doi:10.2307/1555691

Loucks-Horsley, S., Love, N., Stiles, K. E., Mundry, S., & Hewson, P. W. (2003). *Designing professional development for teachers of science and mathematics* (2nd ed.). Thousand Oaks, CA: Corwin Press, Inc.

Lowe, P. D., & Worboys, M. (1975). The teaching of social studies of science and technology in British polytechnics. *Social Studies of Science (Sage), 5*, 177–192. doi:10.1177/030631277500500204

Lynch, K., Bednarz, B., Boxall, J., Chalmers, L., France, D., & Kesby, J. (2008). E-learning for Geography's Teaching and Learning Spaces. *Journal of Geography in Higher Education, 32*, 135–149. doi:10.1080/03098260701731694

Mabry, J. B. (1998). Pedagogical variations in service-learning and student outcomes: How time, Contact, and reflection matter. *Michigan journal of community service learning, 5*, 32-47.

MacLachlan, K. (1996). Web Evaluation. *WWW Cyberguides web site*. Retrieved from http://www.cyberbee.com/guides.html

Main, L. (1998). WOOing the millennium. *Journal of Education for Library and Information Science, 39*, 339–342.

Malloy, J. A., & Gambrell, L. B. (2006). Approaching the unavoidable: Literacy instruction and the Internet. *The Reading Teacher, 59*, 482–484. doi:10.1598/RT.59.5.8

Mangos, P. M., & Steele-Johnson, D. (2001). The role of subjective task complexity in goal orientation, self-efficacy, and performance relations. *Human Performance, 14*(2), 169–186. doi:10.1207/S15327043HUP1402_03

Mann, C., & Stewart, F. (2000). *Internet communication and qualitative research: A handbook for researching online*. London: Sage Publications.

Markel, S. (2001). Technology and Education Online Discussion Forums: It's in the Response. *Online Journal of Distance Learning Administration, 4*(2), 63–74.

Marks, R. (1990). Pedagogical content knowledge: From a mathematical case to a modified conception. *Journal of Teacher Education, 41*, 3–11. doi:10.1177/002248719004100302

Marratech AB. (1998-2008). *Marratech (version 6.1.2)*. Stockholm, Sweden: Marratech AB.

Marshall, J. C., Horton, B., Igo, B. L., & Switzer, D. M. (in press). K-12 science and mathematics teachers' beliefs about and use of inquiry in the classroom. *International Journal of Science and Mathematics Education*.

Martin, A. (1967). Industrial training: Current research and future needs. *Occupational Psychology, 41*, 109–119.

Martin, H. E. (1996). Tracking weather satellites. *Science Teacher (Normal, Ill.), 63*, 30–32.

Mashup (Music). (2009). Retrieved June 2, 2009 from http://www.mashupshub.com/music/

Mason, C., Berson, M., Diem, R., Hicks, D., Lee, J., & Dralle, T. (2000). Guidelines for using technology to prepare social studies teachers. *Contemporary Issues in Technology & Teacher Education, 1*(1). Retrieved from http://www.citejournal.org/vol1/iss1/currentissues/socialstudies/article1.htm.

Massey, A. P., Ramesh, V., & Khatri, V. (2006). Design, development, and assessment of mobile applications: The case for problem-based learning. *IEEE Transactions on Education, 49*, 183–192. doi:10.1109/TE.2006.875700

Mathews, B. (2009). Web design matters. [from Academic Search Premier database.]. *Library Journal, 134*(3), 24–25. Retrieved April 7, 2009.

Matthews, D. (1999). The origins of distance education and its use in the United States. *T.H.E. Journal, 27*(2), 54–67.

Maxymuk, J. (2007). Whose space? *The Bottom, 20*(1), 54–57. doi:10.1108/08880450710747461

Mayer, R. E. (2001). *Multimedia Learning* (1st ed.). New York: Cambridge University Press.

Mayer, R. E. (2009). *Multimedia Learning* (2nd ed.). New York: Cambridge University Press.

Mayer, R. E., & Moreno, R. (2003). Nine ways to reduce cognitive load in multimedia learning. *Educational Psychologist, 38*(1), 43–52. doi:10.1207/S15326985EP3801_6

Mayer, R. E., & Moreno, R. (2003). Nine ways to reduce cognitive load in multimedia learning. In Bruning, R., Horn, C. A., & Pytlik Zillig, L. M. (Eds.), *Web-based learning: What do we know? Where do we go?* (pp. 23–44). Greenwich, CT: Information Age Publishing.

Mayer, R. E., & Wittrock, M. C. (1996). Problem-solving transfer. In Calfee, R., & Berliner, R. (Eds.), *Handbook of educational psychology* (pp. 47–62). New York: Macmillan.

McCoy, N. L. (1998). Methodological problems in the study of sexuality and the menopause. *Maturitas, 29*, 51–60. doi:10.1016/S0378-5122(98)00028-0

McGee, P., & Diaz, V. (2007, September/October). Wikis and Podcasts and Blogs! Oh, My! What is a Faculty Member Supposed to Do? *EDUCAUSE Review*, •••, 2007.

McIntyre, J. D., & Paper, S. (1993). Using video protocols to enhance teacher reflective thinking. *Teacher Educator, 28*(3), 2–10. doi:10.1080/08878739309555031

McIntyre, J., Byrd, D., & Foxx, S. (1997). Field and laboratory experiences. In Sikula, J. (Ed.), *Handbook of research on teacher education* (pp. 171–193). New York: Simon and Schuster Macmillan.

McLaughlin, J. (2006a). The CHANCE program: Promoting learning for teachers and students through experiences and inquiry. *The American Biology Teacher, 68*(4), 17–24. Retrieved from https://royercenter.cwc.psu.edu/CHANCE/press/NABT-CHANCE-04-2006.pdf. doi:10.1662/0002-7685(2006)68[e17:TCPPLF]2.0.CO;2

McLaughlin, J. S. (2006b). Using technology to blend teaching and basic research. *Science Teacher (Normal, Ill.), 73*(8), 48–53.

McLaughlin, J. S. (2010) Re-imagining Science Education and New Pedagogical Tools: Blending Research with Teaching. *Educause Quarterly*, 33 (1). Online at http://www.educause.edu/eq.

McLaughlin, J. S., & Fadigan, K. A. (2010). The CHANCE (Connecting Humans and Nature Through Conservation Experiences) Program: Transitioning from Simple Inquiry-based Learning to Professional Science Practice. In Yager, R. (Ed.), *Exemplary Science Programs: Science for Resolving Issues/Problems*. Arlington, VA: NSTA Press.

McLaughlin, J. S., Arbeider, D. A., Stine, J. L., Dugan, T. R., & Besong, P. J. (2008a). *CHANCE (Online)*. Retrieved from http://chance.psu.edu/

McLaughlin, J., & Arbeider, D. A. (2008b). Evaluating multimedia-learning tools based on authentic research data that teach biology concepts and environmental stewardship. *Contemporary Issues in Technology & Teacher Education, 8*(1), 1–19. Retrieved from http://www.citejournal.org/tempcite/vol8/iss1/science/article1.cfm.

McLoughlin, C. (2002). Learner support in distanceand networked learning environments: Ten dimensions for successful design. *Distance Education, 23*(2), 149–162. doi:10.1080/0158791022000009178

McNeely, B. (2009). Using technology as a learning tool, not just the cool new thing. *Educause*. Retrieved May 2009, from http://www.educause.edu/Resources/EducatingtheNetGeneration/UsingTechnologyasaLearningTool/6060

Means, B., Wagner, M., Haertel, G. D., & Javitz, H. S. (2003). Studying the cumulative impacts of educational technology. In Haertel, G. D., & Means, B. (Eds.), *Evaluating educational technology: Effective research designs for improving learning* (pp. 230–256). New York: Teachers College Press.

Mehlinger, H. D., & Powers, S. M. (2002). *Technology and teacher education: A guide for educators and policymakers*. Boston: Houghton Mifflin.

Menchaca, M., & Bekele, T. A. (2008). Learner and instructor identified success factors in distance education. *Distance Education*, *29*(3), 231–253. doi:10.1080/01587910802395771

Merrill, D. (2006). *Mashups: The new breed of Web app.* Retrieved February 18, 2008 from http://www.ibm.com/developerworks/xml/library/x-mashups.html

Mervielde, I. (1977). Methodological problems of research about attitude-behavior consistency. *Quality & Quantity*, *11*, 259–281. doi:10.1007/BF00138839

Miller, D., & Glover, D. (2007). Into the unknown: The professional development induction experience of secondary mathematics teachers using interactive whiteboard technology. *Learning, Media and Technology*, *32*, 319–331. doi:10.1080/17439880701511156

Mimirinis, M., & Bhattacharya, M. (2007). Design of virtual learning environments for deep learning. *Journal of Interactive Learning Research*, *18*, 55–64.

Min, L. (2005). The effect of a hypermedia learning environment on middle school students' motivation, attitude, and science knowledge. *Computers in the Schools*, *22*, 159–171.

Mintz, S. D., & Hesser, G. W. (1996). Principles of good practice in service-learning. In Jacoby, B. (Eds.), *Service-Learning in Higher Education: Concepts and Practices.* San Francisco: Jossey-Bass.

Mirchin, D. M. (1998, October). Can you be held legally liable for hypertext linking? *Corporate Legal Times*, 22.

Mishra, P., & Koehler, M. J. (2006). Technological pedagogical content knowledge: A framework for teacher knowledge. *Teachers College Record*, *108*, 1017–1054. doi:10.1111/j.1467-9620.2006.00684.x

Mishra, P., & Koehler, M. J. (2008, March). *Introducing Technological Pedagogical Content Knowledge.* Paper presented at the Annual Meeting of the American Educational Research Association, New York City, NY.

Moller, L., Foshay, W. R., & Huett, J. (2008). The Evolution of Distance Education: Implications for Instructional Design on the Potential of the Web. *TechTrends*, *52*(3), 70-76. Retrieved April 2009, from http://ncolr.org/jiol/issues/viewarticle.cfm?volID=4&IssueID=15&ArticleID=73

Moore, G. E. (2003). *No exponential is forever...but we can delay forever.* Presentation to the International Solid State Circuits Conference. Retrieved from http://download.intel.com/research/silicon/Gordon_Moore_ISSCC_021003.pdf

Moreno, R., & Mayer, R. E. (2005). Role of guidance, reflection, and interactivity in an agent-based multimedia game. *Journal of Educational Psychology*, *97*, 117–128. doi:10.1037/0022-0663.97.1.117

Morgridge Center for Public Service. (2008, June). *Faculty introduction to service-learning/community-based research.* University of Wisconsin Madison. Retrieved February 18, 2009, from http://www.morgridge.wisc.edu/faculty/facultyservicelearning.html

Moursund, D. G. (1995). Site-based management: Saving our schools. *Association for Computing Machinery. Communications of the ACM*, *38*, 15–17. doi:10.1145/203241.203243

Mulac, A., & Lundell, T. L. (1986). Linguistic contributors to the gender-linked language effect. *Journal of Language and Social Psychology*, *5*(2), 91–101. doi:10.1177/0261927X8652001

Mulac, A., Bradac, J. J., & Mann, S. K. (1985). Male/female language differences and attributional consequences in children's television. *Human Communication Research*, *11*(4), 481–506. doi:10.1111/j.1468-2958.1985.tb00057.x

Mulcahy, M. D. (1998). Designing the user/using the design: The shifting relations of a curriculum technology change. *Social Studies of Science (Sage)*, *28*, 5–38. doi:10.1177/030631298028001001

Murphy, J., & Lebans, R. (2008). Unexpected outcomes: Web2.0 in the secondary school classroom. *International Journal of Technology in Teaching and Learning, 4*(2), 134-147. Retrieved April 2009, from http://www.sad61.k12.me.us/Web2.0/

Murphy, K. L., Harvell, T. J., Sanders, B., & Lu Epps, M. (1999). *Students as designers and teachers of their courses via computer-mediated communication.* Paper presented at the Annual Convention of the Association for Educational Communications and Technology, Houston, TX, February. Retrieved, December 14, 2008, from http://www.coe.tamu.edu/~kmurphy/writings/aect99webdesign.html

Nag, R. (1999, February). Parody or parasite? A copyright fair use analysis. *Intellectual Property Today*, 36.

Nastri, J., Peña, J., & Hancock, J. T. (2006). The construction of away messages: A speech act analysis. *Journal of Computer-Mediated Communication, 11*(4). Retrieved June 6, 2008, from http://jcmc.indiana.edu/vol11/issue4/nastri.html

National Council for Accreditation of Teacher Education. (2008). *NCATE handbook.* Washington, DC: NCATE. Retrieved from http://www.ncate.org/documents/handbook/handbook.pdf

National Research Council. (1996). *The National Science Education Standards.* Washington, DC: The National Research Council.

National Service-Learning Clearinghouse. (n.d.). *History.* Retrieved February 17, 2009, from http://www.servicelearning.org/what_is_service-learning/history/index.php

Navarro, P., & Shoemaker, J. (2000). Performance and perceptions of distance learners in cyberspace. *American Journal of Distance Education, 14*(2), 15–35. doi:10.1080/08923640009527052

NCATE. 2004. *Professional Standards for the Accreditation of Teacher Preparation Institutions* (2008). Washington: National Council for Accreditation of Teacher Education (NCATE). Retrieved September 13, 2008, from http://www.NCATE.org/institutions/process.asp?ch=4.

NEA. (n.d.). *NCLB/ESEA: It's Time for a Change – Voices from America's Classrooms.* Retrieved from http://www.nea.org/esea/nclbstories/images/classroomvoices.pdf

Neal, J. G. (2006). The research and development imperative in the academic library: Path to the future. *Portal: Libraries & the Academy, 6*, 1–3. doi:10.1353/pla.2006.0007

New Media Consortium. (2009). Horizon report: 2009 K-12 Ed. *The New Media Consortium.* Retrieved on March 30, 2009, from http://www.nmc.org/pdf/2009-Horizon-Report-K12.pdf

Niess, M. L. (2005a). Preparing teachers to teach science and mathematics with technology: Developing a Technology Pedagogical Content Knowledge. *Teaching and Teacher Education, 21*, 509–523. doi:10.1016/j.tate.2005.03.006

Niess, M. L. (2005b). Scaffolding math learning with spreadsheets. Learning connections--mathematics. *Learning and Leading with Technology, 32*, 24–25.

Niess, M. L. (2006). Preparing Teachers to Teach Mathematics With Technology. *Contemporary Issues in Technology and Mathematics Teacher Education, 6*, 195–203.

Niess, M. L. (2007, June). *Mathematics teachers developing Technology, Pedagogy and Content Knowledge (TPCK).* Paper presented at the Informatics, Mathematics, Information and Communication Technology (IMICT) conference, Boston, MA.

Niess, M. L. (2008). Knowledge needed for teaching with technologies — Call it TPACK. *AMTE Connections, 17*, 9–10.

Niess, M. L., Lee, K., & Sadri, P. (2007). *Dynamic spreadsheets as learning technology tools: developing teachers' technology pedagogical content knowledge (TPCK).* Paper presented at the annual meeting of the American

Educational Research Association, Chicago, IL.

Niess, M. L., Lee, K., Sadri, P., & Suharwoto, G. (2006). *Guiding inservice mathematics teachers in developing a Technology Pedagogical Knowledge (TPCK).* Paper presented at the annual meeting of the American Educational Research Association, San Francisco, CA.

Niess, M., Ronau, R. N., Shafer, K. G., Driskell, S. O., Harper, S. R., & Johnston, C. (2009). Mathematics teacher TPACK standards and development model. *Contemporary Issues in Technology and Mathematics Teacher Education*, *9*, 4–24.

No Child Left Behind Act of 2002, 20 U.S.C. § 6301 et seq. (West, 2002). Retrieved on February 1, 2009, from http://www.ed.gov/policy/elsec/leg/esea02/107-110.pdf

No Child Left Behind Act. (2001). Retrieved November 15, 2006, from http://www.ed.gov/nclb

Norman, D. A. (1993). *Things that make us smart.* Reading, MA: Addison-Wesley.

Northedge, A. (2002). Teaching by Distance Learning. In McKeachie, W. J. (Ed.), *Teaching Tips* (11th ed., pp. 258–267). Boston, MA: Houghton-Mifflin.

Novak, J., & Voigt, B. (2008). *Mashing-up mashups: from collaborative mapping to community innovation toolkits.* Retrieved April 5, 2009 from http://www.ifi.uzh.ch/im/fileadmin/user_upload/personen_downloads/MCIS06.MashingUpMashups.Study.FullPaper.pdf

Nowak, S. (1969). Methodological dilemmas. *Studia Socjologiczne*, *3*, 29–44.

O'Connell, J., & Phye, G. (2005). Creating strategies for improved teaching and learning. *T.H.E. Journal*, *32*, 26–29.

O'Donnell, S. (2005). IT education and training for disadvantaged students: Lessons from Europe. *IEEE Technology and Society Magazine*, *24*, 23–31. doi:10.1109/MTAS.2005.1507537

O'Hanlon, C. (2007). The teacher becomes the student. *T.H.E. Journal*, *34*(11), 21–22.

O'Lawrence, H. (2006). The influence of distance learning on adult learners. *Techniques*, *81*(5), 47–49.

O'Reilly, T. (2005, September 30). *What Is Web 2.0 Design Patterns and Business Models for the Next Generation of Software.* Retrieved January 31, 2007, from http://www.oreillynet.com/lpt/a/6228

O'Reilly, T. (2007). Pipes and filters for the Internet. *O'Reilly Radar.* Retrieved February 6, 2008 from http://radar.oreilly.com/archives/2007/02/pipes-and-filte.html.

O'Reilly, T., & Battelle, J. (2009). *Web Squared: Web 2.0 five years on.*

Oblinger, D. G. (2004). The next generation of educational engagement. *Journal of Interactive Media in Education*, *8*, 1–18.

Oblinger, D., & Hawkins, B. (2008). We don't Need to Worry about E-Learning Anymore. *EduCause Review*, *40*(4), 14-15. Retrieved September 30, 2008 from http://connect.educause.edu/Library/EDCAUSE+REVIEW/The MythaboutELearning/40560?time=1237616004

Oblinger, D., & Oblinger, J. (2009). Is it age or IT: First steps toward understanding the net generation. *Educause.* Retrieved May 2009, from http://www.educause.edu/Resources/EducatingtheNetGeneration/IsItAgeorIT-FirstStepsTowardUnd/6058

Office of Science Education. (2006). Curriculum supplement series. *National Institutes for Health web site.* Retrieved from http://science-education.nih.gov/customers.nsf/Supplements

Ohio Department of Education. (n.d.). *District report cards* [Data file]. Retrieved from http://ilrc.ode.state.oh.us/Districts/Default.asp

Oman, R. (1999, January). US enacts new law on Internet copyright. *IP Worldwide.*

Ortiz-Rodriguez, M., Teig, R. W., Irani, T., Roberts, T. G., & Rhoades, E. (2005). College students' perceptions of quality in distance education: The importance of communication. *Quarterly Review of Distance Education*, *6*, 97–184.

Osterman, K. F. (2000). Students' need for belonging in

the school community. *Review of Educational Research, 70*(3), 323–367.

Ouzts, K. (2006). Sense of community in online courses. *The Quarterly Review of Distance Education, 7*, 285–296.

Paas, F. G. W. C., & Van Merrienboer, J. J. G. (1994). Variability of worked examples and transfer of geometrical problem solving skills: A cognitive load approach. *Journal of Educational Psychology, 86*(1), 122–133. doi:10.1037/0022-0663.86.1.122

Pajares (2002). Overview of social cognitive theory and of self-efficacy. Retreived 3/3/2010, from http://www.emory.edu/EDUCATION/mfp/eff.html

Palfrey, J., & Gasser, U. (2008). *Born Digital*. New York: Basic Books.

Pallof, R., & Pratt, K. (2003). *The virtual student: A profile and guide to working with online learners*. San Francisco, CA: Jossey-Bass Publishers.

Palloff, R., & Pratt, K. (1999). *Building learning communities in cyberspace*. San Francisco: Jossey-Bass Publishers.

Panyametheekul, P., & Herring, S. (2003). Gender and turn allocation in a Thai chat room. *Journal of Computer-Mediated Communication, 9*(1). Retrieved June 6, 2008, from http://jcmc.indiana.edu/vol12/issue2/waldvogel.html

Papert, S. (1993). *The Children's Machine: Rethinking School in the Age of the Computer*. New York: Basic Books.

Parker, J., Cordes, D., Laurie, C., Hopenwasser, A., Izatt, J., & Nikles, D. (1995, November). *Curriculum integration in the freshman year at the University of Alabama-foundation coalition program*. Paper presented at the Frontiers in Education Conference, Atlanta, GA.

Parr, J., & Ward, L. (2006). Building on foundations: Creating an online community. *Journal of Technology and Teacher Education, 14*(4), 775–793.

Pasley, J. D. (1998). *APS Frontiers in Physiology Final Evaluation Report*. Chapel Hill, NC: Horizon Research Inc.

Patrick, H., Ryan, A. M., & Pintrich, P. R. (2000). The differential impact of extrinsic and mastery goal orientations on males' and females' self-regulated learning. *Learning and Individual Differences, 11*(2), 153–171. doi:10.1016/S1041-6080(00)80003-5

Patton, M. Q. (2002). *Qualitative research and evaluation methods* (3rd ed.). Thousand Oaks: Sage.

Pawley, D., Ayres, P., Cooper, M., & Sweller, J. (2005). Translating words into equations: A cognitive load theory approach. *Educational Psychology, 25*(1), 75–97. doi:10.1080/0144341042000294903

Pedersen, S., & Macafee, C. (2007). Gender differences in British blogging. *Journal of Computer-Mediated Communication, 12*(4). Retrieved December 23, 2009, from http://jcmc.indiana.edu/vol12/issue4/pedersen.html

Penny, C., & Kinslow, J. (2006). Faculty perceptions of electronic portfolios in a teacher education program. *Contemporary Issues in Technology & Teacher Education, 6*(4), 418–435.

Peressini, D., Borko, H., Romagnano, L., Knuth, E., & Willis, C. (2004). A conceptual framework for learning to teach secondary mathematics: A situative perspective. *Educational Studies in Mathematics, 56*, 67–96. doi:10.1023/B:EDUC.0000028398.80108.87

Perez Cereijo, M. V. (2006). Attitude as predictor of success in online training. *International Journal on E-Learning, 5*, 623–639.

Perry, N. E., & Winne, P. H. (2006). Learning from learning kits: gStudy traces of students' self-regulated engagements with computerized content. *Educational Psychology Review, 18*(3), 211–228. doi:10.1007/s10648-006-9014-3

Phipps, R., & Merisotis, J. (1999). *What's the difference? A review of contemporary research on the effectiveness of distance learning in higher education*. Washington, DC: Institute for Higher Education Policy. Retrieved April 3, 2009 from http://www2.nea.org/he/abouthe/distance.html

Piaget, J. (1973). *To Understand is to Invent*. New York: Grossman. *Professional Standards Accreditation of Teacher Preparation Institutions*. (2008). Retrieved from http://www.ncate.org/institutions/publicationsbooks.asp?ch=49&book=standards

Picciano, A. G., & Seaman, J. (2007). *K-12 online learning: A survey of U.S. school district administrators*. Retrieved April 2, 2009, from http://www.sloan-c.org/publications/survey/pdf/K-12_Online_Learning.pdf

Picciano, A. G., & Seaman, J. (2009). *K-12 online learning: A 2008 follow-up survey of U.S. school district administrators*. Retrieved April 2, 2009, from http://www.sloan-c.org/publications/survey/pdf/k-12_online_learning_2008.pdf

Pintrich, P. R. (1995). Understanding self-regulated learning. In P. R. Pintrich (Ed.), New Directions for Teaching and Learning: Vol. 63. Understanding Self-regulated Learning. San Fransisco: Jossey-Bass.

Pintrich, P. R. (2000a). Multiple goals, multiple pathways: The role of goal orientation in learning and achievement. *Journal of Educational Psychology*, *92*(3), 544–555. doi:10.1037/0022-0663.92.3.544

Pintrich, P. R. (2000b). The Role of Goal Orientation in Self-Regulated Learning. In Pintrich, P. R., & Zeidner, M. (Eds.), *Handbook of Self Regulation*. San Diego, CA: Academic Press. doi:10.1016/B978-012109890-2/50043-3

Plough, C. (2008). Web 2.0 tools motivate student creativity. *Tech and Learning*. Retrieved April 2009, from http://www.techlearning.com/article/8534

Porter Honnet, E., & Poulsen, S. J. (1989). *Principles of good practice for combining service and learning*. Retrieved February 10, 2009, from http://www.johnsonfdn.org/principles.html

Pransky, K., & Bailey, F. (2002/2003). To meet your students where they are, first you have to find them: Working with culturally and linguistically diverse at-risk students. *The Reading Teacher*, *56*, 370–383. doi:10.1598/RT.56.4.3

Prensky, M. (2001). *Digital natives, digital immigrants*. Retrieved February 19, 2004 from http://www.marcprensky.com

Prensky, M. (2005). Engage me or enrage me: What today's learners demand. *Educause Review*. Retrieved January 2009 from http://net.educause.edu/ir/library/pdf/ERM0553.pdf

Prensky, M. (2005/2006). Listen to the natives. *Educational Leadership*, *63*(4), 8–13.

Prensky, M. (2008a, November/December). The role of technology in teaching and the classroom. *Educational Technology*.

Prensky, M. (2008b, June). Young minds, fast times: The twenty-first century digital learner. *Edutopia*.

Prensky, M. (2009, February/March). H. Sapiens digital: From Digital Immigrants and Digital Natives to Digital Wisdom. *Innovate*.

Prerna, R. (2007). Skype as a language-learning tool. *Student Newspaper: The Hatchet*. George Washington University. Retrieved December 2008, from http://media.www.gwhatchet.com/media/storage/paper332/news/2007/01/29/Life/Skype.As.A.LanguageLearning.Tool-2682418.shtml?sourcedomain=www.gwhatchet.com&MIIHost=media.collegepublisher.com

Professional standards for the accreditation of teacher preparation institutions (2008). Washington: National Council for Accreditation of Teacher Education (NCATE).

Putnam, R. T., & Borko, H. (1997). Teacher learning: Implications of new views of cognition. In Biddle, B. J., Good, T. L., & Goodson, I. F. (Eds.), *International Handbook of Teachers and Teaching* (*Vol. 2*, pp. 1223–1296). Dordrecht, The Netherlands: Kluwer Academic Publishers.

Quina, K., Wingard, J. A., & Bates, H. G. (1987). Language style and gender stereotypes in person perception. *Psychology of Women Quarterly*, *11*(1), 111–122. doi:10.1111/j.1471-6402.1987.tb00778.x

Raul, A. C., & Gomez, M. A. (1999). Internet legislation in the 106th Congress, Several issues will vie for the limelight. *The Internet Newsletter: Legal & Business Aspects*, *3*(10), 3.

Raysman, R., & Brown, P. (1998, December). The Digital Millennium Copyright Act. *New York Law Journal*.

Raysman, R., & Brown, P. (1999, March). Developments in trademark and domain-name disputes. *New York Law Journal*, 3–11.

Reed, M., & Mitchell, B. (2001). Using information technologies for collaborative learning in geography: A case study from Canada. *Journal of Geography in Higher Education, 25*, 321–339. doi:10.1080/03098260120067619

Reeves, D. B. (2008). *Reframing Teacher Leadership to Improve Your School*. Alexandria, VA: ASCD.

Reinthaler, J. (1990). Just teach them the basics and leave the applications to us. *Communications Magazine, IEEE, 28*, 56–57. doi:10.1109/35.61723

Reynolds, A., & Lennex, L. (2009). Can you read this? 508 compliance among Kentucky schools? *TechTrends, 53*(3), 61–66.

Rhoads, T. R. (2001, October). *Will you throw out the baby with the bathwater?* Paper presented at the 31st annual Frontiers in Education Conference, Reno, NV.

Rice, K. L. (2006). A comprehensive look at distance education in the K-12 context. *Journal of Research on Technology in Education, 38*(4), 425–448.

Rice, W. R., Beg, Y., Waters, C., Bokreta, M. K., & Santiago-Aviles, J. J. (1999, November). *New pedagogical approaches to computer science education: A case study in peer learning.* Paper presented at the 29th annual Frontiers in Education Conference, San Juan, Puerto Rico.

Richards, K., & Wrigley, N. (1996). Geography in the United Kingdom 1992-1996. *The Geographical Journal, 162*, 41–62. doi:10.2307/3060215

Richman, W. (2007, February). *A psychologist's walk through NCATE: successful creation and implementation of a truly comprehensive database system.* Paper presented at the annual meeting of the American Association of Colleges for Teacher Education, New York, NY.

Riggs, H. (2006). Technology-supported mathematics learning environments: Sixty-seventh yearbook of the National Council of Teachers of Mathematics. *Teaching Children Mathematics, 12*, 333–333.

Ring, G. L., & Foti, S. L. (2003). Addressing standards at the program level with electronic portfolios. *TechTrends, 47*(2), 28–32. doi:10.1007/BF02763422

Risco, V. (1995). *Using videodisc based cases to promote pre-service teachers problem solving and mental model building.* In W. M.

Riva, G., & Galimberti, C. (1998). Computer-mediated communication: Identity and social interaction in an electronic environment. *Genetic, Social, and General Psychology Monographs, 124*(4), 434–464.

Roach, S. (2001, October). *The impact of technology on engineering and computer science education in the 21st century: Changing classroom instructional methods.* Paper presented at the 31st annual Frontiers in Education Conference, Reno, NV.

Robert, H., Evans, W., Honemann, D., Balch, T., & Robert, S. (2000). *Robert's Rules of Order* (10th ed.). New York: New York City.

Rodgers, G., & Jones, G. (1997, November). *Science and technology in the workplace: A decade of experimentation with post-calculus H. S. Math.* Paper presented at the 27th annual Frontiers in Education Conference, Pittsburg, PA.

Rodriguez, C. M. (1998). Commentary on: 'Technology in the classroom: Teaching business marketing in the 21st century,' by Richard P. Vlosky and David T. Wilson. *Journal of Business-To-Business Marketing, 5*, 157–160. doi:10.1300/J033v05n01_15

Ronau, R. N., Niess, M. L., Browning, C. A., Pugalee, D., Driskell, S. O., & Harrington, R. (2008). Framing the research on digital technologies and student learning in mathematics. In Bell, L., Thompson, E. A., & Schrum, L. (Eds.), *Framing research on technology and student learning in the content areas* (pp. 13–31). Charlotte, NC: Information Age Publishing.

Ronau, R. N., Taylor, P. M., Dougherty, B. J., Pyper, J., Wagener, L. L., & Rakes, C. R. (2009). *A comprehensive framework for teacher knowledge: A lens for examining research.* Manuscript in preparation.

Rosaen, C. L., Lundeberg, M., Cooper, M., Fritzen, A., & Terpstra, M. (2008). Noticing noticing: How does investigation of video records change how teachers reflect on their experiences? *Journal of Teacher Education, 59*(4), 347–360. doi:10.1177/0022487108322128

Roschelle, J., Tatar, D., Shechtman, N., & Knudsen, J. (2008). The role of scaling up research in designing for and evaluating robustness. *Educational Studies in Mathematics, 68*, 149–170. doi:10.1007/s10649-008-9119-3

Roseman, J. E., Caldwell, A., Kurth, L., & Stern, L. (2000). *High School Biology Textbooks: A Benchmark-Based Evaluation.* AAAS Project 2061 Textbook Evaluations Reports. Retrieved from http://www.project2061.org/about/press/pr000627.htm

Rosenfeld, E. (2008). Expanding your professional network with Nings. *Teacher Librarian, 35*(3), 60–65.

Rosenthal, L. (1974). A course in technology for artists. *Leonardo, 7*, 27–29. doi:10.2307/1572733

Ross, C., & Banister, S. (2004). From high school to college: How prepared are teacher education candidates for technology integration? In C. Crawford et al. (Eds.), *Proceedings of Society for Information Technology and Teacher Education International Conference 2004* (pp. 228).

Rossi, R. J., & Stringfield, S. C. (1995a). Education reform and students at risk. Volume I: Findings and recommendations. Studies of education reform. Baltimore, MD: John Hopkins University, Center for Research on the Education of Students Placed At Risk & American Institutes for Research in the Behavioral Sciences. (ERIC Document Reproduction Service No. ED397541)

Rossi, R. J., & Stringfield, S. C. (1995b). Education reform and students at risk. Volume II: Case study descriptions. Studies of education reform. Baltimore, MD: John Hopkins University, Center for Research on the Education of Students Placed At Risk & American Institutes for Research in the Behavioral Sciences. (ERIC Document Reproduction Service No. ED397542)

Rourke, L., Anderson, T., Garrison, D., & Archer, W. (1999). Assessing social presence in asynchronous text-based computer conferencing. *Journal of Distance Education, 14*(2), 14-28. Retrieved November 1, 2008, from http://cade.athabascau.ca/vol14.2/rourke_et_al.html

Roush, W. (2005, October 7). 'Web 2.0' has arrived. *Technology Review – MIT.* Retrieved on January 10, 2008, from http://www.techreview.com/Infotech/14869/?a=f

Rovai, A. P., & Lucking, R. (2003). Sense of community in a higher education television-based distance education program. *Educational Technology Research and Development, 51*(2), 5–16. doi:10.1007/BF02504523

Rudd, E. (1986). The value of a Ph.D. in science or technology in Britain. *European Journal of Education, 21*, 223–250. doi:10.2307/1503069

Rudnick, M., & O'Flavahan, L. (2000). *Four fatal errors of Web writing or how to keep your content from crashing.* Retrieved October 10, 2008 from http://www.powerhomebiz.com/vol8/fourfatal.htm

Ryan, R. M., & Deci, E. L. (2000). Intrinsic and extrinsic motivations: Classic definitions and new directions. *Contemporary Educational Psychology, 25*(1), 54–67. doi:10.1006/ceps.1999.1020

Sankaran, S. R., & Bui, T. (2001). Impact of learning strategies and motivation on performance: A study in web-based instruction. *Journal of Instructional Psychology, 28*, 191–199.

Sasaki, M., Oguchi, T., Okabe, A., & Sadahiro, Y. (2008). GIS education at geographical departments in Japanese universities in relation to the Japan standard GIS core curriculum. *International Research in Geographical and Environmental Education, 17*, 298–306. doi:10.1080/10382040802401540

Savery, J. R. (2008). BE VOCAL: Characteristics of Successful Online Instructors. [from http://www.ncolr.org/jiol]. *Journal of Interactive Online Learning, 4*(2), 141–159. Retrieved October 15, 2008.

Schmelzer, R. (2008). *Data mashups: Enabling ad hoc composite, headless, information services.* Retrieved

June 26, 2009, from http://www.zapthink.com/report.html?id=ZAPFLASH-20081107

Schwartz, E. J., & Metalitz, S. J. (1998). The Digital Millennium Act: Why it is important. *The Intellectual Property Strategist, 5*(3).

Scribner, J. P. (1999). Professional development: Untangling the influence of work Context on teacher learning. *Educational Administration Quarterly, 35*, 238–266.

Seago, N. (2004). Using video as an object of inquiry for mathematics teaching and learning. In Brophy, J. (Ed.), *Using video in teacher education* (pp. 259–286). Oxford, UK: Elsevier.

Section 508. (2006). *General Services Administration*. Retrieved November 20, 2006 from http://www.section508.gov/index.cfm?FuseAction=Content&ID=131

Segrave, R. (2004). Communication technologies and knowledge building in agriculture. *Australian Journal of Adult Learning, 44*, 27–43.

Selwyn, N. (2007). Curriculum online? Exploring the political and commercial construction of the UK digital learning marketplace. *British Journal of Sociology of Education, 28*, 223–240. doi:10.1080/01425690701192729

Senge, P., Cambron-McCabe, N., Lucas, T., Smith, B., Dutton, J., & Kleiner, A. (2000). *Schools that learn: A fifth discipline fieldbook for educators, parents, and everyone who cares about education*. New York: Doubleday.

Senge, P., Scharmer, C. O., Jaworski, J., & Flowers, B. S. (2004). Presence: Human purpose and the field of the future. Cambridge, MA: SoL (The Society for Organizational learning, Inc.).

Shadish, W. R. (1995). The logic of generalization: Five principles common to experiments and ethnographies. *American Journal of Community Psychology, 23*, 419–428. doi:10.1007/BF02506951

Shadish, W. R., Cook, T. D., & Campbell, D. T. (2002). *Experimental and quasi-experimental design*. Boston: Houghton Mifflin Company.

Sharp, B. D. (2007). Making the most of digital imagery. *Mathematics Teacher, 100*, 590–593.

Shea, V. (2004). Netiquette. *Albion Books*. Retrieved November 15, 2008 from http://www.albion.com/cat-Netiquette.html

Sherin, M. G. (2004). New perspectives on the role of video in teacher education. In Brophy, J. (Ed.), *Using video in teacher education* (pp. 1–28). Oxford, UK: Elsevier Ltd.

Sherin, M. G., & van Es, E. A. (2005). Using video to support teachers' ability to notice classroom interactions. *Journal of Technology and Teacher Education, 13*(3), 475–491.

Shimony, R., Russo, J. W., Ciaccio, L., Sanders, J. W., Rimpici, R., & Takvorian, P. M. (2002). Medical laboratory technology: A New York state tech-prep model that improves academic skills. *The Journal of Educational Research, 95*, 300–307. doi:10.1080/00220670209596603

Shulman, L. S. (1986). Those who understand: A conception of teacher knowledge. *American Educator, 10*, 9–15.

Shymansky, J. A., Yore, L. D., Annetta, L. A., & Everett, S. A. (2008). Missouri-Iowa science cooperative (science co-op): Rural schools-rrban rniversities collaborative project. *Rural Educator, 29*(2), 1–3.

Siegel, M. (2006). Rereading the signs: Multimodal transformations in the field of literacy education. *Language Arts, 84*, 65–77.

Siemens, G. (2004). Connectivism: A learning theory for the digital age. *Elearnspace*. Retrieved February 2008, from http://www.elearnspace.org/Articles/connectivism.htm

Sigmon, R. L. (1979, Spring). Service-learning: Three principles. *Synergist, 8*(1), 9–11.

Silver, E. A., & Stein, M. K. (1996). The QUASAR Project: The Revolution of the Possible in mathematics instructional reform in urban middle schools. *Urban Education, 30*(4), 476–521. doi:10.1177/0042085996030004006

Simon, M. A., & Tzur, R. (2004). Explicating the role of

mathematical tasks in conceptual learning: An elaboration of the hypothetical learning trajectory. *Mathematical Thinking and Learning, 6*(2), 91–104. doi:10.1207/s15327833mtl0602_2

Singer, S. R., Hilton, M. L., & Schweingruber, H. A. (2005). *America's Lab Report: Investigations in High School Science.* Washington, DC: National Academy of Science. Retrieved from http://books.nap.edu/catalog.php?record_id=11311

Sinkinson, A. J. (2006). The impact of specialist school status: A case study of two contrasting mathematics and computing colleges. *Educational Studies, 32,* 87–99. doi:10.1080/03055690500416041

Slater, J. (2009). *42 things about Web 2.0 in 2008.* Retrieved June 26, 2009 from http://www.jasonslater.co.uk/2008/04/14/42-things-about-web-20-in-2008-part-1-of-3/

Slator, B. M., Clark, J., Juell, P., McClean, P., Saini-Eidukat, B., Schwert, D. P., & White, A. R. (2001, August). *Research on role-based learning technologies.* Paper presented at the IEEE International Conference on Advanced Learning Technologies, Madison, WI.

Slay, H., Siebörger, I., & Hodgkinson-Williams, C. (2008). Interactive whiteboards: Real beauty or just lipstick? *Computers & Education, 51,* 1321–1341. doi:10.1016/j.compedu.2007.12.006

Slough, S. W., & Chamblee, G. E. (2007). Technology as an innovation in science and mathematics teaching. *International Journal of Instructional Media, 107,* 222–224.

Smith, C. (2009). *Urban outreach report.* Unpublished raw data.

Smith, P. S., Banilower, E. R., McMahon, K. C., & Weiss, I. R. (2002). *The National Survey of Science and Mathematics Education: Trends from 1977 to 2000.* Chapel Hill, NC: Horizon Research.

Smith, R. (n.d.). *Fair use: An online guide for educators.* Retrieved March 24, 1999 from http://www.fairuse.com

Solomon, G., & Schrum, L. (2007). *Web 2.0: New Tools, New Schools.* Eugene, OR: International Society for Technology in Education.

Spector, B. S., & Burkett, R. S. (2003). MSTS inquiry for career-change teachers. *Bulletin of Science, Technology & Society, 23,* 297–301. doi:10.1177/0270467603256080

Spellman, K. (2004). A national Sufi Order with trans-national dimensions: The Maktab Tarighat Oveyssi Shahmaghsoudi Sufi Order in London. *Journal of Ethnic and Migration Studies, 30,* 945–960. doi:10.1080/1369183042000245633

Spradlin, L., & Parsons, R. (2008). *Diversity matters: understanding diversity in schools.* Belmont, CA: Thomson Higher Education.

Stanford University. (n.d.). *Copyright law and fair use.* Retrieved March 24, 1999 from http://www.stanford.edu/group/CDL/copyright.html

Steele-Johnson, D., Beauregard, R. S., Hoover, P. B., & Schmidt, A. M. (2000). Goal orientation and task cemand effects on motivation, affect, and performance. *The Journal of Applied Psychology, 85*(5), 724–738. doi:10.1037/0021-9010.85.5.724

Stein, M. K., & Smith, M. S. (1998). Mathematical tasks as a framework for reflection: From research to practice. *Mathematics Teaching in the Middle School, 3*(4), 268–275.

Stein, M. K., Smith, M. S., Henningsen, M. A., & Silver, E. A. (2000). *Implementing standards based mathematics instruction: A casebook for professional development.* New York: Teachers College Press.

Steinkuehler, C., & Duncan, S. (2008). Scientific habits of mind in virtual worlds. *Journal of Science Education and Technology, 17,* 530–543. doi:10.1007/s10956-008-9120-8

Steinman, D. (2007). Educational experiences and the online student. *TechTrends, 51*(5), 46–52. doi:10.1007/s11528-007-0069-x

Stephens, M. (2007). Tools from web 2.0 & libraries: Best practices for social software revisited. *Library Technology Reports, 43*(5), 15–32.

Steve, W. (2005). Learning in school, home and community: ICT for early and elementary education. *Cambridge Journal of Education, 35*, 282.

Stevens, K. K., & Schlossberg, S. (1997, November). *Connection technology.* Paper presented at the 27th annual Frontiers in Education Conference, Pittsburg, PA.

Stockero, S. (2008). Differences in pre-service mathematics teachers' reflective abilities attributable to use of a video case curriculum. *Journal of Technology and Teacher Education, 16*(4), 433–458.

Stringfield, S. (1995). Attempting to enhance students' learning through innovative programs: The case for schools evolving into high reliability organizations. *School Effectiveness and School Improvement, 6*, 67–96. doi:10.1080/0924345950060104

Strudler, N., & Wetzel, K. (2005). The diffusion of electronic portfolios in teacher education: Issues of initiation and implementation. *Journal of Research on Technology in Teacher Education, 37*(4), 411–433.

Strudler, N., & Wetzel, K. (2008). Costs and benefits of electronic portfolios in teacher education: faculty perspectives. *Journal of Computing in Teacher Education, 24*(4), 135–142.

Stuhlmann, J. M. (1998). A model for infusing technology into teacher training programs. *Journal of Technology and Teacher Education, 6*(2-3), 125–139.

Suh, J., & Moyer, P. S. (2007). Developing students' representational fluency using virtual and physical algebra balances. *Journal of Computers in Mathematics and Science Teaching, 26*, 155–173.

Suharwoto, G., & Lee, K. H. (2005, March). *Assembling the pieces together: What are the most influential components in mathematics preservice teachers' development of Technology Pedagogical Content Knowledge (TPCK)?* Paper presented at the annual meeting of the Society for Information Technology & Teacher Education (SITE), Phoenix, AZ.

Sutin, A. N., & Goldberg, E. (1998, December). High-tech agenda in Congress. *New York Law Journal*, S3.

Svetcov, D. (2000). The virtual classroom vs. the real one. *Forbes, 166*(7), 50–52.

Swan, B., & Dixon, J. (2006). The effects of mentor-supported technology professional development on middle school mathematics teachers' attitudes and practice. *Contemporary Issues in Technology & Teacher Education, 6*, 67–86.

Swan, K. (2004). Relationships between Interactions and Learning in Online Environments. *Sloan-C Effective Practices Site*. Retrieved October 4, 2008, from http://www.aln.org/effective/index.asp

Swartz, E. (2003). Teaching white preservice teachers. *Urban Education, 38*(3), 255–278. doi:10.1177/0042085903038003001

Sweller, J. (1988). Cognitive load during problem solving: Effects on learning. *Cognitive Science, 12*(2), 257–285.

Tabatabaei, M., Schrottner, B., & Reichgelt, H. (2006). Target populations for online education. *International Journal on E-Learning, 5*, 401–414.

Tall, D. (2008). James J. Kaput (1942-2005), Imagineer and futurologist of mathematics education. *Educational Studies in Mathematics, 68*, 185–193. doi:10.1007/s10649-008-9121-9

Tankersley, M., Landrum, T. J., & Cook, B. G. (2004). How research informs practice in the field of emotional and behavioral disorders. In Rutherford, R. B., Quinn, M. M., & Mathur, S. R. (Eds.), *Handbook of research in emotional and behavioral disorders* (pp. 98–116). New York: Guilford Press.

Tannen, D. (1991). *You Just Don't Understand: Men and Women in Conversation.* New York: Ballantine Books.

Tashakkori, A., & Teddlie, C. (1998). *Mixed methodology: Combining qualitative and quantitative approaches.* Thousand Oaks, CA: Sage Publications.

Teddlie, C., & Stringfield, S. (1985). A differential analysis of effectiveness in middle and low socioeconomic status schools. *Journal of Classroom Interaction, 20*, 38–44.

Terrell, S. (2008). Consider Learner Characteristics, Learning Conditions in Course Design. *Magna Resources for Higher Education September*. Retrieved November 30, 2008, from http://www.magnapubs.com/issues/magnapubs_ff/5_22/news/601829-1.html

Thomas, L. G., & Livingston, M. (2004). Using video exhibits to support technology integration in teacher preparation and P-12 student learning. *Digitial Edge Project*. International Society for Technology in Education. Retrieved from http://cnets.iste.org/dedge/docs/FinalReport_DE_BellSouth.pdf

Thompson, A. D., & Mishra, P. (2007). Breaking news: TPCK becomes TPACK! *Journal of Computing in Teacher Education, 24*, 38, 64.

Thompson, M., Oakes, W., & Bodner, G. (2005, October). *A qualitative investigation of students in a first-year engineering learning community*. Paper presented at the 35th annual Frontiers in Education Conference, Indianapolis, IN.

Thoms, L., & Thelwall, M. (2005). Academic home pages: Reconstruction of the self. *First Monday, 12* 10). Retrieved September 14, 2006.from,http://firstmonday.org/issues/issue10_12/thoms/index.html

TK20 Campuswide. (2009). Retrieved April 2, 2009, from http://www.tk20.com/

Toots, A., & Lanpere, M. (2004). Tiger in focus -- A national survey of ICT in Estonian schools. *Educational Media International, 41*, 7–18. doi:10.1080/0952398032000105049

Triandis, H. C. (1976). Methodological problems of comparative research. *International Journal of Psychology, 11*, 155–159. doi:10.1080/00207597608247355

Trucano, M. (2005). *Knowledge Maps: ICTs in Education*. Washington, DC: infoDev / World Bank. Retrieved from http://www.infodev.org/en/Publication.8.html

TrueOutcomes Assessment Manager. (2009). Retrieved April 2, 2009, from http://www. trueoutcomes.com/

U. S. Congress. (1995). *Teachers and technology: Making the connections (GPO #052-003-0149-2). Office of Technology Assessment*. Washington, DC: U.S. Government Printing Office.

U.S. Department of Education. (2001). *Enhancing Education Through Technology Act of 2001*. Retrieved March 8, 2009, from http://www.ed.gov/policy/elsec/leg/esea02/pg34.html

United States Copyright Office. *Section 102*. (n.d.). Retrieved March 24, 1999 from http://lcweb.loc.gov/copyright/fls102/fl102.pdf

Universal Services Administrative Company. (2007). USAC provides demand estimate for funding year 2007 to FCC. *Schools and Libraries USAC web site*. Retrieved from http://www.universalservice.org/sl/tools/latest-news.aspx#030907

University of Texas. (n.d.). *Getting permission*. Retrieved February 3, 1999 from http://www.utsystem.edu/OGC/IntellectualProperty/permissn.htm

University of Texas. (n.d.). *Will we need fair use in the twenty-first century?* Retrieved February 3, 1999 from http://www.utsystem.edu/OGC/IntellectualProperty/fair_use.htm

US Department of Education. (2009). Retrieved April 7, 2009 from http://www.ed.gov

Van de Walle, D., Brown, S. P., Cron, W. L., & Slocum, J. W. (1999). The Influence of goal orientation and self-regulation tactics on sales performance: A longitudinal field test. *The Journal of Applied Psychology, 84*(2), 249–259. doi:10.1037/0021-9010.84.2.249

Van Horn, R. (2003). Web page accessibility. [from EBSCOhost database.]. *Phi Delta Kappan, 103*, 173. Retrieved September 26, 2007.

Van Merrienboer, J. J. G., Kirschnet, P. A., & Kester, L. (2003). Taking the load off a learner's mind: Instructional design for complex learning. *Educational Psychologist, 38*(1), 5–13. doi:10.1207/S15326985EP3801_2

Vanderburg, W. H. (1992). Education for sustainability: A report card on engineering. *Technology and Society Magazine, IEEE, 11*, 26–31. doi:10.1109/44.141672

Vella, M. (2008, June 24). The 10 commandments of Web design. *Business Week Online*. Retrieved April 7, 2009, from Academic Search Premier database.

Vonderwell, S., Liang, X., & Alderman, K. (2007). Asynchronous Discussions and Assessment in Online Learning. *Journal of Research on Technology in Education, 39*(3), 309–329.

Vygotsky, L. (1978). *Mind in Society: The Development of Higher Psychological Processes*. Cambridge, MA: Harvard University Press.

Walters, M. D. (1998, October). Cyber-pirates beware. *Intellectual Property Magazine*.

Walther, J. B. (1992). Interpersonal effects in computer-mediated interaction: A relational perspective. *Communication Research, 19*(1), 52–90. doi:10.1177/009365092019001003

Waltonen-Moore, S., Stuart, D., Newton, E., Oswald, R., & Varonis, E. (2006). From virtual strangers to a cohesive online learning community: The evolution of online group development in a professional development community. *Journal of Technology and Teacher Education, 14*(2), 287–311.

Wang, L. (2005). The advantages of using technology in second language education: Technology integration in foreign language teaching demonstrates the shift from a behavioral to a constructivist learning approach. *T.H.E. Journal, 32*(10), 38.

Wayman, J. C., Stringfield, S., & Yakimowski, M. (2004). Software enabling school improvement through analysis of student data (Rep. No. 67). Baltimore, MD: John Hopkins University, Center for Research on the Education of Students Placed at Risk (CRESPAR). (ERIC Document Reproduction Service No. EJ330697)

Weaver, G. C., Russell, C. B., & Wink, D. J. (2008). Inquiry-based and research-based laboratory pedagogies in undergraduate science. *Nature Chemical Biology, 4*(10), 577–580. doi:10.1038/nchembio1008-577

Web Access Initiative. (2001). Retrieved January 21, 2007, from_http://www.w3.org/WAI/quicktip

Webb, M. E. (2005). Affordances of ICT in science learning: Implications for an integrated pedagogy. *International Journal of Science Education, 27*, 705–735. doi:10.1080/09500690500038520

Weiant, C. L. (1999, January). When computers cause mischief. *Legal Times*, S32.

Wells, J., & Lewis, L. (2006). *Internet access in U.S. public schools and classrooms: 1994-2005 (NCES 2007020)*. U.S. Department of Education. Washington, DC: National Center for Education Statistics. Retrieved November 1, 2007, from http://jtc.colstate.edu/vol2_2/pelling.htmhttp://nces.ed.gov/pubsearch/pubsinfo.asp?pubid=2007020.

Welsch, R. G., & Devlin, P. A. (2007). Developing preservice teachers' reflection: Examining the use of video. *Action in Teacher Education, 28*(4), 53–61.

Wenglinsky, H. (2005). *Using technology wisely: The keys to success in schools*. New York: Teachers College Press.

Wetzel, K. (1993). Models for achieving computer competencies in preservice education. *Journal of Computing in Teacher Education, 9*(4), 4–6.

Whitehurst, G. J. (2002, October). *Evidence-based education*. Presentation given at the annual meeting of the School Accountability Conference, Orlando, FL. Retrieved on May 5, 2006 from http://www.ed.gov/offices/OERI/presentations/evidencebase.html

Whitehurst, G. J. (2003). *Identifying and implementing educational practices supported by rigorous evidence: A user-friendly guide*. Washington, D.C.: U. S. Department of Education, Institute of Education Sciences, National Center for Education Evaluation and Regional Assistance. Retrieved on June 1, 2009 from http://www.ed.gov/rschstat/research/pubs/rigorousevid/rigorousevid.pdf

Wijekumar, K. (2005). Creating Effective Web-Based learning Environments: Relevant Research and Practice. *Innovate, 1*(5). Retrieved, December 29, 2008, from http://www.innovateonline.info/index.php?view=article&id=26

Wilhelm, L., Puckett, K., Beisser, S., Wishart, W., Merideth, E., & Sivakumaran, T. (2006). Lessons Learned from the Implementation of Electronic Portfolios at Three Universities. *Curriculum Journal*, *17*(4), 397–411.

Willis, J. W., & Mehlinger, H. D. (1996). Information technology and teacher education. In Sikula, J., Buttery, T., & Guyton, E. (Eds.), *Handbook of research on teacher education* (2nd ed., pp. 978–1029). New York: Macmillan.

Willis, J., & Mehlinger, H. (1996). Information technology and teacher education. In Sikula, J., Buttery, T., & Guyton, E. (Eds.), *Handbook of research on teacher education* (2nd ed., pp. 978–1029). New York: MacMillan.

Winne, P. H., & Hadwin, A. F. (1998). Studying as self-regulated learning. In Hacker, D. J., Dunlosky, J., & Graesser, A. C. (Eds.), *Metacognition in educational theory and practice* (pp. 277–304). Manwah, NJ: Erlbaum.

Winne, P. H., & Perry, N. E. (2000). Measuring self-regulated learning. In Pintrich, P. R., & Zeidner, M. (Eds.), *Handbook of self-regulation* (pp. 531–566). San Diego, CA, US: Academic Press. doi:10.1016/B978-012109890-2/50045-7

Witmer, D. F., & Katzman, S. L. (1997). On-Line smiles: Does gender make a difference in the use of graphic accents? *Journal of Computer-Mediated Communication*, *2*(4). Retrieved March 6, 2009, from http://jcmc.indiana.edu/vol2/issue4/witmer1.html

Wittmann, E. C. (1998). Mathematics education as a 'design science. In Sierpinska, A., & Kilpatrick, J. (Eds.), *Mathematics education as a research domain: A search for identity*. Dordrecht: Kluwer Academic Publishers.

Wojciechowski, A., & Palmer, L. B. (2005). Individual Student Characteristics: Can Any Be Predictors Of Success In Online Classes? *Online Journal of Distance Learning Administration*, *8*(2). Retrieved December 20, 2008, from http://www.westga.edu/~distance/ojdla/summer82/wojciechowski82.htm

Wolf, M. A. (2008). High schools: An equation that works. *T.H.E. Journal*, *35*, 24–26.

Wolsey, T. (2008). Efficacy of Instructor Feedback on Written Work in an Online Program. *International Journal on E-Learning*, *7*(2), 311–330.

Wolters, C. A., Yu, S. L., & Pintrich, P. R. (1996). The relation between goal orientation and students' motivational beliefs and self-regulated learning. *Learning and Individual Differences*, *8*(3), 211–238. doi:10.1016/S1041-6080(96)90015-1

Wong, A. (2007). *Adapting to the E-world*. Retrieved June 15, 2009, from http://www.lawcrossing.com/article/1429/Adapting-to-the-E-world/

Wong, P. (2005). Online and face-to-face students' perceptions of teacher-learner interactions: A preliminary examination. *Distance Leanring*, *2*(5), 1–7.

Woodgate, D., & Fraser, D. S. (2006, December). *EScience, science education and technology integration in the classroom: Some practical considerations*. Paper presented at the IEEE International Conference on e-Science and Grid Computing, Amsterdam, The Netherlands.

Woody, K. (2006). Designs for learning with new technologies. *Peer Review*, *8*, 23–25.

Wu, C. C., & Kao, H. C. (2008). Streaming video in peer assessment to support training pre-service teachers. *Educational Technology & Society*, *11*(1), 45–55.

Yoder, M. (1994). Preferred learning style and educational technology: Linear vs. interactive video. *Nursing & Health Care*, *15*(3), 128–132.

Young, D. (1999). Congress modifies copyright protection for the digital age. *Legal Backgrounder*, *14*(6).

Young-Suk, S. (2004). Virtual experiment environment's design for science education. *International Journal of Distance Education Technologies*, *2*, 62–76.

Yung, B. H. W., Wong, S. L., & Cheng, M. W. (2007). Tracking pre-service teachers' changing conceptions of good science teaching: The role of progressive reflection with the same video. *Research in Science Education*, *37*(3), 239–259. doi:10.1007/s11165-006-9024-7

Zeichner, K. M. (1996). *Reflective teaching: An introduction.* Mahwah, NJ: L. Erlbaum Associates

Zhu, E. (1996). Meaning negotiation, knowledge construction, and mentoring in a distance learning course. In *Proceedings of Selected Research and Development Presentations at the 1996* (pp. 821–844). Indianapolis, IN: National Convention of the Association for Educational Communications and Technology.

Zhu, E. (1998). Learning and mentoring: Electronic discussions in a distance learning course. In Bonk, C. J., & King, K. S. (Eds.), *Electronic collaborators: Learner-centered technologies for literacy, apprenticeship, and discourse* (pp. 233–259). Mahwah, NJ: Lawrence Erlbaum Associates.

Zia, L. L., & Mulder, M. C. (1996). NSF workshop on information technology and undergraduate science, mathematics, engineering, and technology education: Challenges and opportunities. *Education. IEEE Transactions on, 39*, 452–454.

Zimmerman, B. J. (1990). Self-regulated learning and academic achievement: An overview. *Educational Psychologist, 25*(1), 3–17. doi:10.1207/s15326985ep2501_2

Zimmerman, B. J., & Bandura, A. (1994). Impact of self-regulatory influences on writing course attainment. *American Educational Research Journal, 31*(4), 845–862.

Zucker, A. A., & Hug, S. (2008). Teaching and learning physics in a 1:1 laptop school. *Journal of Science Education and Technology, 17*, 586–594. doi:10.1007/s10956-008-9125-3

Zucker, A. A., Tinker, R., Staudt, C., Mansfield, A., & Metcalf, S. (2008). Learning science in grades 3-8 using probeware and computers: Findings from the TEEMSS II project. *Journal of Science Education and Technology, 17*, 42–48. doi:10.1007/s10956-007-9086-y

Zurita, G., & Nussbaum, M. (2007). A conceptual framework based on activity theory for mobile CSCL. *British Journal of Educational Technology, 38*, 211–235. doi:10.1111/j.1467-8535.2006.00580.x

About the Contributors

Junko Yamamoto teaches Instructional Technology, World Language Teaching Methodology, and English Language Learners Teaching Methodology at Secondary Education/ Foundations of Education Department, Slippery Rock University. She also supervises student teachers. She earned her doctorate degree in Instructional Technology from Duquesne University. She is a reviewer for the American Council on the Teaching of Foreign Languages / National Council for Accreditation of Teacher Education institutional accreditation for teacher education programs. She also reviews papers for multiple international conferences.

Chris Penny teaches educational technology and curriculum assessment courses at West Chester University of Pennsylvania. He earned his doctor of philosophy in education at the Pennsylvania State University. He evaluates Classrooms for the Future Grants for the Pennsylvania Department of Education.

Joanne Leight teaches instructional technology to physical education majors at Slippery Rock University of Pennsylvania where she serves as Associate Professor. In addition, she teaches classes for the coaching minor (Psychological and Sociological Bases of Sport, Philosophy and Psychology of Coaching, Sports Officiating and Coaching Practicum). She also supervises student teachers and has supervised SRU student teachers in Mexico City, Mexico and Dublin, Ireland. She earned her doctorate degree in education from Duquesne University. She has successfully written numerous technology grants and serves as the technology editor of the Journal of Physical Education, Recreation and Dance.

Sally Winterton, Ed. D. is an associate professor at West Chester University of Pennsylvania. She served as Coordinator of Field Experiences in the Department of Elementary Education, a university supervisor, and as the Interim Director of the Teacher Education Center which is responsible for field placements for the teacher education program. She completed her doctoral work at the University of Pennsylvania in Organizational Leadership, Curriculum, and Instruction. She currently teaches courses, supervises pre-service teacher candidates, and provides professional development for WCU's cooperating teachers and new supervisors on observation and conferencing skills. Prior to joining the university Dr. Winterton taught elementary school, served first as an assistant elementary school principal, a middle school assistant principal, an elementary school principal, and a Director of Personnel in public school districts. Her research interests are learning styles and teacher preparation.

***

Heejung An is an Assistant Professor in the Department of Elementary and Early Childhood Education at the College of Education, William Paterson University, New Jersey, USA and teaches educational technology courses in-person, online, and in blended formats. Her research interests are in the areas of fostering metacognitive knowledge through online group learning, the impact of instructor facilitation approaches on students' interactions in online learning environments, and technology integration in K-16 teaching and learning. She holds an Ed.D from Teachers College, Columbia University.

Jill A. Ashbaugh Earman, Ed.D. is an administrator in the Indiana Area School District in Indiana, PA, where she has served since 2000. Prior to that, she was a secondary mathematics teacher and a computer science instructor at the college level. She earned her doctorate in education at Duquesne University, with an emphasis in instructional technology. She is a Pennsylvania certified instructional technology specialist. She provides professional development and consultation in all areas of instructional technology and education, especially helping teachers to use technology as a tool for learning and increasing student achievement. Jill enjoys traveling, playing classical piano, and spending time with her family.

Ronan S. Bernas is a Professor at the Department of Psychology of Eastern Illinois University. He received his Ph.D. in Psychology (Committee on Human Development) from the University of Chicago in 1995. His research is on argumentative and explanatory discourse. He examines the learning and conceptual changes that occur during argumentative and explanatory discourse.

Kevin Biesinger, Ph.D. is a recent graduate of the Learning & Technology program from the University of Nevada, Las Vegas and currently working as a program evaluator in the Grants Department of the Clark County School District. His dissertation, "The effects of Feedback Protocol and Learning Environment Perceptions on Self-Regulated Learning" investigated the application and effects of worked examples and feedback types on goal orientation, self efficacy, and achievement in a virtual environment undergraduate chemistry assessment system. To date, Dr. Biesinger has had four papers accepted for publication and several additional topics selected for presentation. His professional career accomplishments include assisting the 5th largest K-12 school system in the nation to find, secure, monitor, and evaluate nearly $40M in State and Federal competitive grant funding since 2006.

Christine Browning has authored or co-authored many publications including papers, chapters, and books, along with providing numerous presentations and workshops, with most focusing on the use of technology in the mathematics classroom. She has been the Academic Coordinator for two national professional development workshop prograams supporting the use of hand-held graphing technology in middle school classrooms as well as writing professional development materials supporting the use of graphing calculators for mathematics educators at the collegiate level. Her research interests center on hand-held technology use in the K-16 mathematics classrooms and the mathematical knowledge K-8 teachers need for teaching. Most recently, her work has focused on TPACK and assessment issues.

Howard V. Coleman is an Assistant Professor and Graduate Coordinator for the Doctoral Program in Educational Leadership at University of North Carolina at Wilmington. He received his doctorate in educational administration from University of North Carolina at Chapel Hill. Coleman has served as a public school superintendent, a director of research, and a consultant for public schools, state agencies and corporations. He teaches graduate level courses in leadership, research, program evaluation, curriculum assessment, school law and educational policy. Coleman has published several articles on technology and leadership, co-authored book chapters on professional teaching standards, e-portfolio assessment and organizational health in middle schools. He currently serves as the Executive Director for Consortium for Research on Educational Accountability and Teacher Evaluation, a board member for the National Evaluation Institute and a board member for the North Carolina Association for Research in Education.

Kent Crippen, Ph.D. is an Associate Professor of Science Education and Technology and serves as Associate Director of the Center for Science and Mathematics Education at the University of Nevada Las Vegas. His leadership at UNLV has produced multiple collaborative grant proposals, research projects, and graduate programs between the colleges of science and education. He is an editorial review board member for numerous journals in the field and serves as Associate Editor of the Journal of Science Education and Technology. Dr. Crippen's research involves the design and implementation of Web-based learning systems with a focus on cognitive scaffolds to support self-regulated learning. His interests include the improvement of teaching and learning strategies for general chemistry and in-service science teacher professional development. Dr. Crippen has been recognized by Apple Computer as an Apple Distinguished Educator and as a recipient of the UNLV College of Education's Outstanding Faculty Research Award.

Pru Cuper is an Associate Professor in the Keene State College Education Department. Dr. Cuper earned her doctorate in Curriculum and Instruction from North Carolina State University in 2003 where she started a middle grades literacy-support website, *Literacy Junction.* Dr. Cuper's current research focuses on literacy instruction and the use of technology in teacher education. Dr. Cuper and Dr. Gong's video work was funded by an internal technology grant that has allowed them the resources and time to develop their video-based supervision model. Dr. Cuper and Dr. Gong have also developed a hybrid model for delivering instruction at the student teaching level.

Jeremy Dickerson is an Assistant Professor in the Department of Business and Information Technologies Education in the College of Education at East Carolina University. He holds a Doctoral Degree in Technology Education with a concentration in Training and Development from North Carolina State University and has over ten years experience as an information technology manager, consultant and educator. Dickerson teaches information technology-related courses to undergraduate and graduate students and focuses his research on the integration of emerging technologies in education, business and industry settings. He has presented at national and international conferences and professional meetings across the United States and in countries abroad.

Shannon O. Driskell, Shannon.Driskell@notes.udayton.edu, is an associate professor of mathematics education at the University of Dayton in Dayton, Ohio. Her research interests include the appropriate use of technology to teach K–12 mathematics, the content knowledge of prospective mathematics teachers, and the teaching and learning of geometry.

Julie Faulkner is a Senior Lecturer in Literacy in the School of Education at RMIT University. Her research and publications focus on questions of engagement and poplar culture in relation to teenage learning, as well as the increasingly popular text forms associated with information and multimedia technologies. Her writing includes 'It gives you an image of yourself that you can reflect upon': Literacy, identity and new media in I. Snyder and C. Beavis (Eds) *Doing Literacy Online: Teaching, Learning and Playing in an Electronic World* (Hampton Press), and the co-authored *Learning to teach: New times, new practices* (Latham, G. , Blaise, M., Dole, S., Faulkner, J., Lang, J., Malone, K. (2006). *Learning to teach: New times, new practices.* Melbourne: Oxford University Press).

Heather Flynn is a senior undergraduate student at Morehead State University. She is an English linguistics major, graduating in spring 2010. She has worked as an undergraduate fellow for the university for two and a half year: in the Business Marketing and Management department with Dr. Michelle Kunz, then with Curriculum and Instruction, Dr. Lesia Lennex, and Brianna Swetnam. Ms. Flynn was recently published for research in Web site development of public school teachers. She hopes to pursue a Masters degree in Library Science after finishing her bachelor's degree. She is interested in learning about diverse cultures, especially their languages, history, and literature. In her free time, she enjoys reading classical novels, writing, hiking, and traveling

William J. Gibbs is an Associate Professor in the Journalism and Multimedia Arts Department at Duquesne University where he teaches course in multimedia, instructional design, e-Learning, and human computer interaction. He received his Ph.D. in Instructional Systems from The Pennsylvania State University. His research interests include knowledge acquisition, technology-based learning environments, computer-mediated communication, and human-technology interaction.

Yi Gong is an Assistant Professor in the Keene State College Education Department. Dr. Gong earned his doctorate in Curriculum and Instruction from Indiana University of Pennsylvania in 2005. Dr. Gong's research focuses on assessment, program evaluation, quantitative data analysis, electronic portfolio, and database development. Additionally, Dr. Gong has developed courses and curricular experiences related to technology in teacher education which he has delivered to both pre-service and in-service teacher audiences. Dr. Cuper and Dr. Gong have also developed a hybrid model for delivering instruction at the student teaching level.

Terry L. Herman is an Assistant Professor and Graduate Coordinator in the Visual Communication and Technology Education Department in Bowling Green State University's College of Technology. Her research interests have focused on cloud computing, Web 2.0, virtual and synthetic learning environments, online learning, adaptive educational hypermedia, learning design, digital mashups, and interactive multimedia. She has presented at national and international conferences. Recent articles include *Collaboration beyond the Virtual Classroom through Wikis* for the Journal of Industrial Technology and *Face-to-Face versus Online Coursework: A Comparison of Learning Outcomes and Costs* for Contemporary Issues in Technology and Teacher Education - Current Practices.

Natalie A. Johnson-Leslie (PHD), a Jamaican native, is an assistant professor of teacher education at Arkansas State University (ASU) since fall 2004. She received double doctoral degrees from Iowa State University in the areas of Educational Leadership and Policy Studies (ELPS) as well as Curriculum and Instructional Technology (CIT). She has been involved with training faculty and students to use College LiveText (CLT™). Her main research interests lie in the field of educational leadership, technology integration in the curriculum as well as assessing and evaluating student behavior. In her research she poses difficult questions and solves complex problems using insightful research techniques. Her work has been published in the Journal of Educational Technology (JET), International Journal of Reflection (IJR), Journal of the European Teacher Education Network (JETEN), and the International Journal of Learning (IJL). She served as a reviewer for the Journal of College Student Development for four years.

Elizabeth Juelich-Velotta, M.A., is Director of the Office of Service Learning at Walsh University in North Canton, Ohio. She has been engaged in the service arena for more than a decade and continues to be passionate about the transformational power of service endeavors. Prior to working in higher education, Juelich-Velotta worked in the non-profit sector working in the areas of domestic violence prevention, immigrant civil rights, and women's leadership. She earned her B.A. degree (2003) in English from the College of St. Benedict and her M.A. degree (2007) in college student personnel from Bowling Green State University.

Kioh Kim is an Assistant Professor of Educational Technology at Northwestern State University (NSU) of Louisiana. His teaching and research interests include examining and developing potential applications of emerging technologies in the classroom, improving training which results in teachers' increased use of computer-based technology in their classroom, and developing effective online learning environments. Dr. Kim uses a variety of forms of subtle and obvious positive feedback in hopes that students not only learn better, but adopt similar modeling techniques in their own classrooms. Dr. Kim has considerable teaching experience with technology in South Korea and the United States. Dr Kim's teaching experiences include teaching English at the middle and high school levels, teaching at a college in South Korea, and teaching undergraduate and graduate educational technology courses at the University of Wyoming and NSU. Dr. Kim has written extensively including a book titled *Appreciating Computer-Based Technology Use in Teacher Education Programs: A Case-Study Monograph* (Chicago, IL: Discovery Association Publishing House). He enjoys living in Northwest Louisiana with his wife and two children.

Dennis S. Kubasko, Jr. is an Associate Professor of Secondary Science Education at the University of North Carolina at Wilmington. He received his PhD from the College of Education at the University of North Carolina at Chapel Hill. Kubasko serves as Program Coordinator for the International Field Experience in San Pedro, Belize and as Director of the Wilmington Regional Science Olympiad. He teaches undergraduate and graduate courses in secondary education, curriculum, programs and practices. Kubasko has published widely in the field of secondary education, digital instruction and information technologies. He has presented at international, national and regional conferences on science education, effective instructional practices and digital enhancement in classroom environments.

Gloria Latham is a Senior Lecturer in Literacy in the School of Education at RMIT University. Gloria teaches students in undergraduate and graduate programs and along with Julie Faulkner she created and maintains Lathner Primary (the Virtual School) as part of a Teacher Education text: *Learning to teach: New times, New Practices.* Currently Gloria is working on a research project concerning student feedback. In 2009 Gloria was recognised in the Australian Learning and Teaching Council Citations for Outstanding Contributions to Student Learning for inspiring face-to-face teaching that supports and challenges knowledge creation while using sustained innovative design and application of educational technologies.

Lesia Lennex received her doctorate in curriculum and instruction from the University of Tennessee, Knoxville, in 1995. She is currently an Associate Professor of Education in the department of Middle and Secondary Education at Morehead State University, Morehead Kentucky. Dr. Lennex holds degrees in biology, anthropology, and education. She researches, presents, and publishes in technology issues and integration for P-16 schools, NCATE accreditation Web sites, biology curriculum, and ethnobotany. Dr. Lennex is a former high school science teacher in biology, chemistry, physics, and ecology. She is the Chair of Information Technology Education SIG for the Society for Information Technology and Teacher Education (SITE) 2008-2011.

Ronald Lombard is an assistant professor of education at Chatham University in Pittsburgh, PA. He has eighteen years experience as a secondary social studies teacher and served as both a building level and district level administrator for the remainder of his tenure in the public schools. His interest in the implementation of technology into the classroom grew during his years as an administrator with the realization of the impact technology would have on changing both the teaching and learning processes in schools. This interest led to Dr. Lombard to leaving public education and working with Co-Nect, an organization funded by New American Schools aimed at the effective expansion and implementation of technology in American schools. His work in the Pittsburgh Public Schools led to his current position with Chatham, an adjunct position with Gannon University, both with continued emphasis in technology integration.

Susann M. Mathews is a professor at Wright State University, where she has a joint appointment in the departments of Mathematics and Statistics and Teacher Education. During her career, she has participated in the evolution of technology in the classroom —from scientific calculators and *Logo* to graphing calculators and *Fathom* and *Mathematica*. Her interests lie in helping students learn mathematical modeling, both for applying mathematics to the world and to develop a deeper understanding of the mathematics. Technology has helped her make complicated mathematical modeling accessible to her students and has helped her students explore the mathematics and the models.

Jacqueline S. McLaughlin is an Associate Professor of Biology at Penn State Lehigh Valley. She has spent much of her academic career transforming the textbook method of teaching biology into dynamic pedagogical methods of learning that immerse students in biological concepts and real-world issues by engaging them directly in research. Whether in her "physical classroom/lab" or in her "field classrooms" around the world, she works to build and assess programs and pedagogical tools that connect skilled educators and research scientists with teachers for professional development, and with students for high-impact learning. She is grounded on the belief that in 21st century science classrooms, the power of experiential teaching and learning, in which the use of technology replaces in-class lectures or readings and color-coded diagrams from a textbook as the medium of experience, will prevail. Because of this, science education will be more rigorous, relevant, and based on relationships with stakeholders beyond the confines of academic walls. The flagship element of this teaching method is a professional development program she founded and directs, called CHANCE, for Connecting Humans and Nature through Conservation Experiences. She is currently developing a new multimedia-based product in conjunction with W. H. Freeman Publishers that is specifically geared toward bringing research scientists, their methodologies and published data, directly into our nation's undergraduate biology classrooms.

Jacqueline M. Mumford, Ph.D., is an Assistant Professor in the Division of Education at Walsh University in North Canton, Ohio. Jacqueline teaches undergraduate courses in instructional technology, middle childhood and adolescent to young adult assessment, and pre-clinical teaching methods. Her research interests include educational technology, eLearning, ePortfolios, service learning, assessment, and language learning. She holds a B.A. degree (1993) in Liberal Arts: German and Political Science from Purdue University in West Lafayette, Indiana; a M.S. degree (1995) in Education: Instructional Design and Development from Purdue Calumet in Hammond, Indiana; and, a Ph.D. degree (2005) in Education: Curriculum and Instruction from Purdue University in West Lafayette, Indiana.

Margaret (Maggie) L. Niess is a Professor Emeritus of Mathematics Education at Oregon State University (OSU). At OSU she was Department Chair of the Department of Science and Mathematics Education and Director of Science and Mathematics Teacher Preparation and is currently PI of an Oregon MSP Title IIB grant. Her research efforts focus on the integration of technology in teaching science and mathematics with specific attention to the knowledge teachers need to teach with technology – a technology pedagogical and content knowledge (TPACK). Her research has lead to recognition of teachers' levels of TPACK as they learn more about teaching with technology as well as framing professional development and other educational experiences that support teachers in developing TPACK. She is Vice-President for the Mathematics Teacher Education Committee for the Society of Information Technology and Teacher Education (SITE) and active member of the Association of Mathematics Teacher Educators(AMTE).

Stella Porto is currently the director of the Master of Distance Education and E-Learning program in the Graduate School of Management & Technology at University of Maryland University College. Dr. Porto has BS in Electrical Engineering (1986), a Master's (1991) and Doctoral (1995) degrees in Informatics from the Pontifical Catholic University of Rio de Janeiro (PUC-Rio). She has also a second master's degree in Distance Education (2008) from UMUC. Since 2001, Dr. Porto has worked in the field of distance education. She has published in different conferences, including EDEN Workshop, ALN, DLA, ICDE and UCEA conferences in the past 8 years. Combining her knowledge in information technology and her more recent experience and study in the field of distance education, her research interests include topics related to learning objects, new technologies, multimedia and course development models, as well as education of Information Technology.

David Pugalee is Professor of Education at the University of North Carolina at Charlotte where he is Research Associate in the Center for Mathematics, Science, & Technology Education. He earned his Ph.D. in mathematics education from the University of North Carolina at Chapel Hill. He has taught at the elementary, middle, and secondary levels before moving into higher education. His list of publications includes research articles in *Educational Studies in Mathematics* and *School Science and Mathematics.* His works include several books and book chapters published by the National Council of Teachers of Mathematics. His research interest is the relationship between language and mathematics teaching and learning.

Christopher R. Rakes is a doctoral candidate at the University of Louisville, where he is studying Curriculum and Instruction in Secondary Mathematics Education. Over the last eight years, he has taught secondary mathematics in both urban and rural settings. His research interests center on teacher knowledge, instructional improvement in algebra and geometry, and addressing misconceptions in mathematics. Currently, he is preparing his dissertation proposal, *Misconceptions in rational numbers, probability, algebra, and geometry* under the directorship of Dr. Robert N. Ronau. He expects to complete his degree in May 2010.

Robert N. Ronau is a Professor of Mathematics Education and Associate Dean for Research at the University of Louisville whose research interests and publications include the implementation of instructional technology, teacher knowledge, teacher preparation and assessment. Over the last fifteen years, he has played a critical role in numerous state-wide and local grant efforts including development of State Wide Mathematics Core-Content and Assessments, LATTICE (Learning Algebra Through Technology, Investigation, and Cooperative Experience), the Secondary Mathematics Initiative (SMI) of PRISM (Partnership for Reform Initiatives in Science and Mathematics), Kentucky's state-wide systemic reform initiative, Technology Alliance, Teaching K-4 Mathematics in Kentucky, the Park City/IAS Geometry Project, and U2MAST. He currently serves as a Co-PI on the NSF Funded project, Geometry Assessments for Secondary Teachers (GAST), an initiative to determine critical geometry knowledge for secondary teachers and to design assessments to measure levels of teacher knowledge.

Shari L. Stockero received her Ph.D. from Western Michigan University in 2006 and is an Assistant Professor of Mathematics Education at Michigan Technological University. Her research focuses on understanding how to best support teacher learning and help teachers become reflective practitioners, both during initial teacher preparation and in professional development contexts. A former rural high school mathematics teacher herself, Dr. Stockero recognized a need to make high-quality professional development available to teachers who do not typically have access to such opportunities, and has made providing such opportunities an integral part of her work. Her interest in online teacher education has developed through her work on professional development projects focused on providing such opportunities to rural secondary mathematics teachers.

Brianna Swetnam was born in 1985 in the small town of Morehead, Kentucky, where she still lives with her husband and two dogs. After completing high school, she enrolled in Morehead State University, where she majored in biology. Upon graduating in 2007, she took a summer off to work as a Cave Guide at Carter Caves State Resort Park, in Olive Hill, Kentucky. It was there that she realized her passion for education. The epiphany prompted her to enter the MAT (Masters in the Art of Teaching) program at Morehead State University. After graduating in May of 2009, she hopes to begin teaching biology at one of the many wonderful high schools in Eastern Kentucky.

Lauren Wagener is a doctoral candidate in Theory and Practice in Teacher Education with a focus in Mathematics Education at the University of Tennessee – Knoxville. In addition to exploring the knowledge for teaching mathematics, her research examines the roles of gender, adaptive expertise, socialization, and transitions on student persistence and attrition from the study of mathematics in higher education. Over the past ten years, she has completed advanced degrees in Mathematics and Mathematics Education and taught mathematics at the high school and university levels. She is currently an instructorin the Mathematics Department at Mars Hill College in Mars Hill, North Carolina.

Hilary Wilder is an Associate Professor in the Department of Educational Leadership and Professional Studies at the College of Education, William Paterson University, New Jersey, USA and teaches educational technology courses there. She also worked for many years as an instructional technologist designing and developing multimedia and web-based corporate training. Her research interests include the use of technology to promote the expression of student ideas, in addition to ways of using technology for collaborative teaching and learning. She is also interested in digital equity and technology possibilities which connect people globally. She holds an Ed.D from Teachers College, Columbia University.

Index

B

C

D

I

J

K

L

M

N

O

P

Q

R

S

T

U